# Asthma: Challenges and Concerns

# Asthma: Challenges and Concerns

Editor: Jordan Long

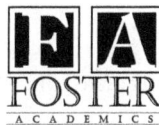

FA
FOSTER
ACADEMICS

www.fosteracademics.com

www.fosteracademics.com

**FA**
**FOSTER**
ACADEMICS

Cataloging-in-Publication Data

Asthma : challenges and concerns / edited by Jordan Long.
    p. cm.
Includes bibliographical references and index.
ISBN 978-1-63242-796-0
1. Asthma. 2. Bronchi--Diseases. 3. Lungs--Diseases, Obstructive.
4. Respiratory allergy. I. Long, Jordan.
RA645.A83 A88 2019
616.238--dc23

Foster Academics,
118-35 Queens Blvd., Suite 400,
Forest Hills, NY 11375, USA

ISBN 978-1-63242-796-0 (Hardback)

# Contents

# Preface

Asthma is a chronic inflammatory condition of the airway of the lungs. It often involves reversible airflow obstruction and bronchospasm. Some of its common symptoms include shortness of breath, coughing, wheezing and chest tightness. The condition of a person having asthma usually becomes worse with exercise. It is caused due to a combination of environmental and genetic factors. Air pollution, smoking during pregnancy, exposure to indoor volatile organic compounds and exposure to indoor allergens, like cockroaches and dust mites, are the common environmental factors contributing to asthma. Spirometry is the recommended test to diagnose asthma. Bronchodilators, leukotriene antagonists and mast cell stabilizers are some of the most commonly used treatment methods. This book unravels the recent studies in the management of asthma. It strives to provide a fair idea about asthma and the challenges and concerns related to it. This book includes contributions of experts and scientists which will provide innovative insights into this disease.

The information contained in this book is the result of intensive hard work done by researchers in this field. All due efforts have been made to make this book serve as a complete guiding source for students and researchers. The topics in this book have been comprehensively explained to help readers understand the growing trends in the field.

I would like to thank the entire group of writers who made sincere efforts in this book and my family who supported me in my efforts of working on this book. I take this opportunity to thank all those who have been a guiding force throughout my life.

**Editor**

# Complementary Therapy with Traditional Chinese Medicine for Childhood Asthma

Bei-Yu Wu, Chun-Ting Liu, Yu-Chiang Hung and Wen-Long Hu

## Abstract

Asthma is a heterogeneous disease that is typically characterized by chronic airway inflammation and obstruction of airflow; it frequently presents in early childhood and is the leading chronic disease in children in the western world. This review presents a brief description of the pathophysiology of asthma and summarizes recent research results on the mechanisms of action of anti-asthma Chinese herbal medicine commonly used in clinical practice. Other interventions of traditional Chinese medicine (TCM), such as acupuncture, tai chi, and meditation are also briefly discussed. We believe that this contribution is theoretically and practically relevant because the prevalence of asthma is increasing and, in addition to standard treatment, the use of complementary therapy is increasing and there is increasing scientific evidence demonstrating that TCM has potential for the treatment of childhood asthma.

**Keywords:** Childhood asthma, traditional Chinese medicine, Acupuncture, complementary and alternative medicine

## 1. Introduction

Asthma is a heterogeneous disease that is typically characterized by chronic airway inflammation and obstruction of airflow. Asthma is defined by a history of respiratory symptoms such as wheezing, shortness of breath, chest tightness, and cough [1]. Both these symptoms and airflow limitation characteristically vary over time as well as in intensity. These variations are often triggered by external factors, such as exercise, allergen or irritant exposure, change in the weather, or viral respiratory infections [2]. Symptoms and airway limitation may resolve with or without medication and may sometimes be absent for weeks or months at a time.

Asthma, a life-long condition, frequently presents in early childhood and is the leading chronic disease in children in the Western world. Although the prevalence of childhood varies widely across the world as described in the Phase III ISAAC study [3], most studies have reported that this prevalence has increased in recent decades [4–6]. This increase has been associated with a rise in atopic sensitization and other allergic disorders, such as eczema and rhinitis [6]. Approximately 25.9 million Americans (including 7.1 million children) had asthma in 2011, which equates to a rate of 84.8 per 1,000 in the population. The highest prevalence rate was seen in those in the 5–17 years of age bracket (105.5 per 1,000). Overall, the rate in those under the age of 18 years (94.9 per 1,000) was significantly greater than that in those over 18 years (81.6 per 1,000). The current asthma prevalence rate for boys under 18 years (101.7 per 1,000) was 16% higher than the rate among similarly aged girls (87.8 per 1,000) [7]. In 2008, the condition accounted for an estimated 14.4 million lost school days in children and 14.2 million lost work days in adults. Asthma is thus a leading cause of activity limitation and amounts to $56.0 billion in health care costs annually in the United States [7].

Approximately 80 percent of children with asthma develop symptoms before 5 years of age, but the disease is frequently misdiagnosed or not suspected, particularly in infants [8]. Coughing and wheezing are the most common symptoms of childhood asthma. Breathlessness, chest tightness or pressure, and chest pain have also been reported [1, 2]. Descriptors may vary between cultures and by age; for example, children may be described as having heavy breathing [2]. Confirmation of the diagnosis of asthma in children requires a careful review of a child's current and past medical history, family history, as well as a physical examination.

Asthma is characterized by variable expiratory airflow limitation. Pulmonary function tests are sometimes needed to diagnose asthma and to rule out other possible causes of the symptoms. Spirometry is the most common pulmonary function test; it measures the flow and volume of air blown out after a child takes a very deep breath and then forcefully exhales. The important parameters derived from spirometry include forced expiratory volume in 1 s ($FEV_1$), forced vital capacity (FVC), flow between 25% and 75% of the vital capacity (FEF 25–75%), and peak expiratory flow rate (PEFR) [9]. The greater the variation in lung function, or the more times excess variation is seen in a patient with respiratory symptoms, the more likely the diagnosis is to be one of asthma. The $FEV_1$/FVC ratio is normally >0.75–0.80 and usually exceeds 0.90 in children [10]. In asthma, at least once during diagnostic process, the $FEV_1$ is low, confirming that the $FEV_1$/FVC ratio is reduced. Generally, an increase in $FEV_1$ of >12% of that predicted after inhalation of a rapid-acting bronchodilator and/or average daily diurnal peak expiratory flow (PEF) variability exceeding 13% indicates that a child has asthma [2]. In young children, in whom lung function testing is not feasible, including most preschool children, asthma is defined by the presence of variable respiratory symptoms.

Traditional Chinese medicine (TCM), particularly herbal medicine, has been used for the treatment of asthma for hundreds of years, as documented in the *Yellow Emperor's Inner Canon* (*Huangdi Neijing*) and the *Essential Prescriptions from the Golden Cabinet* (*Jin Gui Yao Lue*). In Taiwan, Chinese herbal medicine is commonly used as complementary and alternative therapy for the treatment of atopic diseases such as asthma, allergic rhinitis, and atopic dermatitis. The medicines used for the prevention and treatment of asthma have received much attention in recent years. The cellular and molecular details of the underlying mechanisms of action of Chinese herbal medicine efficacious for treating asthma are just beginning to be understood.

This chapter presents a brief description of the pathophysiology of asthma and summarizes recent research results on the mechanisms of action of anti-asthma Chinese herbal medicine commonly used in clinical practice. Other interventions of TCM, such as acupuncture, *tai chi*, and meditation, are also briefly discussed.

# 2. Pathophysiology and pathogenesis of asthma

Asthma can be classified as atopic/allergic (extrinsic), which is the most common form, or nonatopic/nonallergic (intrinsic) asthma, which is more rare, has a later onset, and tends to be more severe than atopic asthma [11]. Atopic asthma involves inflammation mediated by specific IgE antibodies directed against common environmental allergens, whereas nonatopic asthma involves inflammation and airway constriction mediated by local production of IgE antibodies that are possibly directed at bacterial or viral antigens. The pathophysiology of nonatopic asthma is very similar to that of atopic asthma, but it is not caused by exposure to an allergen [2, 11].

The gross pathology of asthma reveals significant overinflation of the lungs [12]. Microscopically, this overinflation of lungs is manifest as marked distension of the alveoli. Notable airway smooth muscle (ASM) hyperplasia, basement membrane thickening, mucous gland hyperplasia, mucosal epithelium sloughing, and tissue edema are also seen [12]. This increase in muscle mass, mucous gland tissues, and tissue edema leads to a thickened airway wall, with a resultant decrease in airway caliber [12, 13]. These structural changes have been described as remodeling, a term used to define complex morphological changes that involve all of the structures of the bronchial wall [12, 13].

The initiation of bronchial epithelial damage by environmental agents (allergens, viruses, irritants, etc.) or their inflammatory products activates a sequence of events that amplify the inflammation and induce airway remodeling [13, 14]. Bousquet et al. suggested that asthma pathophysiology involved overlapping interactions of smooth muscle dysfunction, airway inflammation, and airway remodeling [13]. The inflammatory, physiological, and structural factors that contribute to the pathogenesis of asthma will be described below.

## 2.1. Airway inflammation

Inflammation plays a central role in the pathophysiology of asthma [15]. Airway inflammation remains a consistent pattern throughout the distinct phenotypes of asthma (e.g., intermittent, persistent, exercise-associated, aspirin-sensitive, or severe asthma) [16]. Airway inflammation involves an interaction of many cell types and multiple mediators with the airway, which eventually results in the characteristic pathophysiological features of asthma. The principal cells involved in airway inflammation are mast cells, eosinophils, epithelial cells, macrophages, and activated T lymphocytes [12, 13].

T lymphocytes play an important role in the regulation of airway inflammation through the release of numerous cytokines. Airway inflammation in asthma may indeed represent a loss of the normal balance between Th1 and Th2 lymphocytes [12, 16]. Th1 cells produce interleukin (IL)-2 and interferon gamma (IFN-$\gamma$), which are critical in the defense mechanisms of cells in response to infection. Th2 cells, in contrast, generate a family of cytokines (IL-4, IL-5, IL-6, IL-9, and IL-13) that can stimulate the growth, differentiation, and recruitment of mast cells, basophils, eosinophils, and B-cells, all of which are involved in humoral immunity and in the allergic response [13, 14, 16].

IgE plays an essential role in type I hypersensitivity, which results in various allergic diseases, such as allergic asthma, most types of sinusitis, allergic rhinitis, food allergies, and specific types of chronic urticaria and atopic dermatitis [17]. Antigen-specific IgE is partly responsible for the initiation of an allergic response in asthma. IgE primes the IgE-mediated allergic response by binding to Fc receptors expressed on the surface of mast cells, basophils, eosinophils, monocytes, macrophages, or platelets in humans [18]. Antigens cross-link to the IgE on mast cells, which then release bronchoconstricting mediators (histamine, cysteinyl-leukotrienes, prostaglandin D2) and further amplify the inflammatory response by damaging local tissue and attracting other lymphocytes [17]. IL-4 produced by Th2 cells stimulates IgE production in B-lymphocytes and expression of vascular cell adhesion molecule 1 (VCAM-1) on endothelial cells, whereas IL-5 stimulates eosinophil differentiation and mobilization to inflammatory sites [13, 16]. Circulating eosinophils enter the area of allergic inflammation and begin migrating to the lung by rolling, through interactions with selectins, and eventually adhere to the endothelium by means of binding between integrins and members of the immunoglobulin superfamily of adhesion proteins, namely VCAM-1 and intercellular adhesion molecule 1 (ICAM-1) [13, 16]. As the eosinophils enter the matrix of the airway through the influence of various chemokines, such as monocyte chemotactic protein (MCP-1), macrophage inflammatory protein (MIP-1$\alpha$), eotaxin or RANTES, and cytokines, their survival is prolonged by IL-4 and granulocyte-macrophage colony–stimulating factor (GM-CSF) [13, 16]. Upon activation, the eosinophils release inflammatory mediators, such as leukotrienes and granule proteins, which injure airway tissues [19]. In addition, eosinophils can generate GM-CSF to prolong and potentiate their survival and thereby contribute to persistent airway inflammation [16]. Eosinophils are the most characteristic cells accumulated in asthma and allergic inflammation; their presence is often related to disease severity. Eosinophils are recruited or activated by IL-5, the eotaxin family of chemokines, via the eosinophil-selective chemokine receptor CCR3, and by Toll-like receptors (TLRs). Activated eosinophils produce lipid mediators, such as leukotrienes and platelet-activating factor, which mediate smooth muscle contraction; toxic granule products (e.g., major basic protein, eosinophil-derived neurotoxin, eosinophil peroxidase, or eosinophil cationic protein) that can damage airway epithelium and nerves; and cytokines, such as GM-CSF, transforming growth factors (TGF)-$\alpha$ and $\beta$, and interleukins, which may be involved in airway remodeling and fibrosis [13]. Recently, Th regulatory cells that exclusively produce IL-17 cytokines (TH17 cells) have been identified in patients with severe asthma [19]. The involvement of TH17 responses in the pathogenesis of asthma has been shown by the overexpression of IL-17 mRNA in the airways of asthma model mice [19]. It is now suggested that TH17-related cytokines play a critical role in airway remodeling and may be involved in interactions with structural cells [13, 19].

## 2.2. Airway remodeling and ASM dysfunction

The histopathologic changes of airway remodeling include damage or loss of the normal pseudostratified structure of airway epithelium, an increase in the proportion of mucous-producing goblet cells, fibrotic thickening of the subepithelial reticular basement membrane or "lamina reticularis," increased numbers of myofibroblasts, increased vascularity, increased ASM mass, and increased extracellular matrix [20]. These structural changes contribute to bronchial wall thickening, alterations in the physiological consequences of smooth muscle contraction, or loss of airway-parenchymal interdependence [13, 20].

Epithelial alterations in asthma include epithelial shedding, destruction of ciliated cells, goblet cell hyperplasia, upregulation of growth factor release, and overexpression of receptors, such as the epidermal growth factor receptors [21]. Loss of epithelial surface and the resultant denudation of the basement membrane may decrease this protective effect, thereby increasing the propensity for allergic insult to the airway [21]. A second important feature of airway remodeling is subepithelial fibrosis, which has been consistently reported in asthma of all levels of severity, in patients with atopic rhinitis, and even in children with treatment-resistant asthma [21]. Subepithelial fibrosis occurs in the lamina reticularis, immediately below the basement membrane, resulting in thickening of the basement membrane just below the epithelium [22]. In the asthmatic airway, fibroblasts are activated and differentiate into myofibroblasts, which secrete proinflammatory mediators and extracellular matrix proteins, including collagens I, III, and V; fibronectin; tenascin; lumican; and biglycan [21, 22]. Asthmatic airway fibroblasts promote fibrosis though expression of a higher ratio of tissue inhibitor of metalloproteinase (TIMP)-2 to matrix metalloproteinase (MMP)-2, resulting in increased matrix deposition [21]. MMPs are a family of proteases implicated in collagen degradation. MMP-2, MMP-3, MMP-8, and MMP-9 have been associated with asthma [20]. Among these, MMP-9 levels have been reported to be significantly higher in the sputum of patients with asthma than in that of control subjects [20–23].

Respiratory ASM cells are the critical effector cells that modulate airway tone [22]. In asthmatic airways, smooth muscle mass is increased due to a coordinated increase in the size (hypertrophy) and number (hyperplasia) of ASM cells [21, 22]. ASM remodeling is considered to be the primary cause of airway obstruction [21]. ASM cells participate in the inflammatory and remodeling process through the expression of cellular adhesion molecules, receptors for cytokines (e.g., TNF-$\alpha$), chemokines (RANTES, eotaxin, MIP-1$\alpha$, and IL-8), and TLRs [21]. Additionally, the migration of ASM cells toward the epithelium contributes to remodeling. A wide range of inflammatory mediators, such as TNF-$\alpha$, IL-1b, and IFN-$\gamma$, have been shown to induce the expression of ICAM-1 and VCAM-1 on cultured ASM cells [21]. The surface expression of cellular adhesion molecules by ASM cells might be pivotal in regulating interactions with a variety of inflammatory cells, including eosinophils and T cells [21].

Additionally, accumulating evidence has indicated an abnormal increase in the number and size of microvessels within bronchial tissue in remodeled airways [21]. This occurs mainly below the basal lamina, in the space between the muscle layer and the surrounding parenchyma [21]. An imbalance between vascular endothelial growth factor (VEGF) and angiopoietin-1 has been shown to be involved in these abnormalities [21]. In fact, VEGF acts by increasing the permeability of these abnormal blood vessels, resulting in vessel dilation and edema, which contribute to airway narrowing [21, 22]. In addition to providing nutrition to the airways, these vessels are the source of inflammatory cells and plasma-derived mediators and cytokines [21].

## 3. Conventional treatment of childhood asthma

The optimal treatment of childhood asthma depends upon a number of factors, including the child's age, the severity and frequency of asthma attacks, and the ability to properly use the prescribed medications [2]. For the vast majority of children, asthma treatment can control symptoms, allowing the child to participate fully in all activities, including sports. Identifying and avoiding asthma triggers, the factors that set off or worsen asthma symptoms, are essential for preventing asthma flare-ups [2]. Common asthma triggers generally include allergens (such as dust, pollen, and furred animals), respiratory infections, irritants (such as tobacco smoke, chemicals, and strong odors or fumes), physical activity, certain medicines (such as beta blockers, aspirin, or other nonsteroidal anti-inflammatory medications), and emotional stress [2]. After identifying potential triggers of asthma, the parent and health care provider should develop a plan to deal with the triggers. If possible, the child should completely avoid or limit exposure to the trigger [2].

The long-term goals of asthma management are to achieve good symptom control and to minimize future risk of exacerbation, fixed airflow limitation, and side effects of treatment [2]. In control-based asthma management, pharmacological and nonpharmacological treatment is adjusted continuously in a cycle that involves assessment, treatment, and review of the response [2]. Asthma severity is determined by considering the following factors: the symptoms reported over the previous 2 to 4 weeks, the current level of lung function ($FEV_1$ and $FEV_1$/FVC values), and the number of instances of exacerbation requiring oral glucocorticoids per year [2]. The classification of severity in children aged 5–11 years or in adolescents over the age of 12 years is similar to that in adults [2]. The severity in children under the age of 4 years, however, is classified somewhat differently and includes intermittent, mild persistent, moderate persistent, and severe persistent asthma [2].

### 3.1. Categories of asthma medications

Medication for asthma is mainly divided into two categories: controller medications and reliever (rescue) medications [2]. Controller medications, such as inhaled corticosteroids (ICS) and long-acting beta-adrenoceptor agonists (LABA), are used for regular maintenance treatment [24–26]. These medications reduce airway inflammation, control symptoms, and reduce future risks, such as exacerbations and decreased lung function. Reliever medications, such as short-acting beta-2-adrenoceptor agonists (SABA), are provided to all patients for as-needed relief of breakthrough symptoms, including during worsening of asthma or exacerbations [24–26]. They are also recommended for short-term prevention of exercise-induced bronchoconstriction [2]. Reducing and, ideally, eliminating the need for reliever treatment are both an important goal in asthma management and a measure of the success of asthma treatment. Add-on therapies for patients with severe asthma may be considered when patients have persistent symptoms and/or exacerbations, despite optimized treatment with high-dose controller medications (usually a high-dose ICS and a LABA) and treatment of modifiable risk factors [2].

The initiation of asthma therapy in a stable patient who is not already receiving medications is based upon the severity of asthma in the individual. Patients with mild intermittent asthma are best treated with an inhaled SABA, which should be taken as needed for the relief of symptoms [2]. Patients in whom triggering of asthmatic symptoms can be predicted (e.g., exercise-induced bronchoconstriction) are encouraged to use their inhaled beta agonist approximately 10 min prior to exposure, to prevent the onset of symptoms [2]. For mild persistent asthma, the preferred long-term controller is a low-dose ICS [2]. Regular use of ICS reduces the frequency of symptoms (and the need for SABAs for symptom relief), improves the overall quality of life, and decreases the risk of serious exacerbations [2]. Alternative strategies for treatment of mild persistent asthma include leukotriene receptor antagonists, theophylline, and cromoglycate [2, 26].

For moderate persistent asthma, the preferred therapy is low doses of ICS plus an inhaled LABA, or medium doses of ICS [2]. Alternative strategies include adding a leukotriene modifier (leukotriene receptor antagonist or lipoxygenase inhibitor) or theophylline to low-dose ICS [2]. For severe persistent asthma, the preferred treatments are medium (Step 4) or high (Step 5) doses of ICS, in combination with an inhaled LABA [2]. In addition, for patients who are inadequately controlled on high-dose ICS and LABAs, the anti-IgE therapy omalizumab may be considered, if there is objective evidence of sensitivity to a perennial allergen (by allergy skin tests or in vitro measurements of allergen-specific IgE) and if the serum IgE level is within the established target range [2].

## 4. Status and purpose

Currently, according to the guidelines published by the Global Initiative for Asthma (GINA), conventional medicines are the mainstay for managing asthma; these include steroids, beta-2 adrenergic agonists, leukotriene modifiers, theophylline, and anti-IgE therapies [2]. However, current conventional medications for childhood asthma are not yet satisfactory. The side effects of long-term use of steroids and beta-2 adrenergic agonists are major concerns for parents, in that growth, bone turnover, and adrenal gland function may be suppressed under, particularly higher doses of steroids [24, 25]. Due to the chronic and potentially life-threatening nature of asthma, and the lack of definitive preventive and curative therapies, many families look to complementary and alternative medicine (CAM) for treatment. CAM is popular in the treatment of asthma and encompasses many therapies, including mind–body techniques, nutritional manipulation, dietary and herbal supplements, TCM (including acupuncture), exercise, manual therapies, and homeopathy [26]. Reportedly, CAM is commonly used in children who have mild or moderate persistent asthma, those receiving high-dose ICS, and patients who experience poor symptom control or require frequent physician visits, including emergency room visits [26]. One retrospective longitudinal cohort study showed that initiation of CAM treatment does not decrease future adherence to conventional asthma medications, suggesting that alternative or integrative medicine use does not necessarily compete with conventional asthma therapies [27]. As CAM use becomes more prevalent, it will become increasingly important for physicians attending to asthmatic children to be aware of CAM use. TCM is the major component of CAM therapies used in the United States and Taiwan. TCM is one of the oldest medical practices in the world and has played an important role in preventing and treating diseases in China for centuries, where it is still used as a monotherapy or as part of an integrated medicine approach. Evidence has increased showing the efficacy of TCM for the treatment of childhood asthma. Below, we explore complementary therapy, involving TCM therapy for childhood asthma.

## 5. Chinese herbal formulas use in children with asthma

TCM formulas have been used to treat asthma for centuries. A number of well-controlled clinical studies of several TCM formulas, including modified Mai-Men-Dong-Tang (mMMDT, five herbs), Ding-Chuan-Tang (DCT, nine herbs), and STA-1 (the combination of Mai-Men-Dong-Tang and Liu-Wei-Di-Huang-Wan, 10 herbs), and anti-asthma herbal medicine intervention (ASHMI, three herbs) provided evidence of clinical efficacy, safety, and immunomodulatory effects [24]. Typically, the traditional TCM formulas that are prescribed combine several single herbs to treat a specific disease. Recent research [25] from the National Health Insurance Research Database (NHIRD) in Taiwan has revealed the core herbal treatments for children with asthma. The most commonly used herbal formulas for the treatment of childhood asthma are Ma-Xing-Gan-Shi-Tang and Xiao-Qing-Long-Tang; the former is used for excess heat congested in the lung, whereas the latter is used for the exterior wind-cold with internal accumulation of retained fluid in the lung. These herbal formulas (shown in Table 1) and several single herbs commonly used for the treatment of childhood asthma are described below. The immunomodulatory effects of suppressing Th2 cells and decreasing subsequent cytokine secretion of these herbal remedies will also be investigated. Other commonly prescribed formulas that are used mainly to relieve asthma-related symptoms, such as productive cough (Xing-Su-San, Zhi-Sou-San), coughing with a sore throat (Yin-Qiao-San), and nasal congestion (Xin-Yi-Qing-Fei-Tang, Cang-Er-Zi-San, Shin-Yi-San), do not fall within the scope of this review.

### 5.1. ASHMI

ASHMI is the first herbal medicine to receive approval for phase I and II clinical trials as a US Food and Drug Administration investigational new drug (IND No. 71526) for treating asthma.

| Formula | Composition | Possible mechanisms |
| --- | --- | --- |
| ASHMI | Ling Zhi (*Ganoderma Lucidum*), Ku Shen (*Radix Sophorae Flavescentis*), and Gan Cao (*Radix Glycyrrhizae*) | Decreases Th2 response; increases IFN-γ levels; decreases IL-4, IL-5, IL-13, eotaxin, TNF-α, total and specific IgE levels; reduces AHR, mucous production, neutrophilic and eosinophilic inflammation; improves FEV$_1$ and PEF [24, 28–30] |
| Modified Mai-Men-Dong-Tang (mMMDT) | Mai Men Dong (*Radix Ophiopogonis*), Ban Xia (*Rhizoma Pinelliae*), American Ren Shen (*Radix Panacis Quinquefolii*), Gan Cao (*Radix Glycyrrhizae*), and Lantern Tridax (*Herba Tridacis procumbentis*) | Antitussive effect, bronchial dilation via beta-2 adrenergic effect; decreases IL-4, total IgE, and specific IgE; reduces AHR; improves FEV$_1$ [24, 31–33] |
| STA-1 | Mai Men Dong (*Radix Ophiopogonis*), Ban Xia (*Tuber Pinellia*), American Ren Shen (*Radix Panacis Quinquefolii*), Gan Cao (*Radix Glycyrrhizae*), Shu Di Huang (*Radix Rehmanniae Preparata*), Mu Dan Pi (*Cortex Moutan Radicis*), Shan Zhu Yu (*Fructus Corni*), Fu Ling (*Poria*), Ze Xie (*Rhizoma Alismatis*), and Shan Yao (*Radix Dioscoreae*) | Reduces symptom scores, systemic steroid dose, airway inflammation, AHR, total IgE, and specific IgE; improves FEV$_1$ [34, 35] |
| Ma-Xing-Gan-Shi-Tang | Ma Huang (*Herba Ephedrae*), Xing Ren (*Semen Armeniacae Amarum*), Shi Gao (*Gypsum Fibrosum*), and Gan Cao (*Radix Glycyrrhizae*) | Antitussive effect, beta-2 adrenergic effect; reduces neutrophilic inflammation [36, 37] |
| Xiao-Qing-Long-Tang | Ma Huang (*Herba Ephedrae*), Gui Zhi (*Ramulus Cinnamomi*), Ban Xia (*Rhizoma Pinelliae*), Gan Jiang (*Rhizoma Zingiberis*), Xi Xin (*Herba Asari*),Wu Wei Zi (*Fructus Schisandrae*), Bai Shao Yao (*Radix Paeoniae*), and Gan Cao (*Radix Glycyrrhizae*) | Decreases Th2 response; increases IFN-γ; decreases IL-4, IL-5, IL-10, IL-13, IgE, RANTES, eotaxin, and MCP-1 levels; suppresses histamine release, reduces airway inflammation, remodeling, and immunomodulation; bronchial dilation, partial beta-2 adrenergic effect [38–40] |
| Ding-Chuan-Tang | Ma Huang (*Herba Ephedrae*), Gan Cao (*Radix Glycyrrhizae*), Ban Xia (*Rhizoma Pinelliae*), Bai Guo (*Semen Ginkgo*), Kuan Dong Hua (*Flos Farfarae*), Sang Bai Pi (*Cortex Moris*), Su Zi (*Fructus Perillae*), Xing Ren (*Semen Armeniacae Amarum*), and Huang Qin (*Radix Scutellariae*) | Improves AHR, symptoms, and medication; reduces eosinophilic inflammation; beta-2 adrenergic effect [41, 42] |

**Table 1.** Herbal formulas frequently used for asthmatic children

ASHMI is composed of the aqueous extracts of Ling Zhi (*Ganoderma lucidum*), Ku Shen (*Sophora flavescens*), and Gan Cao (*Glycyrrhiza uralensis*) [24]. ASHMI improved lung function ($FEV_1$), reduced symptom scores, and decreased beta-2-adrenoceptor agonist use, to a degree similar as that achieved by prednisone in adults with moderate to severe asthma, but without the adverse effect of prednisone on adrenal function and with no overall immune suppression. Individually, Ling Zhi, Ku Shen, and Gan Cao extracts and ASHMI (the combination of individual extracts) inhibited production of IL-4 and IL-5 by murine memory Th2 cells and that of eotaxin-1 by human lung fibroblast cells [28]. ASHMI synergistically inhibited eotaxin-1 production as well as Th2 cytokine production. In another mouse model of asthma, ASHMI also reduced the levels of ovalbumin (OVA)-specific IgE and Th2 cytokines, including IL-4, IL-5, and IL-13 in the lung, and increased IFN-$\gamma$ secretion [29]. Moreover, ASHMI markedly reduced airway hyperresponsiveness (AHR), mucous production, neutrophilic inflammation, and TNF-$\alpha$, IL-8, and IL-17 levels and also decreased eosinophilic inflammation and Th2 responses in vivo [30].

## 5.2. Modified Mai-Men-Dong-Tang

Mai-Men-Dong-Tang is a herbal TCM that has been used for the treatment of bronchitis, bronchial asthma, and cough. The compositions of Mai-Men-Dong-Tang are Mai Men Dong (*Ophiopogon japonicus*), Ban Xia (*Pinellia ternata*), Ren Shen (*Panax ginseng*), Gan Cao (*Glycyrrhiza uralensis*), Da Zao (*Ziziphus jujuba*), and Geng Mi (*Oryza sativa*). Mai-Men-Dong-Tang was shown to have an antitussive effect, based on improved airway clearance. The pharmacological effect of this antitussive effect is suggested to involve the inhibition of C-fibers, bronchodilation, anti-inflammatory effects, suppression of mucosal excretion, and augmentation of surfactant secretion [31]. Mai-Men-Dong-Tang was shown to potentiate beta-adrenergic function in ASM, which may reflect the efficacy on AHR and asthma [32]. mMMDT contains five herbs, including Mai Men Dong (*Radix Ophiopogonis*), Ban Xia (*Rhizoma Pinelliae*), American Ren Shen (*Radix Panacis Quinquefolii*), Gan Cao (*Radix Glycyrrhizae*), and Lantern Tridax (*Herba Tridacis procumbentis*) [33]. mMMDT was shown to decrease serum total IgE and house dust mite-specific IgE significantly and downregulate the expression of IL-4 in allergen-sensitized mice. The effect of mMMDT on changes in $FEV_1$ was studied as the first efficacy end point, given its validity for monitoring airway obstruction, which showed significant improvement in $FEV_1$ in patients treated with mMMDT [33]. Moreover, mMMDT also relieved asthma symptoms, including coughing, wheezing, and breathlessness [33].

## 5.3. STA-1

STA-1 is a combination of mMMDT (four herbs) and Lui-Wei-Di-Huang-Wan (six herbs) [34]. The four herbs of mMMDT comprise Mai Men Dong (*Radix Ophiopogonis*), Ban Xia (*Tuber Pinellia*), American Ren Shen (*Radix Panacis Quinquefolii*), and Gan Cao (*Radix Glycyrrhizae*) without Lantern Tridax (*Herba Tridacis procumbentis*). The six herbs of Lui-Wei-Di-Huang-Wan are Shu Di Huang (*Radix Rehmanniae Preparata*), Mu Dan Pi (*Cortex Moutan Radicis*), Shan Zhu Yu (*Fructus Corni*), Fu Ling (*Poria*), Ze Xie (*Rhizoma Alismatis*), and Shan Yao (*Radix Dioscoreae*). STA-1 was able to inhibit mite-induced IgE synthesis, reduce inflammation-associated accumulation of eosinophils and neutrophils in the airway, and relieve AHR in a murine model [35]. Clinical evaluation of STA-1 in the treatment of mild-to-moderate chronic asthma revealed a significant reduction of symptom scores, systemic steroid dose, total IgE, and specific IgE in patients treated with STA-1 [34]. Furthermore, STA-1 also improved lung function (FEV$_1$) as compared with placebo after 6 months' treatment and with only minimal side effects [34].

## 5.4. Ma-Xing-Gan-Shi-Tang

Ma-Xing-Gan-Shi-Tang, a TCM, has been used in the treatment of bronchial asthma for several centuries. Ma-Xing-Gan-Shi-Tang consists of Ma Huang (*Herba Ephedrae*), Xing Ren (*Semen Armeniacae Amarum*), Shi Gao (*Gypsum Fibrosum*), and Gan Cao (*Radix Glycyrrhizae*). A murine cough model, induced by sulfur dioxide gas, was used to investigate the antitussive effect of Ma-Xing-Gan-Shi-Tang [36]. Both Ma Huang and Xing Ren inhibited cough induction in a dose-dependent manner. However, Ma-Xing-Gan-Shi-Tang, which contains Ma Huang and Xing Ren, showed stronger antitussive effects than the individual crude drugs [36]. In a guinea pig model of allergic asthma, Ma-Xing-Gan-Shi-Tang was efficacious in stimulation of beta-2-adrenoceptors on bronchial smooth muscle and had an anti-inflammatory effect, involving inhibition of neutrophil infiltration into the airway [37]. Ma-Xing-Gan-Shi-Tang is typically indicated in syndromes involving wind-heat on the lung or stagnated wind-cold that has turned into heat and that stayed in the lung. In Taiwan, asthma triggered by respiratory tract infection among asthmatic children is much more common than that triggered by cold exposure and weather change. Asthma triggered by respiratory tract infection is the most important indication for Ma-Xing-Gan-Shi-Tang [25].

## 5.5. Xiao-Qing-Long-Tang

Xiao-Qing-Long-Tang (XQLT) has been widely used clinically for the treatment of allergic diseases, including bronchial asthma and allergic rhinitis. XQTL consists of Ma Huang (*Herba Ephedrae*), Gui Zhi (*Ramulus Cinnamomi*), Ban Xia (*Rhizoma Pinelliae*), Gan Jiang (*Rhizoma Zingiberis*), Xi Xin (*Herba Asari*), Wu Wei Zi (*Fructus Schisandrae*), Bai Shao Yao (*Radix Paeoniae*), and Gan Cao (*Radix Glycyrrhizae*).

XQLT was shown to reduce bronchial inflammatory cell infiltration and airway remodeling in repetitive *Dermatogoides pteronyssinus*-challenged mouse model of chronic asthma [38]. XQLT inhibited *D. pteronyssinus*-induced total IgE and *D. pteronyssinus*-specific IgG1 in serum and changed the Th2-bios in bronchoalveolar lavage fluid (BALF) by inhibiting the activation of nuclear factor-Kappa B (NF-κB). The same study also showed that XQLT treatment increased the protein levels of IL-12, but decreased that of TNF-α, TGF-β1, IL-5, IL-6, and IL-13 by inhibiting expression of the genes including IL-10, IL-13, eotaxin, RANTES, and MCP-1 in the lung. Moreover, collagen assays and histopathology indicated that XQLT reduces airway remodeling in the lung [38]. XQLT treatment could inhibit the secretion of IL-5 in the serum and downregulate mRNA expression of genes encoding eotaxin, RANTES, and MCP-1 in lung tissues, which may contribute to a reduction in eosinophils and monocytes recruited to the airway.

Studies on the OVA-sensitized allergic airway inflammation model in mice revealed that XQLT significantly inhibited the antigen-induced immediate asthmatic response and late asthmatic response in actively sensitized mice. XQLT was shown to reduce the production of Th2-associated cytokines, IL-4 and IL-5, and to restore the production of the Th1 cell-associated cytokine, IFN-$\gamma$ [39]. Anti-OVA IgE antibody levels were reduced in the BALF of sensitized mice after oral administration of XQLT [39]. Furthermore, XQLT was shown to have an anti-asthmatic effect, which is partly mediated by stimulation of beta-2-adrenoceptors, leading to bronchorelaxation; furthermore, XQLT inhibits the infiltration of eosinophils into the airway [40].

### 5.6. Ding-Chuan-Tang

Ding-Chuan-Tang (DCT), another TCM, has been used in the treatment of bronchial asthma for several centuries. DCT is composed of nine herbs, including Ma Huang (*Herba Ephedrae*), Gan Cao (*Radix Glycyrrhizae*), Ban Xia (*Rhizoma Pinelliae*), Bai Guo (*Semen Ginkgo*), Kuan Dong Hua (*Flos Farfarae*), Sang Bai Pi (*Cortex Mori*), Su Zi (*Fructus Perillae*), Xing Ren (*Semen Armeniacae Amarum*), and Huang Qin (*Radix Scutellariae*). According to TCM principles, this decoction is frequently prescribed for children with coughing, wheezing, and chest tightness.

One study of a murine OVA-sensitized allergic airway inflammation model revealed that DCT significantly inhibited the increase of eosinophils in the airway and caused concentration-dependent bronchorelaxation via a beta-2 adrenergic effect [41]. A randomized, double-blind clinical trial [42] conducted to assess the add-on effect of DCT showed that AHR significantly improved after weeks of DCT treatment compared with that after placebo use. In addition, patients in the DCT group also showed superior clinical improvement and used less medication than in the placebo group. This study suggested that addition of DCT to conventional treatment could further improve AHR, even in patients with well-controlled asthma. However, this study did not find a significant reduction in IgE levels and $FEV_1$ with DCT treatment, as compared to placebo [42].

## 6. Chinese single herbs use in children with asthma

We described several single herbs frequently used for asthmatic children in Taiwan (shown in Table 2), including Zhe Bei Mu (*Fritillaria thunbergii*), Xing Ren (*Semen Armeniacae Amarum*), Huang Qi (*Astragalus membranaceus*), Qian Hu (*Peucedanum praeruptorum Dunn*), Gan Cao (*Glycyrrhiza uralensis*), Sang Bai Pi (*Cortex mori radicis*), Ban Xia (*Pinellia ternate*), Bo He (*Mentha haplocalyx*), Da Huang (*Rheum palmatum*), Jie Geng (*Platycodon grandiflorum*), Huang Qin (*Scutellaria baicalensis*), and Yu Xing Cao (*Houttuynia cordata Thunb.*).

### 6.1. Zhe Bei Mu

Zhe Bei Mu is used as an antitussive therapy and expectorant in TCM. Its extract inhibited histamine release from rat peritoneal mast cells in a concentration-dependent manner. Moreover, it also inhibits the production of inflammatory cytokines (IL-6, IL-8, and TNF-$\alpha$) in human mast cell line-1 (HMC-1) cells and components of the mitogen-activated protein kinase (MAPK) pathway in mast cells [43].

## 6.2. Xing Ren

Xing Ren has long been used in TCM to control acute lower respiratory tract infection and asthma as a result of its expectorant and anti-asthmatic activities. Xing Ren was shown to have anti-asthmatic activity and selectively inhibit the Th2 response in a mouse model by decreasing eosinophils and IL-4 in the airway [44].

## 6.3. Huang Qi

Huang Qi has a long history of medicinal use for asthma treatment in China. It increases metabolism and stimulates tissue regeneration, and it is used to treat colds, allergies, digestive problems, and fatigue in TCM. Huang Qi was shown to inhibit the Th2 response. It significantly reduced AHR, eosinophil counts, and IL-4, IL-5, and IL-13 levels and increased INF-$\gamma$ levels in BALF. Histological studies showed that Huang Qi markedly decreased inflammatory infiltration, mucus secretion, and collagen deposition in lung tissues. CD4$^+$CD25$^+$Foxp3$^+$ regulatory T cells (Tregs) play a significant role in the regulation of asthma, and the induction of allergen-specific Tregs has become one appealing strategy for asthma therapy [45–47]. Huang Qi was shown to increase the population of CD4$^+$CD25$^+$Foxp3$^+$ Tregs and promote Foxp3 mRNA expression in a rat model of asthma [47]. This suggests that the anti-asthmatic effects of Huang Qi are at least partially associated with CD4$^+$CD25$^+$Foxp3$^+$ Tregs.

## 6.4. Qian Hu

Qian Hu is a TCM commonly used for the treatment of asthma. Its major constituents, coumarins, were presumed to be responsible for its efficacy. Qian Hu was shown to reduce AHR and airway eosinophilic inflammation significantly, improve pathologic lesions of the lungs, reduce levels of IL-4, IL-5, and IL-13 in BALF and OVA-specific IgE in serum, inhibit the expression of TGF-$\beta$1 in lungs, and upregulate levels of IL-10 and IFN-$\gamma$ in BALF, as well as the percentage of CD4$^+$CD25$^+$Foxp3$^+$ regulatory T cells in the spleen [48, 49]. This suggests that Qian Hu has great therapeutic potential for the treatment of allergic asthma.

## 6.5. Gan Cao

Gan Cao, commonly called "licorice," is one of the most commonly used herbs in TCM. Airway eosinophilic inflammation is a major feature of allergic asthma. Eotaxin-1 is involved in the recruitment of eosinophils to sites of antigen-induced inflammation in asthmatic airways. Licorice flavonoids can inhibit eotaxin-1 secretion by human fetal lung fibroblasts in vitro [50]. Licorice flavonoids also significantly reduced eosinophilic pulmonary inflammation, serum IgE, IL-4, and IL-13 levels but also increased IFN-$\gamma$ production in lung cell cultures in response to antigen stimulation [51]. Glycyrrhizic acid is the main bioactive ingredient of licorice and has been shown to exert anti-asthmatic effects by modulating Th1/Th2 cytokines (IL-4, IL-5, IL-13 inhibition, IFN-$\gamma$ increase in BALF) and enhancing CD4$^+$CD25$^+$Foxp3$^+$ Tregs in OVA-sensitized mice [52]. Histological studies demonstrated that glycyrrhizic acid substantially inhibited OVA-induced eosinophilia in lung and airway tissues [52].

### 6.6. Sang Bai Pi

Sang Bai Pi (*Cortex mori radicis*), the root epidermis of *Morus alba* L., has been traditionally used for cough treatment in TCM. In OVA-induced asthma model mice [53], Sang Bai Pi significantly reduced AHR, inhibited the production of histamine and IgE in serum, and decreased airway eosinophil infiltration in BALF and lung tissue. Sang Bai Pi significantly attenuated the secretion and mRNA levels of Th2 cytokines, such as IL-4, IL-5, and IL-13. In addition, Sang Bai Pi significantly increased mRNA expression of IFN-$\gamma$, a Th1 cytokine. Furthermore, Sang Bai Pi can exert anti-asthmatic effects by enhancing $CD4^+CD25^+Foxp3^+$ Tregs.

### 6.7. Ban Xia

Ban Xia is a commonly used Chinese herb, with high bioactivity against cough and vomiting, and eliminating the stagnation of phlegm. Ban Xia significantly attenuated OVA-induced influx of the total number of leukocytes, eosinophils, neutrophils, macrophages, and lymphocytes into the lungs, decreased airway mucus production, and attenuated levels of IL-4, IL-5, IL-13, and TNF-$\alpha$, in a dose-dependent manner. Ban Xia also significantly reduced the plasma levels of histamine, total IgE and OVA-specific IgE [54, 55].

### 6.8. Bo He

Bo He has been reported to have pharmacological effects, including the lowering of body temperature and relaxation of the muscles of the digestive tract. The herb is traditionally used for the treatment of high fever, mild chills, cough, thirst, and sore throat and to combat nausea, vomiting, and flatulence. Bo He significantly inhibited eosinophils, neutrophils, lymphocytes, macrophages, and total cells in BALF of OVA-challenged mice. Bo He also decreased specific IgE and Th2 cytokines, such as IL-4 and IL-5, in BALF and lung tissue. Airway inflammation and hyperreactivity in asthma are likely to involve oxidative stress to the lung, and excess production of reactive oxygen species (ROS) by immune cells may play an important role in airway injury. An increase in the generation of ROS in the airway and BALF has been noted in OVA-induced asthma models. Bo He has been shown to reduce the ROS in the BALF of asthmatic model mice, as did montelukast, which has been used widely as an anti-asthmatic drug [56].

### 6.9. Da Huang

Da Huang is used to cure stomach illness and as a "cathartic" to relieve severe constipation as well as a poultice for fevers and edema caused by inflammation. Emodin, one of the major compounds of Da Huang, displays a number of biological activities, such as anti-microbial, immunosuppressive, anti-inflammatory, anti-tumor, and anti-atherosclerotic activities. Moreover, emodin attenuates mast cell-dependent passive anaphylactic reactions in IgE-sensitized mice. Emodin has also been shown to reduce IgE and Th2 cytokine levels in OVA-induced asthma mice. The inhibition of AHR by emodin may be associated with the reduction of IL-4, IL-5, and IL-13 production and eosinophilia aggregation into the lungs [57].

## 6.10. Jie Geng

Jie Geng is commonly used as a cough suppressant and expectorant for treatment of common colds, cough, sore throat, tonsillitis, and chest congestion. An aqueous extract of Jie Geng inhibited OVA-specific IgE levels in BALF. Inflammatory cell infiltration and mucus hyper-secretion were also inhibited by Jie Geng extracts. Furthermore, Jie Geng extracts decreased the generation of ROS in BALF, as well as NF-κB nuclear translocation in OVA-induced asthma mouse model [58]. Jie Geng is abundant in saponins, which inhibit IgE antibody-induced increases in IL-4 and TNF-$\alpha$ expression in RBL-2H3 cells. Saponins suppressed dinitrophenyl (DNP)–IgE antibody–induced phosphorylation of Syk, and further downstream, Changkil saponins (CKS) also inhibited the phosphorylation of Akt and MAPKs [59].

## 6.11. Huang Qin

Huang Qin is one of the most widely used medicinal herbs for the treatment of inflammation. Ethanol extracts of Huang Qin may effectively suppress inflammation by downregulating the expression of various inflammatory mediators (such as histamine) and reducing the production of inflammatory cytokines (such as IL-8 and TNF-$\alpha$) as well as MAPK activation [60]. Skullcapflavone II is a flavonoid derived from Huang Qin (*Scutellaria baicalensis*). Skullcapflavone II significantly reduced AHR, airway eosinophilia, Th2 cytokine production, and TGF-$\beta$1 levels in BALF and lungs in an OVA-induced asthma mouse model [61].

## 6.12. Yu Xing Cao

Yu Xing Cao is also used in folk medicine for diuresis and detoxification and for its anti-viral, anti-bacterial, and anti-leukemic activities. It has been used for the treatment of cough, pneumonia, bronchitis, uteritis, eczema, herpes simplex, acne, and chronic sinusitis. Ethanol extracts of Yu Xing Cao downregulate the expression of IL-4, IL-5, thymus and activation-regulated chemokine (TARC), and CCR4 receptor but do not have the same effect on IFN-$\gamma$ [62].

| Herbal name (Latin name) | Pictures | Possible mechanisms |
| --- | --- | --- |
| **Zhe Bei Mu** (*Fritillaria thunbergii*) | | Inhibits mast cell recruitment; decreases serum IL-6, IL-8, and TNF-$\alpha$; and inhibits MAPK pathway [43] |

| Herbal name (Latin name) | Pictures | Possible mechanisms |
| --- | --- | --- |
| **Xing Ren** (*Semen Armeniacae Amarum*) | | Decreases Th2 response; reduces IL-4 levels, eosinophilic inflammation, and AHR [44] |
| **Huang Qi** (*Astragalus membranaceus*) | | Decreases Th2 response; increases IFN-γ level; decreases IL-4, IL-5, IL-13, and TGF-β1 levels; reduces eosinophilic and neutrophilic inflammation; reduces AHR, collagen deposition, and mucus secretion; increases $CD4^+CD25^+FoxP3^+$ regulatory T cells [45–47] |
| **Qian Hu** (*Peucedanum praeruptorum Dunn*) | | Decreases Th2 response; increases IFN-γ and IL-10 levels; decreases IL-4, IL-5, IL-13, specific IgE, and TGF-β1 levels; reduces AHR, eosinophilic inflammation; increases $CD4^+CD25^+FoxP3^+$ regulatory T cells [48, 49] |
| **Gan Cao** (*Glycyrrhiza uralensis*) | | Decreases Th2 response; increases IFN-γ; decreases IL-4, IL-5, IL-13, specific IgE, and eotaxin-1 levels; reduces eosinophilic inflammation; increases $CD4^+CD25^+FoxP3^+$ regulatory T cells [50–52] |
| **Sang Bai Pi** (*Cortex mori radicis*) | | Decreases Th2 response; decreases IL-4, IL-5, IL-13, and specific IgE levels; reduces AHR, eosinophilic inflammation, and histamine release; increases $CD4^+CD25^+FoxP3^+$ regulatory T cells [53] |

| Herbal name (Latin name) | Pictures | Possible mechanisms |
| --- | --- | --- |
| **Ban Xia** (*Pinellia ternate*) | | Reduces IL-4, IL-5, IL-13, specific IgE, and TNF-$\alpha$ levels; reduces eosinophilic inflammation and mucus production [54, 55] |
| **Bo He** (*Mentha haplocalyx*) | | Decreases Th2 responses; decreases IL-4, IL-5, and specific IgE levels; reduces eosinophilic inflammation and mucus production [56] |
| **Da Huang** (*Rheum palmatum*) | | Decreases IL-4, IL-5, IL-13, and specific IgE levels; reduces eosinophilic inflammation [57] |
| **Jie Geng** (*Platycodon grandiflorum*) | | Decreases serum IgE, ROS scavenger; decreases IL-4 and TNF-$\alpha$; decreases Syk-dependent cascades; inhibits MAPK and Akt pathways [58, 59] |
| **Huang Qin** (*Scutellaria baicalensis*) | | Restores serum IL-8 and TNF-$\alpha$; inhibits MAPK pathways; decreases Th2 response; decreases IL-4, IL-5, IL-13, specific IgE, and TGF-$\beta$1 levels; reduces AHR and eosinophilic inflammation [60, 61] |

| Herbal name (Latin name) | Pictures | Possible mechanisms |
|---|---|---|
| **Yu Xing Cao** (*Houttuynia cordata Thunb.*) | | Decreases Th2 response; decreases IL-4, IL-5, and TARC levels [62] |

**Table 2.** Single herbs frequently used for asthmatic children

## 7. Acupuncture use in children with asthma

Acupuncture is a TCM therapeutic approach involving the stimulation of points on the body by using needles. For thousands of years, acupuncture has been used to treat several conditions, including asthma. Other methods of stimulation are traditionally used, such as electroacupuncture, laser acupuncture, and transcutaneous electrical nerve stimulation. There is evidence that acupuncture can reduce eosinophils in peripheral blood and decrease secretory IgA (sIgA) and total IgA levels in the saliva and nasal secretions of patients with allergic asthma [63]. The role of eosinophil activation in asthma has been well documented. sIgA is a potent stimulus for eosinophils and represents the main trigger for eosinophil degranulation. After acupuncture treatment, the reduction of sIgA levels and the decrease in the numbers of eosinophils may be associated with the amelioration of eosinophilic inflammation in patients with allergic asthma [63]. The numbers of CD3+, CD4+, and CD8+ T lymphocytes in the peripheral blood were significantly increased, without significant cortisol changes, in patients with allergic asthma treated by acupuncture [63]. It has been shown that electroacupuncture is prominent in promotion of CD4+CD25+FoxP3+ Tregs in an OVA-induced experimental model [64]. Furthermore, acupuncture has also been shown to inhibit AHR, eosinophils, neutrophils, specific IgE, Th1 cytokines, and the NF-κB pathway in OVA-induced experimental asthma [65].

## 8. Acupuncture point application

Acupuncture point application therapies, combining Chinese herbal medicine and acupuncture points, have been extensively applied for the treatment of allergic rhinitis (AR) and asthma [66]. Summer acupuncture point application treatment, also known as San-Fu-Tie or San-Fu-Jiu, is one type of direct moxibustion administered in the summer through the direct application of an irritating herbal paste to acupuncture points. The basic herbal prescription of San-Fu-Tie is usually composed of Bai Jie Zi (*Semen Sinapis Albae*), Xi Xin (*Herba Asari*), Gan Sui

(*Radix Kansui*), and Yan Hu Suo (*Rhizoma Corydalis*) [66, 67]. These herbs are ground into a powder, mixed, and made into paste using stale ginger juice. The standard acupoints include Fei-shu (BL-13) and Feng-men (BL-12), the meridians named Taiyang Bladder Meridian of Foot [67]. Numerous studies have shown significant efficacy through acupoint stimulation in treatment of asthma, such as improvement of lung function, a decrease in cytokines (IL-4, IL-6, IL-8, and IL-10), and restoring the Th1/Th2 balance toward Th1 [66, 67]. Few adverse effects have been reported, except for mild skin allergy, or local swelling and blisters.

## 9. Mind–body exercise

Mind–body exercise, such as *tai chi*, yoga, and meditation, may benefit people with chronic diseases. *Tai Chi Chuan* (*tai chi*), a Chinese traditional mind–body exercise with low-to-moderate exercise intensity, is thought to improve cardiopulmonary function in patients with chronic disease. *Tai Chi Chuan* has been shown to improve pulmonary function of asthmatic children [68]. Yoga training was reported to improve pulmonary function tests ($FEV_1$ and PEFR), quality of life, and decrease in the weekly number of asthma attacks, scores for drug treatment, and peak flow rate [69–71]. Meditation has also been shown to be a useful adjunct for treating asthma [72].

## 10. Further research

There is increasing evidence for the efficacy of TCM or other complementary therapies in the treatment of children with asthma, but this is still insufficient evidence for making recommendations about the value of TCM as an asthma treatment, as well-designed double-blind, randomized clinical trials are lacking.

## 11. Conclusion

Asthma is the leading cause of chronic illness and missed school days among childhood. In addition to standard treatment, the use of complementary therapy is increasing. TCM is a popular CAM in East Asia and throughout the world. There is increasing scientific evidence demonstrating that TCM has potential for the treatment of childhood asthma.

## 12. Abbreviations

AHR: airway hyperresponsiveness

ASM: airway smooth muscle

BALF: bronchoalveolar lavage fluid(s)

$FEV_1$: forced expiratory volume in 1 second

FVC: forced vital capacity

GM-CSF: granulocyte-macrophage colony-stimulating factor

ICAM-1: intercellular adhesion molecule 1

ICS: inhaled corticosteroids

IFN-$\gamma$: interferon gamma

IL: interleukin

LABA: long-acting beta-adrenoceptor agonists

MAPK: mitogen-activated protein kinases

MCP: monocyte chemotactic protein

MIP: macrophage inflammatory protein

MMP: matrix metalloproteinase

NF-$\kappa$B: nuclear factor-Kappa B

OVA: ovalbumin

PEFR: peak expiratory flow rate

RANTES: regulated on activation, normal T cell expressed and secreted

SABA: short-acting beta-2-adrenoceptor agonists

TARC: thymus and activation-regulated chemokine

TCM: Traditional Chinese medicine

TGF: transforming growth factors

TLRs: Toll-like receptors

TNF: tumor necrosis factor

VCAM-1: vascular cell adhesion molecule 1

VEGF: vascular endothelial growth factor

## Author details

Bei-Yu Wu[1], Chun-Ting Liu[1], Yu-Chiang Hung[1,2] and Wen-Long Hu[1,3,4*]

*Address all correspondence to: oolonghu@gmail.com

1 Department of Chinese Medicine, Kaohsiung Chang Gung Memorial Hospital and School of Traditional Chinese Medicine, Chang Gung University College of Medicine, Kaohsiung, Taiwan

2 School of Chinese Medicine for Post Baccalaureate, I-Shou University, Kaohsiung, Taiwan

3 Kaohsiung Medical University College of Medicine, Kaohsiung, Taiwan

4 Fooyin University College of Nursing, Kaohsiung, Taiwan

# References

[1] P.L. Brand, M.J. Makela, S.J. Szefler, T. Frischer, and D. Price. Monitoring asthma in childhood: symptoms, exacerbations and quality of life, *Eur Respir Rev, vol.* 24, no. 136, pp. 187–193, 2015.

[2] Global Initiative for Asthma. Global Strategy for Asthma Management and Prevention, 2015. Available from: www.ginasthma.org, accessed November 17, 2015.

[3] C.K. Lai, R. Beasley, J. Crane, S. Foliaki, J. Shah, and S. Weiland. Global variation in the prevalence and severity of asthma symptoms: phase three of the International Study of Asthma and Allergies in Childhood (ISAAC), *Thorax, vol.* 64, no. 6, pp. 476–483, 2009.

[4] N. Pearce and J. Douwes. The global epidemiology of asthma in children, *Int J Tuberc Lung Dis, vol.* 10, no. 2, pp. 125–132, 2006.

[5] C. Anandan, U. Nurmatov, O.C. van Schayck, and A. Sheikh. Is the prevalence of asthma declining? Systematic review of epidemiological studies, *Allergy, vol.* 65, no. 2, pp. 152–167, 2010.

[6] M. Masoli, D. Fabian, S. Holt, and R. Beasley. The global burden of asthma: executive summary of the GINA Dissemination Committee report, *Allergy, vol.* 59, no. 5, pp. 469–478, 2004.

[7] American Lung Association. Trends in Asthma Morbidity and Mortality, 2012. www.lung.org/assets/documents/research/asthma-trend-report.pdf, accessed November 1, 2015.

[8] A.N. Speight, D.A. Lee, and E.N. Hey. Underdiagnosis and undertreatment of asthma in childhood, *Br Med J (Clin Res Ed), vol.* 286, no. 6373, pp. 1253–1256, 1983.

[9] M.L. Levy, P.H. Quanjer, R. Booker, B.G. Cooper, S. Holmes, and I. Small. Diagnostic spirometry in primary care: Proposed standards for general practice compliant with American Thoracic Society and European Respiratory Society recommendations: a General Practice Airways Group (GPIAG)1 document, in association with the Association for Respiratory Technology & Physiology (ARTP)2 and Education for Health3 1

www.gpiag.org 2 www.artp.org 3 www.educationforhealth.org.uk, *Prim Care Respir J*, vol. 18, no. 3, pp. 130–147, 2009.

[10] P.H. Quanjer, S. Stanojevic, T.J. Cole, et al. Multi-ethnic reference values for spirometry for the 3-95-yr age range: the global lung function 2012 equations, *Eur Respir J*, vol. 40, no. 6, pp. 1324–1343, 2012.

[11] E.H. Bel. Clinical phenotypes of asthma, *Curr Opin Pulm Med*, vol. 10, no. 1, pp. 44–50, 2004.

[12] P. Fireman. Understanding asthma pathophysiology, *Allergy Asthma Proc*, vol. 24, no. 2, pp. 79–83, 2003.

[13] M. Frieri. Asthma concepts in the new millennium: update in asthma pathophysiology, *Allergy Asthma Proc*, vol. 26, no. 2, pp. 83–88, 2005.

[14] L. Maddox and D.A. Schwartz. The pathophysiology of asthma, *Annu Rev Med*, vol. 53, pp. 477–498, 2002.

[15] R. Djukanovic. Airway inflammation in asthma and its consequences: implications for treatment in children and adults, *J Allergy Clin Immunol*, vol. 109, no. 6 Suppl, pp. S539–548, 2002.

[16] National Asthma Education and Prevention Program, Third Expert Panel on the Diagnosis and Management of Asthma. Expert Panel Report 3: Guidelines for the Diagnosis and Management of Asthma. Bethesda (MD): National Heart, Lung, and Blood Institute (US); 2007 Aug. Section 2, Definition, Pathophysiology and Pathogenesis of Asthma, and Natural History of Asthma. Available from: www.ncbi.nlm.nih.gov/books/NBK7223/.

[17] S. Hall and D.K. Agrawal. Key mediators in the immunopathogenesis of allergic asthma, *Int Immunopharmacol*, vol. 23, no. 1, pp. 316–329, 2014.

[18] K.D. Stone, C. Prussin, and D.D. Metcalfe. IgE, mast cells, basophils, and eosinophils, *J Allergy Clin Immunol*, vol. 125, no. 2 Suppl 2, pp. S73–80, 2010.

[19] K. Nakagome and M. Nagata. Pathogenesis of airway inflammation in bronchial asthma, *Auris Nasus Larynx*, vol. 38, no. 5, pp. 555–563, 2011.

[20] C. Bergeron, M.K. Tulic, and Q. Hamid. Airway remodelling in asthma: from benchside to clinical practice, *Can Respir J*, vol. 17, no. 4, pp. e85–93, 2010.

[21] S. Al-Muhsen, J.R. Johnson, and Q. Hamid. Remodeling in asthma, *J Allergy Clin Immunol*, vol. 128, no. 3, pp. 451–462; quiz 463–454, 2011.

[22] A. Shifren, C. Witt, C. Christie, and M. Castro. Mechanisms of remodeling in asthmatic airways, *J Allergy (Cairo)*, vol. 2012, Article ID 316049, 2012.

[23] S. Saglani and C.M. Lloyd. Novel concepts in airway inflammation and remodelling in asthma, *Eur Respir J*, vol. 46, no. 6, pp. 1796–1804, 2015.

[24] X.M. Li. Complementary and alternative medicine in pediatric allergic disorders, *Curr Opin Allergy Clin Immunol*, vol. 9, no. 2, pp. 161–167, 2009.

[25] H.Y. Chen, Y.H. Lin, P.F. Thien, et al. Identifying core herbal treatments for children with asthma: implication from a chinese herbal medicine database in Taiwan, *Evid Based Complement Alternat Med*, vol. 2013, Article ID 125943, 2013.

[26] J.D. Mark. Pediatric asthma: an integrative approach to care, *Nutr Clin Pract*, vol. 24, no. 5, pp. 578–588, 2009.

[27] J.C. Philp, J. Maselli, L.M. Pachter, and M.D. Cabana. Complementary and alternative medicine use and adherence with pediatric asthma treatment, *Pediatrics*, vol. 129, no. 5, pp. e1148–1154, 2012.

[28] B. Jayaprakasam, N. Yang, M.C. Wen, et al. Constituents of the anti-asthma herbal formula ASHMI(TM) synergistically inhibit IL-4 and IL-5 secretion by murine Th2 memory cells, and eotaxin by human lung fibroblasts in vitro, *J Integr Med*, vol. 11, no. 3, pp. 195–205, 2013.

[29] P.J. Busse, B. Schofield, N. Birmingham, et al. The traditional Chinese herbal formula ASHMI inhibits allergic lung inflammation in antigen-sensitized and antigen-challenged aged mice, *Ann Allergy Asthma Immunol*, vol. 104, no. 3, pp. 236–246, 2010.

[30] K.D. Srivastava, D. Dunkin, C. Liu, et al. Effect of Antiasthma Simplified Herbal Medicine Intervention on neutrophil predominant airway inflammation in a ragweed sensitized murine asthma model, *Ann Allergy Asthma Immunol*, vol. 112, no. 4, pp. 339–347, 2014.

[31] K. Irifune, H. Hamada, R. Ito, et al. Antitussive effect of bakumondoto a fixed kampo medicine (six herbal components) for treatment of post-infectious prolonged cough: controlled clinical pilot study with 19 patients, *Phytomedicine*, vol. 18, no. 8–9, pp. 630–633, 2011.

[32] J. Tamaoki, A. Chiyotani, K. Takeyama, T. Kanemura, N. Sakai, and K. Konno. Potentiation of beta-adrenergic function by saiboku-to and bakumondo-to in canine bronchial smooth muscle, *Jpn J Pharmacol*, vol. 62, no. 2, pp. 155–159, 1993.

[33] C.H. Hsu, C.M. Lu, and T.T. Chang. Efficacy and safety of modified Mai-Men-Dong-Tang for treatment of allergic asthma, *Pediatr Allergy Immunol*, vol. 16, no. 1, pp. 76–81, 2005.

[34] T.T. Chang, C.C. Huang, and C.H. Hsu. Clinical evaluation of the Chinese herbal medicine formula STA-1 in the treatment of allergic asthma, *Phytother Res*, vol. 20, no. 5, pp. 342–347, 2006.

[35] T.T. Chang, C.C. Huang, and C.H. Hsu. Inhibition of mite-induced immunoglobulin E synthesis, airway inflammation, and hyperreactivity by herbal medicine STA-1, *Immunopharmacol Immunotoxicol*, vol. 28, no. 4, pp. 683–695, 2006.

[36] M. Miyagoshi, S. Amagaya, and Y. Ogihara. Antitussive effects of L-ephedrine, amygdalin, and makyokansekito (Chinese traditional medicine) using a cough model induced by sulfur dioxide gas in mice, *Planta Med*, no. 4, pp. 275–278, 1986.

[37] S.T. Kao, T.J. Yeh, C.C. Hsieh, H.B. Shiau, F.T. Yeh, and J.G. Lin. The effects of Ma-Xing-Gan-Shi-Tang on respiratory resistance and airway leukocyte infiltration in asthmatic guinea pigs, *Immunopharmacol Immunotoxicol*, vol. 23, no. 3, pp. 445–458, 2001.

[38] S.D. Wang, L.J. Lin, C.L. Chen, et al. Xiao-Qing-Long-Tang attenuates allergic airway inflammation and remodeling in repetitive Dermatogoides pteronyssinus challenged chronic asthmatic mice model, *J Ethnopharmacol*, vol. 142, no. 2, pp. 531–538, 2012.

[39] T. Nagai, Y. Arai, M. Emori, et al. Anti-allergic activity of a Kampo (Japanese herbal) medicine "Sho-seiryu-to (Xiao-Qing-Long-Tang)" on airway inflammation in a mouse model, *Int Immunopharmacol*, vol. 4, no. 10–11, pp. 1353–1365, 2004.

[40] S.T. Kao, C.S. Lin, C.C. Hsieh, W.T. Hsieh, and J.G. Lin. Effects of xiao-qing-long-tang (XQLT) on bronchoconstriction and airway eosinophil infiltration in ovalbumin-sensitized guinea pigs: in vivo and in vitro studies, *Allergy*, vol. 56, no. 12, pp. 1164–1171, 2001.

[41] S.T. Kao, C.H. Chang, Y.S. Chen, S.Y. Chiang, and J.G. Lin. Effects of Ding-Chuan-Tang on bronchoconstriction and airway leucocyte infiltration in sensitized guinea pigs, *Immunopharmacol Immunotoxicol*, vol. 26, no. 1, pp. 113–124, 2004.

[42] C.K. Chan, M.L. Kuo, J.J. Shen, L.C. See, H.H. Chang, and J.L. Huang. Ding Chuan Tang, a Chinese herb decoction, could improve airway hyper-responsiveness in stabilized asthmatic children: a randomized, double-blind clinical trial, *Pediatr Allergy Immunol*, vol. 17, no. 5, pp. 316–322, 2006.

[43] I.H. Cho, M.J. Lee, J.H. Kim, et al. Fritillaria ussuriensis extract inhibits the production of inflammatory cytokine and MAPKs in mast cells, *Biosci Biotechnol Biochem*, vol. 75, no. 8, pp. 1440–1445, 2011.

[44] J.S. Do, J.K. Hwang, H.J. Seo, W.H. Woo, and S.Y. Nam. Antiasthmatic activity and selective inhibition of type 2 helper T cell response by aqueous extract of semen armeniacae amarum, *Immunopharmacol Immunotoxicol*, vol. 28, no. 2, pp. 213–225, 2006.

[45] X. Yuan, S. Sun, S. Wang, and Y. Sun. Effects of astragaloside IV on IFN-gamma level and prolonged airway dysfunction in a murine model of chronic asthma, *Planta Med*, vol. 77, no. 4, pp. 328–333, 2011.

[46] H.H. Shen, K. Wang, W. Li, et al. Astragalus Membranaceus prevents airway hyper-reactivity in mice related to Th2 response inhibition, *J Ethnopharmacol*, vol. 116, no. 2, pp. 363–369, 2008.

[47]  H. Jin, Q. Luo, Y. Zheng, et al. CD4+CD25+Foxp3+ T cells contribute to the antiasthmatic effects of Astragalus membranaceus extract in a rat model of asthma, *Int Immunopharmacol, vol.* 15, no. 1, pp. 42–49, 2013.

[48]  Y.Y. Xiong, J.S. Wang, F.H. Wu, J. Li, and L.Y. Kong. The effects of (±)-Praeruptorin A on airway inflammation, remodeling and transforming growth factor-beta1/Smad signaling pathway in a murine model of allergic asthma, *Int Immunopharmacol, vol.* 14, no. 4, pp. 392–400, 2012.

[49]  Y.Y. Xiong, F.H. Wu, J.S. Wang, J. Li, and L.Y. Kong. Attenuation of airway hyperreactivity and T helper cell type 2 responses by coumarins from Peucedanum praeruptorum Dunn in a murine model of allergic airway inflammation, *J Ethnopharmacol, vol.* 141, no. 1, pp. 314–321, 2012.

[50]  B. Jayaprakasam, S. Doddaga, R. Wang, D. Holmes, J. Goldfarb, and X.M. Li. Licorice flavonoids inhibit eotaxin-1 secretion by human fetal lung fibroblasts in vitro, *J Agric Food Chem, vol.* 57, no. 3, pp. 820–825, 2009.

[51]  N. Yang, S. Patil, J. Zhuge, et al. Glycyrrhiza uralensis flavonoids present in antiasthma formula, ASHMI, inhibit memory Th2 responses in vitro and in vivo, *Phytother Res, vol.* 27, no. 9, pp. 1381–1391, 2013.

[52]  C. Ma, Z. Ma, X.L. Liao, J. Liu, Q. Fu, and S. Ma. Immunoregulatory effects of glycyrrhizic acid exerts anti-asthmatic effects via modulation of Th1/Th2 cytokines and enhancement of CD4(+)CD25(+)Foxp3+ regulatory T cells in ovalbumin-sensitized mice, *J Ethnopharmacol, vol.* 148, no. 3, pp. 755–762, 2013.

[53]  H.J. Kim, H.J. Lee, S.J. Jeong, H.J. Lee, S.H. Kim, and E.J. Park. Cortex Mori Radicis extract exerts antiasthmatic effects via enhancement of CD4(+)CD25(+)Foxp3(+) regulatory T cells and inhibition of Th2 cytokines in a mouse asthma model, *J Ethnopharmacol, vol.* 138, no. 1, pp. 40–46, 2011.

[54]  M.Y. Lee, I.S. Shin, W.Y. Jeon, H.S. Lim, J.H. Kim, and H. Ha. Pinellia ternata Breitenbach attenuates ovalbumin-induced allergic airway inflammation and mucus secretion in a murine model of asthma, *Immunopharmacol Immunotoxicol, vol.* 35, no. 3, pp. 410–418, 2013.

[55]  I.S. Ok, S.H. Kim, B.K. Kim, J.C. Lee, and Y.C. Lee. Pinellia ternata, Citrus reticulata, and their combinational prescription inhibit eosinophil infiltration and airway hyperresponsiveness by suppressing CCR3+ and Th2 cytokines production in the ovalbumin-induced asthma model, *Mediators Inflamm, vol.* 2009, Article ID 413270, 2009.

[56]  M.Y. Lee, J.A. Lee, C.S. Seo, H. Ha, N.H. Lee, and H.K. Shin. Protective effects of Mentha haplocalyx ethanol extract (MH) in a mouse model of allergic asthma, *Phytother Res, vol.* 25, no. 6, pp. 863–869, 2011.

[57] X. Chu, M. Wei, X. Yang, et al. Effects of an anthraquinone derivative from Rheum officinale Baill, emodin, on airway responses in a murine model of asthma, *Food Chem Toxicol*, vol. 50, no. 7, pp. 2368–2375, 2012.

[58] J.H. Choi, Y.P. Hwang, H.S. Lee, and H.G. Jeong. Inhibitory effect of Platycodi Radix on ovalbumin-induced airway inflammation in a murine model of asthma, *Food Chem Toxicol*, vol. 47, no. 6, pp. 1272–1279, 2009.

[59] E.H. Han, J.H. Park, J.Y. Kim, Y.C. Chung, and H.G. Jeong. Inhibitory mechanism of saponins derived from roots of Platycodon grandiflorum on anaphylactic reaction and IgE-mediated allergic response in mast cells, *Food Chem Toxicol*, vol. 47, no. 6, pp. 1069–1075, 2009.

[60] H.S. Jung, M.H. Kim, N.G. Gwak, et al. Antiallergic effects of Scutellaria baicalensis on inflammation in vivo and in vitro, *J Ethnopharmacol*, vol. 141, no. 1, pp. 345–349, 2012.

[61] H.Y. Jang, K.S. Ahn, M.J. Park, O.K. Kwon, H.K. Lee, and S.R. Oh. Skullcapflavone II inhibits ovalbumin-induced airway inflammation in a mouse model of asthma, *Int Immunopharmacol*, vol. 12, no. 4, pp. 666–674, 2012.

[62] J.S. Lee, I.S. Kim, J.H. Kim, J.S. Kim, D.H. Kim, and C.Y. Yun. Suppressive effects of Houttuynia cordata Thunb (Saururaceae) extract on Th2 immune response, *J Ethnopharmacol*, vol. 117, no. 1, pp. 34–40, 2008.

[63] Y.Q. Yang, H.P. Chen, Y. Wang, L.M. Yin, Y.D. Xu, and J. Ran. Considerations for use of acupuncture as supplemental therapy for patients with allergic asthma, *Clin Rev Allergy Immunol*, vol. 44, no. 3, pp. 254–261, 2013.

[64] Y. Kwon, S.H. Sohn, G. Lee, et al. Electroacupuncture attenuates ovalbumin-induced allergic asthma via modulating CD4(+)CD25(+) regulatory T cells, *Evid Based Complement Alternat Med*, vol. 2012, Article ID 647308, 2012.

[65] Y. Wei, M. Dong, H. Zhang, et al. Acupuncture Attenuated Inflammation and Inhibited TH17 and Treg Activity in Experimental Asthma, *Evid Based Complement Alternat Med*, vol. 2015, Article ID 340126, 2015.

[66] C.Y. Wen, Y.F. Liu, L. Zhou, H.X. Zhang, and S.H. Tu. A systematic and narrative review of acupuncture point application therapies in the treatment of allergic rhinitis and asthma during Dog Days, *Evid Based Complement Alternat Med*, vol. 2015, Article ID 846851, 2015.

[67] X. Wu, J. Peng, G. Li, W. Zhang, G. Liu, and B. Liu. Efficacy evaluation of summer acupoint application treatment on asthma patients: a two-year follow-up clinical study, *J Tradit Chin Med*, vol. 35, no. 1, pp. 21–27, 2015.

[68] Y.F. Chang, Y.H. Yang, C.C. Chen, and B.L. Chiang. Tai Chi Chuan training improves the pulmonary function of asthmatic children, *J Microbiol Immunol Infect*, vol. 41, no. 1, pp. 88–95, 2008.

[69] A.J. Bidwell, B. Yazel, D. Davin, T.J. Fairchild, and J.A. Kanaley. Yoga training improves quality of life in women with asthma, *J Altern Complement Med*, vol. 18, no. 8, pp. 749–755, 2012.

[70] R. Nagarathna and H.R. Nagendra. Yoga for bronchial asthma: a controlled study, *Br Med J (Clin Res Ed)*, vol. 291, no. 6502, pp. 1077–1079, 1985.

[71] T. Saxena and M. Saxena. The effect of various breathing exercises (pranayama) in patients with bronchial asthma of mild to moderate severity, *Int J Yoga*, vol. 2, no. 1, pp. 22–25, 2009.

[72] A.F. Wilson, R. Honsberger, J.T. Chiu, and H.S. Novey. Transcendental meditation and asthma, *Respiration*, vol. 32, no. 1, pp. 74–80, 1975.

# 2

# Current and Future Asthma Treatments: Phenotypical Approach on the Path to Personalized Medicine in Asthma

Irina Diana Bobolea, Carlos Melero and
Jesús Jurado-Palomo

### Abstract

Despite widely available and effective treatments, achieving asthma control is still an unmet need for many patients. One of the explanations resides perhaps in the heterogeneity of the disease. Asthma is in fact, as we understand it today, a complex syndrome made up of numerous disease variants or asthma phenotypes; when the different underlying mechanisms are identified, the more ambitious term "endotype" is used, with consequent therapeutic implications. Remarkable efforts have been made to identify the features of difficult-to-control (usually severe) asthma, which are different from those described for mild-to-moderate asthma, setting the stage for the development of new and even individualized therapies. As different drugs target different pathways, it is necessary to determine the individual profile of pathophysiological abnormalities for each patient. The most fascinating options of the new asthma treatments are the monoclonal antibodies targeted against key inflammatory cytokines, and the most proximately available treatments within the next years are discussed here. Also, current evidence and understanding of somehow older therapeutic options, such as anticholinergics, thermoplasty, or omalizumab, are reviewed from a phenotypical approach.

**Keywords:** asthma, mepolizumab, monoclonal antibodies, omalizumab, phenotypes, thermoplasty, tiotropium

## 1. Introduction

International [1] and national [2] guidelines for the management of asthma highlight the importance of finding the effective treatments for achieving and maintaining control. In spite of the existence of uniform treatment guidelines, as well as of quite accessible and effective treatments, achieving asthma control often remains a constant challenge. Recent studies indicate that over 50% of patients with asthma are not controlled [3, 4], not even when receiving a combination of inhaled corticosteroids (ICSs) and a long acting beta-2-agonist (LABA) [5] as controller treatment. These data suggest that the search for alternative treatments is required, particularly for patients with severe uncontrolled a-wrap id="tab1" position="anchor"> sthma.

When searching for new treatment options in asthma, it is important to remember that different drugs, particularly biological agents, act on different pathogenic pathways. So, the individual profile of physiopathological alterations of each patient should be determined to prescribe the most appropriate treatment in each case [6].

Asthma management, from both a current as well as a future risk perspective, must comprehend the stratification of patients into the recently defined phenotypes (such as clinical, inflammatory, and molecular) [7] and endotypes (such as allergic asthma, aspirin-sensitive asthma, late-onset hypereosinophilic asthma) [8], in the attempt to find a more personalized treatment for each patient. Moreover, in the last 10 years, significant efforts have been made to identify the characteristics that differentiate severe asthma from mild to moderate asthma, preparing the ground for the development of new selective treatments.

The main goal of the treatment is to achieve and maintain the control of the disease as soon as possible, to prevent chronic airflow obstruction, and to reduce mortality. The goals of the treatment, both in its current control domain and in preventing exacerbations and accelerated loss of lung function (future risk), could be achieved in most of the patients with appropriate treatment [9, 10].

## 2. New bronchodilators for asthma

### 2.1 Anticholinergics

Maintenance treatment to achieve asthma control currently includes inhaled or systemic glucocorticoids (ICS), leukotriene antagonists, LABAs, theophylline, monoclonal antibodies (mAbs) anti-IgE (omalizumab), and recently, newly included in the latest clinical practice guidelines, tiotropium bromide [1, 2]. The parasympathetic or cholinergic system is the most important bronchoconstrictor and hypersecretory neurological mechanism of the airways [11], and blocking specific muscarinic receptors is a therapeutic alternative to reduce the increase in parasympathetic activity that characterizes the main pulmonary obstructive diseases, such as asthma and chronic obstructive pulmonary disease (COPD). Therefore, the natural alkaloids from the Solanaceae family plants (*Atropa belladonna* and *Datura stramonium*) represent one of the traditional remedies against bronchospasm. Atropine, the prototype nonselective muscarinic receptor antagonist, with "tertiary ammonium" structure, was widely used from the late nineteenth century in oral, parenteral, and inhaled forms for the treatment of asthma; however, its use is constrained by the cardiovascular side effects. Following the introduction of ephedrine and adrenaline, in the early twentieth century, atropine fell into disuse. Later, anticholinergic therapy has returned to the forefront in the treatment of COPD, with the introduction of synthetic quaternary derivatives of atropine, short acting (ipratropium bromide) and long acting (tiotropium, aclidinium, umeclidinium, and glycopyrronium), the latter known under the acronym LAMA (long-acting muscarinic antagonists). The "quaternary ammonium" structure [12] makes them soluble in water and insoluble in lipids, therefore preventing the passage through biological barriers that are easily crossed by "tertiary ammonium" components, such as atropine, hence their lack of central nervous system effects; also they are poorly absorbed from the lung and gastrointestinal tract and do not inhibit the mucociliary clearance [13].

### 2.1.1 Tiotropium

Tiotropium bromide is the first long-acting anticholinergic agent (24 hours action), widely used for treatment of COPD. At the end of 2014, it was also approved by the FDA as an additional treatment of asthma in patients >12 years in the United States and in adult patients with asthma not controlled by the ICS in the European Union (Spiriva® Respimat). Such approval has been obtained based on sound scientific evidence on the effectiveness and safety of treatment with tiotropium in patients with mild-to-moderate and severe asthma. The major evidence is discussed below and is summarized in Table 1 [14].

| Study | Patients' characteristics | Main results and Conclusions |
|---|---|---|
| Park et al. 2009 [15] | One hundred and thirty-eight patients with severe asthma on conventional medications and with decreased lung function. | – Forty-six of the 138 (33.3%) of patients with severe asthma were found to respond to adjuvant tiotropium bromide.<br>– The presence of Arg16Gly in ADRB2 (coding beta-2 adrenoreceptor) may predict response to tiotropium bromide. |
| Peters et al. 2010 [17] | Two hundred and ten patients with poorly controlled asthma with an ICS alone. | – Tiotropium bromide, added to an IC, improved symptoms and lung function in patients with inadequately controlled asthma.<br>– Its effects appeared to be equivalent to those with the addition of salmeterol. |
| Bateman et al. 2011 [16] | Three hundred and eighty-eight patients with asthma with the B16-Arg/Arg genotype whose symptoms were not controlled by ICS (moderate asthma). | – Tiotropium bromide was more effective than placebo and as effective as salmeterol in maintaining improved lung function in B16-Arg/Arg patients with moderate persistent asthma.<br>– Safety profiles were comparable. |
| Kerstjens et al. 2011 [18] | One hundred patients with uncontrolled severe asthma, despite receiving treatment with high-dose ICS plus a LABA. | – The addition of once-daily tiotropium to asthma treatment significantly improved lung function over 24 hours in patients with inadequately controlled, severe, persistent asthma. |

| Study | Patients' characteristics | Main results and Conclusions |
|---|---|---|
| Kerstjens et al. 2012 [19] | Nine hundred and twelve patients (814 finished the study) with uncontrolled asthma in spite of ICS/LABA (studies PrimoTinAsthma 1 and 2). | – The addition of tiotropium (409 patients) compared with placebo (405 patients) significantly increased the time to the first severe exacerbation and provided a modest but sustained bronchodilation. |

*ICS = inhaled corticosteroids; LABA = long-acting beta-2-agonists.*

**Table 1.** Summary of studies that demonstrate the efficiency of tiotropium bromide in asthma [14].

A study published in 2009 [15] showed additional improvement in lung function in patients with severe asthma when tiotropium was added to conventional treatment, according to the guidelines (LABA/ICS, theophylline, antagonists of leukotriene receptor, and oral steroids). A total of 138 severe asthmatics with decreased lung function were recruited. Tiotropium 18 µg (via HandiHaler) was added once a day, and lung function was assessed every 4 weeks. Responders were defined as those with an improvement of ≥15% (or 200 mL) in FEV1 that was maintained for at least 8 successive weeks. Of the 138 people with asthma, 46 (33.3%) responded to tiotropium.

Peters et al. [16] conducted an independent three-way, double-blind, crossover study in 210 patients with asthma to evaluate the effect of the addition of tiotropium to ICS, when compared with doubling the dose of ICS (primary superiority comparison) or adding salmeterol (secondary comparison of non-inferiority). Use of tiotropium was superior when compared with doubling the dose of ICS; it also demonstrated superiority in the secondary endpoints, including evening PEF, the proportion of asthma control days, prebronchodilator FEV1, and daily symptom scores. The addition of tiotropium was not inferior to the addition of salmeterol on all evaluated results and increased FEV1 prebronchodilator more than salmeterol. In summary, when added to an ICS, tiotropium improved symptoms and lung function in poorly controlled patients with asthma, and its effects appear to be equivalent to those obtained with the addition of salmeterol.

Bateman et al. [17] carried out a double-blind, double-dummy, placebo-controlled trial to compare the efficacy and safety profile of tiotropium (Respimat 5 µg, administered daily in the evening with the Respimat device) with that of salmeterol and placebo added to an ICS, in 16-Arg/Arg patients with asthma that was not controlled by ICS alone. The study population comprised patients aged 18–67 years, with reversibility to bronchodilators and symptoms that were not controlled by regular therapy with ICS (400–1000 µg of budesonide or equivalent maintained throughout the trial). Changes in weekly primary endpoint (PEF) from the last week of the run-in period to the last week of treatment showed that tiotropium was not inferior to salmeterol.

It has been also assessed whether tiotropium could be an effective bronchodilator in patients with severe asthma who remain symptomatic and obstructed despite maximum recommended treatment with the combination of ICS and LABA. Kerstjens et al. [18] compared the efficacy and safety profile of two doses of tiotropium (Respimat, 5 and 10 µg daily) with placebo as an add-on therapy in 100 patients with uncontrolled severe asthma despite maintenance treatment with at least a high dose ICS combined with a LABA, in a randomized, double-blind, crossover study with three treatment periods of 8 weeks each. The PEF was peak FEV1 at the end of each treatment period. Peak FEV1 was significantly higher with 5 μg and 10 μg of tiotropium than placebo, whereas there was no significant difference between the two active doses. Domiciliary PEF values were higher with both tiotropium doses. Adverse events were balanced across groups, except for dry mouth, which was more common in patients taking tiotropium 10 μg. This study shows that the addition of once-daily tiotropium for asthma treatment, including a high-dose ICS combined with a LABA, significantly improves lung function over 24 hours in patients with uncontrolled severe asthma.

Subsequently, Kerstjens et al. [19] have evaluated the influence of add-on treatment with tiotropium on exacerbations, an important marker, as is well known, of asthma control. Two parallel, randomized, double-blind placebo-controlled trials (PrimoTinAsthma 1 and PrimoTinAsthma 2) were conducted between October 2008 and July 2011 in 15 countries, involving 912 patients with severe asthma and fixed airflow obstruction, who were randomized for tiotropium (Respimat, 5 μg) or placebo once daily for 48 weeks.

It was concluded that in patients with poorly controlled severe asthma despite the use of ICS and LABA, the addition of tiotropium significantly increased the time to the first severe exacerbation and provided a modest but sustained bronchodilation.

As mentioned in the introduction, we once more insist on the importance of determining the asthma phenotype: a small study (17 patients) showed that tiotropium is more effective in asthmatic smokers or non-smokers treated with medium-to-high doses of ICS if the inflammatory phenotype according to induced sputum is non-eosinophilic [20]. This suggests that perhaps early phenotyping poorly controlled asthmatic patients with high doses of ICS and even systemic corticosteroids (SC) could give tiotropium a corticosteroid-sparing effect in patients who turn out to have steroid-resistant asthma phenotypes. In fact, given its mechanism of action, the bronchodilator additive effect of tiotropium makes most sense in the following circumstances [21]: patients with asthma–COPD overlap syndrome (ACOS) [12], asthma of psychogenic origin, bronchospasm triggered by beta blockers, asthma with chronic airflow limitation, and severe asthmatics with Arg/Gly variation in codon 16 of the ADRB2 gene [15].

However, it seems that the effect of tiotropium goes beyond the bronchodilation because it has significant anti-inflammatory and antiproliferative capacities, such as reduction of hyperplasia of bronchial smooth muscle and inhibition of proliferation of fibroblasts and myofibroblasts [22]. Furthermore, in vitro studies using experimental models of asthma (ovalbumin-sensitized guinea pigs) have shown that tiotropium inhibits airway remodeling induced by allergens in a similar way to budesonide [23, 24], so its role in the management of allergic asthma may be more important than it seems at first glance.

Regarding adverse effects, tiotropium is a safe drug and is generally well tolerated, the most common side effect being dry mouth. The heart rhythm disturbances are rare (atrial fibrillation, atrial sinus, or supraventricular tachycardia). The TIOSPIR [25] study concluded that tiotropium Respimat was safe in COPD patients with ischemic heart disease and/or stable arrhythmias. The study excluded patients with myocardial infarction in the past 6 months, class III–IV NYHA heart failure, potentially fatal arrhythmias, and chronic renal failure.

## 2.2. New combinations: ICS/LABA, LABA/LAMA, and triple therapy LABA/LAMA/ICS

Because combination therapy with ICS and LABA is the usual therapeutic option for the treatment of asthma, there is great interest in developing combinations of administration once a day, in an attempt to simplify treatment and improve treatment compliance [26], a currently achievable challenge with the new ICSs (such as ciclesonide, mometasone, and fluticasone furoate) and the emergence of new ultra-LABAs (such as indacaterol, vilanterol, and olodaterol), which can be administered in a single-daily dose. Currently, new combination therapies of ultra-LABA/ICS have been developed, are in clinical trial phases II–III, or have even recently marketed (vilanterol/fluticasone furoate), like several other LAMA–LABA combinations for the treatment of COPD: tiotropium/ olodaterol, aclidinium/ formoterol, umeclidinium / indacaterol, vilanterol / umeclidinium, and so on [27]. However, the use of some of these drugs in asthma is still being investigated (see also Table **2** ).

---

**Long-acting muscarinic antagonists (LAMA):**

- Aclidinium bromide (approved for treatment of COPD)

**Ultra-long-acting muscarinic antagonists (ultra-LAMA):**

- Tiotropium bromide (approved for treatment of asthma and COPD)

- Glycopyrronium bromide (approved for treatment of COPD)

**Ultra–long-acting beta-2-agonists (ultra-LABA):**

- Indacaterol maleate (approved for treatment of COPD)

- Carmoterol hydrochloride, milveterol hydrochloride, olodaterol hydrochloride

**New combinations of ultra–long-acting beta-2-agonists (ultra-LABA) and inhaled corticosteroids (ICS):**

- Vilanterol trifenatate / fluticasone furoate (approved for treatment of asthma and COPD)

- Indacaterol maleate / mometasone (MGC-149)

- Indacaterol maleate / QAE 397

**New combinations of LAMA or ultra-LAMA and LABA or ultra-LABA:**

- Tiotropium bromide / olodaterol hydrochloride

- Indacaterol maleate / glycopyrronium bromide (QVA149)

- Umeclidinium bromide / vilanterol trifenatate (approved for COPD)

- Formoterol/ aclidinium (approved for COPD)

**Triple therapy of ultra-long-acting beta-2-agonists (ultra-LABA), inhaled corticosteroids (ICS), and ultra–long-acting muscarinic antagonists (ultra-LAMA):**

• Vilanterol trifenatate/fluticasone furoate/umeclidinium bromide

---

*COPD = chronic obstructive pulmonary disease; ICS = inhaled corticosteroids; LABA = long-acting beta-2-agonists; LAMA = long-acting muscarinic antagonists.*

---

**Table 2.** New bronchodilators, either available or under clinical development, with probable upcoming indication for asthma (monotherapy and combinations).

When talking about the triple combination, it refers to ICSs, such as beta-2-agonist and inhaled anticholinergics, but mainly to long-acting drugs (LAMA–LABA–ICS). The possibility of associating these three drugs can contribute to better compliance, better control of the symptoms, and improved quality of life, as well as to a decrease in exacerbations. There are several clinical studies in development: fluticasone/salmeterol/tiotropium and budesonide/formoterol/tiotropium [28]. The first triple combination formoterol/tiotropium/ciclesonide (Triohale®, Cipla) is now available in India [29], and its probable effectiveness in asthma is yet to be proven in future clinical trials.

# 3. Biological and other highly specialized therapies for uncontrolled asthma: Phenotype-oriented present and future options

In the last decade, significant efforts have been made to identify the characteristics of severe asthma, which are different from those described in the mild-to-moderate asthma, setting the stage for the development of new personalized therapies [7, 30]. The most promising options are represented by biological therapies, including mAbs against selective targets [10]. Later, we summarize the evidence of the only mAb that is available today to treat patients with severe asthma (omalizumab) and review those biological treatments that are currently in clinical trials, but in a more advanced stage of development and will be available for the clinical practice in the upcoming years.

## 3.1 Allergic asthma

*3.1.1 Omalizumab: state of the art on long-term efficacy and safety in real life studies.*

Omalizumab is currently approved as an additional treatment in patients older than 6 years with severe allergic asthma [31]. The antibody is an IgG1 kappa that binds to IgE and prevents it binding to FCεRI and FCεRII (IgE receptors of, respectively, high and low affinity), expressed on mast cells, basophils, and dendritic cells [32]. Several post-marketing studies have been conducted in European countries [33–37] to assess the effectiveness of omalizumab: despite obvious differences between countries, all studies confirmed the usefulness and safety of omalizumab in real-life conditions. The discontinuation rate was variable, but the lack of efficacy was less than 20%, whereas in clinical trials, it was 30–40%. A probable explanation is that the "real" patients are more serious and less selected than those included in clinical trials. In Spain, a multicenter study was conducted within the routine clinical practice, in Pulmonology and Allergology departments, to evaluate the efficacy and tolerability of omalizumab [38]. With the participation of 30 centers nationwide, 266 patients who had received at least one dose of omalizumab, with 2 years of follow-up at least, were analyzed. The global evaluation of therapeutic efficacy (GETE) was good or excellent in most treated patients: 74.6% at 4 months, reaching 81.6% of the patients after 2 years, with statistically significant differences from baseline. Significant improvements in asthma control test (ACT), lung function, and exacerbation frequency were also demonstrated. In terms of medication, the doses of ICSs were significantly decreased, and the maintenance treatment with oral corticosteroids was suspended in many patients [38].

### 3.1.2. Current evidence on omalizumab efficacy in off-label uses: Non-allergic asthma, nasal polyps, and allergic broncopulmonary aspergillosis

The interaction between IgE and omalizumab prevents a fundamental step in the inflammatory cascade. The rapid decrease in the free circulating IgE leads to a progressive and significant decrease in the expression of IgE receptors on the inflammatory cells, so it is important to take into consideration certain entities in which IgE may also play a part even if the allergic etiology is not well established, such as nasal polyposis (NP) or non-allergic asthma.

While the inflammation in allergic or "extrinsic" asthma is clearly caused by outdoor allergens (such as dust mites and animal dander), in the intrinsic disease, there is no identifiable allergen, at least not by currently available methods. In this case, an unidentified exogenous antigen (without systemic sensitization), an infectious agent, or an endogenous "allergen" might be responsible for triggering the mechanism of atopy or in this case "entopy" [39]. The finding of specific IgEs against *Staphylococcus aureus* enterotoxins in patients with severe asthma, intolerance to NSAIDs and NP allowed to speculate that they were susceptible of having their airways colonized by *S. aureus*, which through the release of superantigens could trigger an inflammatory response with formation of local IgE [40]. NP may be present in asthma with or without concomitant atopy, but it is particularly associated with non-allergic aspirin-sensitive asthma and is one of the most common comorbid conditions in patients with severe asthma. NP is not a life-threatening condition, but the patients see their quality of life severely compromised and must undergo prolonged treatments with topical and systemic corticosteroids and multiple sinus surgeries in most cases. Over time, the lack of effective alternative treatments and the need to respond to these IgE-mediated diseases led professionals to use omalizumab off-label, with very promising results, as discussed later.

In 2010, a multicenter study performed in Spain described the evolution of nasal polyps in 19 patients with NP and severe asthma treated with omalizumab [41]. The average treatment time was 16 (15–28) months. Thirteen patients (68%) had undergone at least one endoscopic surgery. The size of the polyps (assessed by calculating a score of 0–8 points by means of nasal endoscopy and confirmed by CT scan) diminished significantly in both nasal cavities after the treatment. Later, Bachart et al assessed the usefulness of anti-IgE in severe or recurrent NP associated with asthma, in a prospective double-blind placebo-controlled study (24 patients)

[42]. There was a significant improvement at 16 weeks of treatment in clinical terms: nasal congestion, rhinorrhea, and loss of smell. An overall reduction in polyp size (primary end-point, assessed using the same above-mentioned score) when compared to baseline was observed [41].

As to non-allergic asthma, in Spain it was first demonstrated, in a retrospective observational study [43], the efficacy of omalizumab in 29 patients with "non-atopic" asthma. GETE, ACT, the number of exacerbations and lung function improved significantly after treatment with omalizumab. There was no statistically significant difference in the response of the non-atopic asthmatics when compared with 266 patients with positive prick tests to usual inhalants. These results were subsequently confirmed in a prospective double-blind placebo-controlled trial [44].

Total IgE levels are a marker of immune activity in another severe lung disease, often without any effective therapeutic alternative to systemic corticosteroids: allergic bronchopulmonary aspergillosis (ABPA). The anti-IgE treatment was also evaluated in this pathology (also off-label). In 2011, a multicenter research conducted in Spain included 18 patients with ABPA from 11 hospitals [45]. Patients were followed for a median of 36 (28–42) weeks. In this series, the largest published so far, omalizumab was beneficial in reducing daytime symptoms (44%) and nighttime awakenings (22%), significantly reduced exacerbations and improved FEV1 ($p$ = 0.03), allowing a reduction or even discontinuance of systemic corticosteroids.

### 3.1.3. New anti-IgE agents: ligelizumab and quilizumab

The inverse correlation between free IgE levels and asthma control, found in several studies [46], suggests that a more profound suppression of free IgE could lead to an even more marked clinical improvement, so new, more potent anti-IgE mAbs are currently being assessed in clinical trials.

### 3.1.3.1. Ligelizumab

QGE031B (ligelizumab) is a new anti-IgE mAb (Novartis). It is a humanized IgG1 that binds with higher affinity to the Ce3 region of IgE. QGE031 is designed for greater suppression of IgE, with a dissociation constant (Kd) of 139 pM, representing an increase in almost 50 times of the affinity for IgE when compared with omalizumab (Kd = 6–8 nM). This is hypothesized to overcome some of the limitations associated with the dosage of omalizumab and lead to better clinical outcomes in asthma.

Up to date, December 2015, we have only data from preclinical experiments, and the results of two phase I, randomized, double-blind placebo-controlled studies investigating the pharmacokinetics, pharmacodynamics, and safety of ligelizumab in atopic but otherwise healthy subjects [47]. Ligelizumab was superior to omalizumab in the suppression of free IgE and FceRI expression on surface of basophils. These effects resulted in the almost complete suppression of skin response to allergens, which was higher in extent and duration when compared with omalizumab. In the 156 patients who completed the study, no serious adverse effects were reported, and only one patient developed urticaria accompanied by systemic symptoms. QGE031B's effectiveness is currently being evaluated in patients with allergic asthma (GINA step 4/5) in a phase IIa clinical trial, with omalizumab as an active comparator.

# Quilizumab

Quilizumab (MEMP1972A, Genentech/Roche), another mAb anti-IgE, is being studied now in a phase IIb, randomized, double-blind, placebo-controlled clinical trial aimed to evaluate the efficacy and safety of three different doses (150, 300, and 450 mg, subcutaneously) in adults with allergic asthma not controlled with ICS and a second controller (NCT01582503). Quilizumab already has been proven effective in decreasing total and specific IgE in patients with allergic rhinitis (NCT01160861) and mild allergic asthma (NCT01196039), with a good safety profile [48].

## 3.2. Eosinophilic and Th2 high asthma

### 3.2.1. Anti IL-5 monoclonal antibodies: mepolizumab, reslizumab, and benralizumab

Interleukin-5 (IL-5) is a hematopoietic cytokine produced by various cells such as Th2 lymphocytes, eosinophils, basophils, mast cells, and natural killer T-cells, and it is the main eosinophil modulator cytokine [49] because it enhances eosinophil chemotaxis, activation, and degranulation, while reducing apoptosis and prolonging eosinophils' survival. The IL-5 receptor (IL-5R), expressed on both basophils and eosinophils, is made up of two subunits: an $\alpha$-subunit (IL-5R$\alpha$) that is IL-5-specific and a $\beta$c-subunit (IL-5R$\beta$c) that is responsible for signal transduction and is shared with the specific $\alpha$-receptor subunits of IL-3 receptors and granu-locyte–macrophage colony–stimulating factor (GM-CSF).

Two mAbs (mepolizumab and relizumab) that neutralize IL-5 and another mAb (benralizu-mab) that blocks the IL-5R$\alpha$ have been developed and are currently being evaluated in clinical trials [50].

### 3.2.1.1 Mepolizumab

Mepolizumab in a fully humanized anti-IL-5 IgG1 mAb that binds to the free IL-5 with high affinity and specificity, thus preventing its binding to the $\alpha$ chain of the IL-5R on the eosinophil cell surface. It was the first IL-5 antagonist used in randomized, controlled trials in patients with mild asthma [51, 52] and with moderate uncontrolled persistent asthma [53]. A reduced eosinophil count was observed in both sputum and peripheral blood asthma in biopsies of bronchia and bone marrow, but with no effect on bronchial hyperresponsiveness (BHR), late asthmatic response, lung function, symptoms, or use of rescue medication whatsoever [51–53]. The reduction in the percentage of exacerbations [53] did not reach statistical significance though.

In these studies, patients were not selected according to the presence of eosinophilic airway inflammation, and the number of exacerbations, a parameter directly and causally related with eosinophilic airway inflammation, was not evaluated as a principal variable of the response to treatment [49]. Two new trials were subsequently performed in patients with refractory severe persistent asthma with recurrent exacerbations, who had bronchial eosinophilic inflammation [54, 55]. Both trials reported a very significant reduction in the number of exacerbations and in the dose of oral corticosteroids in the active group when compared to those in the placebo group, as well as a major improvement in asthma control questionnaire (ACQ) scores. This response was accompanied by a significant reduction in eosinophil numbers in blood and sputum.

A phase IIb multicenter study (GlaxoSmithKline) has also been performed in order to determine the optimal dose of mepolizumab and to confirm its efficacy and safety in patients with severe eosinophilic asthma (the DREAM study) [56]. A total of 621 patients were randomized to placebo or one of three mepolizumab doses (75, 250, or 750 mg respectively) in parallel groups for 1 year. Mepolizumab reduced the number of severe exacerbations by 50% approximately in all the mepolizumab groups when compared with placebo, irrespective of the dose. Also, no dose–response effect was reported. The blood and sputum eosinophil counts were also reduced, and a dose–response effect was observed for eosinophil counts in sputum. On the other hand, no changes in asthma symptoms, quality of life, FeNO or lung function were observed. The drug was safe and effective. A multivariant analysis established that blood eosinophilia and the number of exacerbations in the 12 months prior to the study only were associated with a good response to mepolizumab. A meta-analysis performed on published clinical trials with mepolizumab, including a total of 1131 patients, confirmed that in cases of eosinophilic asthma, mepolizumab reduced the number of exacerbations and improved asthma-related quality of life [57].

### 3.2.1.2 Reslizumab

Reslizumab, a humanized IgG2, is another IL-5 inhibitor that is administered intravenously, although it has not been studied at such extent as mepolizumab. The only published clinical trial in patients with poorly controlled eosinophilic asthma proved that patients treated with reslizumab showed a significant improvement in FEV1 and, interestingly, patients with concomitant polyposis showed better asthma control compared to the placebo group [58].

### 3.2.1.3 Benralizumab

Benralizumab is a humanized IgG1 mAb targeting IL-5Rα, which reduces eosinophilia by antibody-dependent cell-mediated cytotoxicity. Intravenous benralizumab has shown acceptable safety and tolerability in a phase I, dose-escalating study, with a marked reduction in circulating eosinophils [59].

In a phase I, multicenter, double-blind, placebo-controlled study, 13 patients were randomized to receive a single intravenous dose of placebo or 1 mg/kg benralizumab, and other 14 patients were randomized to receive a monthly subcutaneous dose of placebo, or either 100 or 200 mg benralizumab, for 3 months. The study concluded that both the single intravenous dose and the multiple subcutaneous doses of benralizumab reduced the percentage of eosinophils in the bronchial biopsies and in induced sputum and suppressed eosinophil counts in the bone marrow and peripheral blood [60]. Additional studies are further required.

### 3.2.2. Anti IL-13 monoclonal antibodies: Lebrikizumab

IL-4 and IL-13 are key therapeutic targets in Th2 high asthma, due to their significant role in Th2 lymphocyte responses and in B lymphocyte isotype switching for IgE synthesis and also for their intervention in mast cell selection (see Figure 1). The strong evidence existing upon the involvement of this pathogenic pathway in asthma, initially ranging from genetic studies up to convincing data from animal studies, leads to the development of a wide range of biological agents aimed at these targets, including anti-IL-13, anti-IL-4Rα and anti-IL-13Rα1 mAbs, IL-4Rα/IL-13Rα1 fusion protein, IL-4/IL-13 vaccines, anti-IL-4Rα antisense oligonucleotides, and double mutein IL-4 [61]. However, although many of these drugs are under development, to date only a few have been evaluated in patients with asthma [62] (see also Table 3).

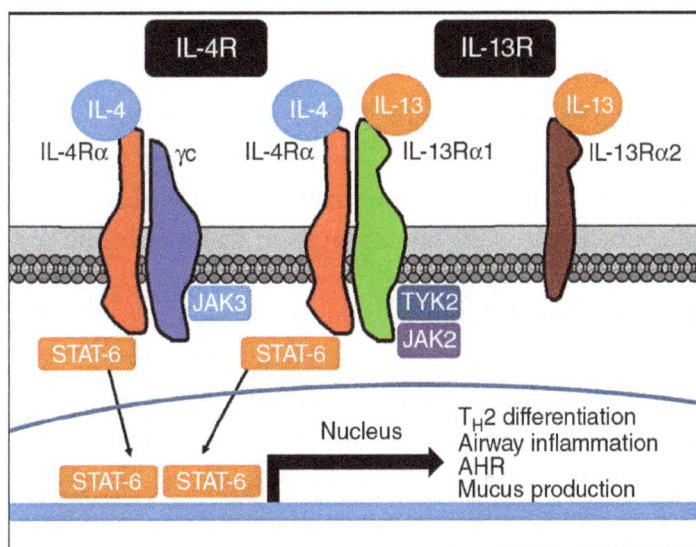

**Figure 1.** The IL-4/ IL-13 receptor.

| | | Drug | Pharmaceutical company |
|---|---|---|---|
| | mAb anti IgE | Quilizumab (MEMP1972A) | Genentech/Roche |
| | | 8D6 | United BioPharma |
| | | Ligelizumab (QGE031B) | Novartis |
| mAb anti IL-5 | IgG1 | Mepolizumab | GlaxoSmithKline |
| | IgG2 | Reslizumab | TEVA |
| mAb anti IL-5 | ASO anti-IL-5Rβc and anti-CCR3 | TPI-ASM8 | BioCentury |

|  | Drug | Pharmaceutical company |
|---|---|---|
| mAb anti IL-5Rα IgG1 | Benralizumab | AstraZeneca |
| mAb anti IL-13 | Lebrikizumab | Roche |
|  | Anrukinzumab | AstraZeneca |
|  | Tralokinumab | AstraZeneca |
| mAb anti IL-4α/IL-13Rα1 | Dupilumab | Sanofi |
| Other IL-4/IL-13 antagonists — mAb anti IL-4 | Pascolizumab | GlaxoSmithKline |
| Recombinant soluble IL-4 receptor (sIL-4 R) | Altrakincept | GlaxoSmithKline |
| AcMo anti IL-4 | Pascolizumab | GlaxoSmithKline |
| IL-4RI-selective mutein (IL-4/Q116E) | Pitrakinra | Aerovance |

*ASO = "anti-sense" oligonucleotide; CCR3 = cysteine–cysteine chemokine receptor-3; IL = interleukin; mAb = monoclonal antibodies; sIL-4 R = recombinant soluble IL-4 receptor.*

**Table 3.** Monoclonal antibodies for the treatment of asthma.

### 3.2.2.1 Lebrikizumab

Corren et al. [30] first studied the effects of lebrikizumab in 219 adults with moderate-to-severe persistent uncontrolled asthma. Lebrikizumab was administered subcutaneously every month for 6 months. A significant improvement in prebronchodilator FEV1 was recorded at 12 weeks in patients treated with lebrikizumab when compared to the placebo group. The study drug was significantly more effective in patients with pretreatment circulating periostin levels above the median and also in those with Th2-high phenotype (total IgE > 100 IU/ml and eosinophilia > 140/mm$^3$), when compared to those with Th2-low phenotype. Exacerbations were not significantly reduced in the active group compared to placebo, but when sub analyzed in the Th2-high subgroup, the rate of exacerbations was 60% lower in patients receiving lebrikizumab compared to placebo. These data suggest that therapy with anti-IL-13 antibodies may be more effective when directed to a selected subgroup of patients (i.e. Th2-high –phenotype).

### 3.2.3. Anti IL4R monoclonal antibodies: Dupilumab

Dupilumab (Sanofi) is a humanized mAb that targets the α-subunit of the IL-4–IL-13 shared receptor. The efficacy and safety of dupilumab in the treatment of patients with persistent eosinophilic asthma were evaluated in a phase IIa, randomized, double-blind, placebo-controlled study [63]. One hundred and five patients with moderate-to-severe persistent asthma and eosinophilia ≥300/mm$^3$ in blood or ≥3% in sputum were included. All patients were on moderate-to-high doses of ICS and LABA. They were randomized to receive either dupilumab 300 mg ($n$ = 52) or placebo ($n$ = 52), subcutaneously, once a week for 12 weeks, or until the development of a moderate or severe exacerbation (primary endpoint).

Asthma exacerbations were reduced by 87% in the active group (6% exacerbations in the patients receiving dupilumab versus 44% in the placebo group), being this difference statistically significant. Significant differences in favor of dupilumab in the time until the first exacerbation and in the risk of exacerbations were also recorded. In the dupilumab patient group, both the morning peak expiratory flow (PEF) and the asthma symptoms evaluated by the ACQ5 improved significantly. Nocturnal awakenings and the use of short-acting beta 2 agonists were also reduced.

Regarding adverse effects, more local reactions at the injection site, nasopharyngitis, nausea, and headache were reported in patients on active treatment, and there was one case of angioedema. The authors of this study emphasize the effect of dupilumab on the reduced frequency of exacerbations, even after withdrawal of ICS and LABA. Nevertheless, they admit that the definition of "exacerbation" used in their protocol does not coincide with that usually employed in clinical practice and, accordingly, recommend that larger studies should be further performed [63].

As we have seen, most new mAbs under development are directed against different targets of the Th2 pathway [62]. A summary of all these drugs is found in Table 3. Figure 2 briefly sketches the allergic inflammatory cascade, so that we might easily visualize these therapeutic targets.

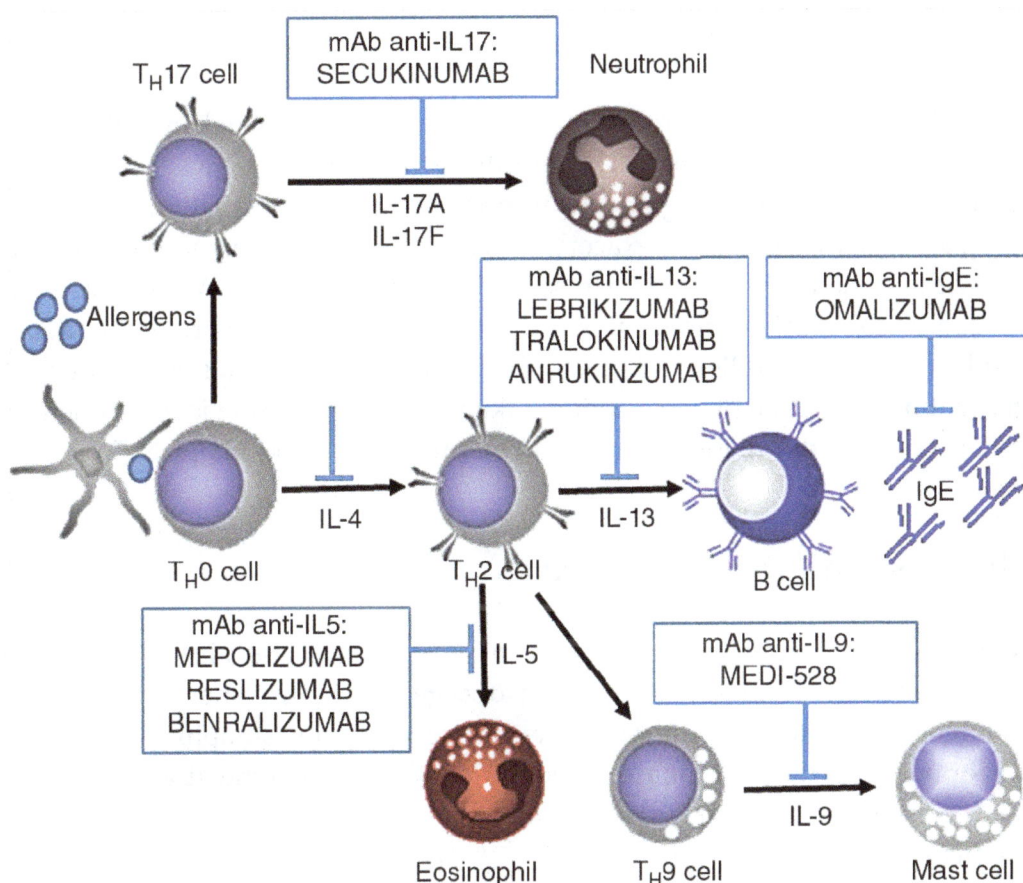

**Figure 2.** Therapeutic targets within the allergic cascade.

## 3.3. Non-eosinophilic asthma: Neutrophilic, Th2-low asthma

### 3.3.1. Anti-tumor necrosis factor-α monoclonal antibodies

Unfortunately, for patients belonging to severe asthma phenotypes other than eosinophilic asthma, current therapeutic options are scarce, and many of these patients are steroid-dependent and even steroid-resistant [2]. Clinical trials with anti-tumour necrosis factor (TNF)-α mAbs (such as infliximab, adalimumab, and golimumab) have been performed with discouraging results. A study including 309 patients with severe persistent asthma, randomized to receive placebo or three different doses of golimumab (50, 100, and 200 mg), showed no significant improvement in any of the efficacy variables [64]. More importantly, the trial had to be prematurely discontinued due to serious adverse events (SAEs), namely infections and malignancies, in the golimumab group. A post-hoc analysis suggested that patients with a prestudy history of sinusitis and FEV1 reversibility (≥12%) who received golimumab (100 and 200 mg) had fewer severe asthma exacerbations, apparently associated with a dose–response effect. Perhaps, if biomarkers were developed for predicting response to anti-TNF-α agents, then they could be used for selected subgroups of patients with severe asthma, but the contradictory efficacy results and especially the potential safety concerns have prevented the performance of any additional clinical trials so far.

### 3.3.2. Bronchial thermoplasty

Thermoplasty is a bronchoscopic procedure that reduces the bronchial smooth muscle layer by applying heat by radiofrequency. The results of the studies showed, in patients with moderate and severe asthma, a significant improvement in their quality of life, increased disease control, and a reduction of exacerbations. These results persist for years after the procedure, without medium- to long-term secondary effects [65–67]. While new evidence is needed to identify the ideal candidate, it is currently considered to be preferably indicated in patients with severe uncontrolled asthma, with chronic airflow limitation (FEV1 > 50% and <80%), and without bronchial hypersecretion. Likewise, its application is recommended to be performed in centers with experienced and sufficiently trained endoscopists [2].

## 4. Conclusions and future perspectives

We are witnessing the rapid development of new molecules and also of promising new combinations in terms of efficacy, safety, and dosage for the treatment of asthma, except perhaps for treatment for a subgroup of patients with severe non-eosinophilic asthma, in which therapeutic options still remain limited. Given the heterogeneity of the disease, we consider it is important to establish the phenotype or endotype as a first step on the road to the "personalized" medicine in asthma.

From a practical point of view, in Table 4 we present the personal opinion of the authors of this chapter on the individualized" utility of the new asthma treatments, already existing or proximally available.

| Asthma phenotype/endotype and its major characteristics | | Therapeutic options |
|---|---|---|
| **1. Extrinsic or allergic asthma** | | – Allergen avoidance, montelukast, allergen-specific immunotherapy, omalizumab<br>– Tiotropium bromide |
| **2. Intrinsic or non-allergic asthma** | | |
| **Eosinophilic, may associate atopy or entopy** | **AERD (or NERD):** Th2-high and extensive eosinophilic infiltration, potentially severe or difficult-to-control asthma, glucocorticoid-dependent/glucocorticoid-resistant asthma | – Montelukast, tiotropium bromide, aspirin desensitization<br>– Omalizumab (anti-Th2 effect, off-label).<br>– In the future: assess new treatments with anti-IL-5 and anti-IL-13 |
| | **Late-onset hypereosinophilic asthma:** similar to AERD, increased airway remodelling, fixed airflow limitation, usually glucocorticoid-dependent asthma | – Tiotropium bromide<br>– Omalizumab (off-label).<br>– Future: anti-IL-5 |
| **Non-eosinophilic, non-atopic** | **Non-eosinophilic asthma:** obese females, neutrophilic or paucigranulocytic inflammation, Th2-low: worse prognosis, glucocorticoid-resistant asthma | – Tiotropium bromide, ultra-LABA/LAMA<br>– Bronchial thermoplasty.<br>– Anti-TNF-$\alpha$???* |

*AERD = aspirin-exacerbated respiratory disease (or Samter's triad); ICS = inhaled corticosteroids; IL = interleukin; LABA = long-acting beta-2-agonists; LAMA = long-acting muscarinic antagonists; NERD = non-steroidal anti-inflammatory drugs-exacerbated respiratory disease; Th2 = helper type 2 lymphocyte; TNF = tumour necrosis factor*
*\* Clinical trials with anti-TNF agents (infliximab, adalimumab, and golimumab) had to be suspended prematurely due to the appearance of serious adverse events, especially severe infections and malignancies [64].*

**Table 4.** The path to personalized treatment of asthma insufficiently controlled with ICS/LABA: Present and future.

# Author details

Irina Diana Bobolea[1,2*], Carlos Melero[2,3] and Jesús Jurado-Palomo[4]

*Address all correspondence to: ibobolea@gmail.com

1 Department of Allergology Hospital Doce de Octubre Institute for Health Research (i+12), Madrid, Spain

2 Highly-specialized Severe Asthma Unit Hospital Doce de Octubre Institute for Health Research (i+12), Madrid, Spain

3 Department of Pulmonology Hospital Doce de Octubre Institute for Health Research (i +12), Madrid, Spain

4 Department of Allergology Nuestra Señora del Prado General Hospital, Talavera de la Reina, Spain

# References

[1] Global Initiative for Asthma (GINA). Global strategy for asthma management and prevention: NHLBI/WHO workshop report. Bethesda: National Institutes of Health, National Heart, Lung and Blood Institute. 2014. Available at http://www.ginasthma.com.

[2] GEMA 4.0. Guía Española para el manejo del asma. 2015. Available at http://www.gemasma.com.

[3] Demoly P, Annunziata K, Gubba E, Adamek L. Repeated cross-sectional survey of patient-reported asthma control in Europe in the past 5 years. Eur Respir Rev 2012; 21: 66–74.

[4] Olaguibel JM, Quirce S, Juliá B, Fernández C, Fortuna AM, Molina J, Plaza V, MAGIC Study Group. Measurement of asthma control according to Global Initiative for Asthma guidelines: a comparison with the Asthma Control Questionnaire. Respir Res 2012; 13: 50.

[5] Quirce S, Bobolea I. Nuevos tratamientos farmacológicos. En: Asma Grave. P Barranco, S Quirce Editors. Luzan 5 S.A. 2013: ISBN 978-84-7989-759-8: 237-54.

[6] Cisneros Serrano C, Melero Moreno C, Almonacid Sánchez C, Perpiñá Tordera M, Picado Valles C, Martínez Moragón E, et al. Guidelines for severe uncontrolled asthma. Arch Bronconeumol 2015; 51(5): 235–46.

[7] Wenzel SE. Asthma phenotypes: the evolution from clinical to molecular approaches. Nat Med 2012; 18: 716–25.

[8] Lötvall J, Akdis CA, Bacharier LB, Bjermer L, Casale TB, Custovic A, et al. Asthma endotypes: a new approach to classification of disease entities within the asthma syndrome. J Allergy Clin Immunol 2011; 127: 355–60.

[9] Kazani S, Wechsler ME, Israel E. The role of pharmacogenomics in improving the management of asthma. J Allergy Clin Immunol 2010; 125: 295–302; quiz 303–304.

[10] Tarantini F, Baiardini I, Passalacqua G, Braido F, Canonica GW. Asthma treatment: 'magic bullets which seek their own targets'. Allergy 2007; 62: 605–10.

[11] Mullol J, Roca Ferrer J. Receptores colinérgicos y la vía muscarinica en las vias respiratorias. Arch Bronconeumol 1997; 33(Suppl. 2): 3–10.

[12] Moulton BC, Freyer A. Muscarinic receptor antagonists, from folklore to pharmacology: finding drugs that actually work in asthma and COPD. Br J Pharmacol 2011; 163: 44–52.

[13] Gross NJ. Ipratropium bromide. N Engl J Med 1988; 319(8): 486–94.

[14] Bobolea I. Utilidad clínica de los anticolinergicos en el asma. En: Reunión anual de la Asociación Aragonesa 2014 de Alergología: "Debates sobre alergología". C. Colas, J

Fraj Lázaro Editors. Sístemas de Impresión Industrias Gráficas SL. ISBN: 978-84-89744-46-8: 28-34

[15] Park HW, Yang MS, Park CS, et al. Additive role of tiotropium in severe asthmatics and Arg16Gly in ADRB2 as a potential marker to predict response. Allergy 2009; 64: 778–83.

[16] Peters SP, Kunselman SJ, Icitovic N, et al. Tiotropium bromide step-up therapy for adults with uncontrolled asthma. N Engl J Med 2010; 363: 1715–26.

[17] Bateman ED, Kornmann O, Schmidt P, et al. Tiotropium is noninferior to salmeterol in maintaining improved lung function in 16-Arg/Arg patients with asthma. J Allergy Clin Immunol 2011; 128: 315–22.

[18] Kerstjens HA, Disse B, Schröder-Babo W, et al. Tiotropium improves lung function in patients with severe uncontrolled asthma: a randomized controlled trial. J Allergy Clin Immunol 2011; 128: 308–14.

[19] Kerstjens HA, Engel M, Dahl R, Paggiaro P, Beck E, Vandewalker M, et al. Tiotropium in asthma poorly controlled with standard combination therapy. N Engl J Med 2012; 367: 1198–207.

[20] Iwamoto H, Yokoyama A, Shiota N, Shoda H, Haruta Y, Hattori N, et al. Tiotropium bromide is effective for severe asthma with noneosinophilic phenotype. Eur Resp J 2008; 31: 1979–82.

[21] Perpiña M. Anticolinergicos en el asma. Espacio Asma 2011; 4(3): 70–5.

[22] Bateman ED, Rennard S, Barnes PJ, Dicpingatis PV, Gosens R, Gross NJ, et al. Alternative mechanisms for tiotropium. Pulm Pharmacol 2006; 533: 36–9.

[23] Boss IST, Gosens R, Zuidhof AB, Schaafsma D, Halayko AJ, Meurs H, et al. Inhibition of allergen-induced airway remodelling by tiotropium and budesonide: a comparison. Eur Resp J 2007: 30: 653–61.

[24] Buels KS, Jacoby DB, Fryer AD. Non-bronchodilating mechanisms of tiotropium prevent airway hyperreactivity in a guinea-pig model of allergic asthma. Br J Pharmacol 2012; 165: 1501–14.

[25] Wise RA, Anzueto A, Cotton D, Dahl R, Devins T, Disse B, et al. Tiotropium Respimat inhaler and the risk of death in COPD. N Engl J Med 2013; 369(16): 1491–501.

[26] Cazzola M, Segreti A, Matera MG. Novel bronchodilators in asthma. Curr Opin Pulm Med 2010; 16: 6–12.

[27] Cazzola M, Page C, Matera MG. Long-acting muscarinic receptor antagonists for the treatment of respiratory disease. Pulm Pharmacol Ther 2013; 26(3): 307–17.

[28] Baloira A. Triple terapia en el tratamiento de la EPOC. Arch Bronconeumol 2010; 46(Suppl. 8): 25–30.

[29]  Barnes P. Triple inhalers for obstructive airways disease: will they be useful? Expert Rev Respir Med 2011; 5(3): 297–300.

[30]  Corren J, Lemanske RF, Hanania NA, Korenblat PE, Parsey MV, Matthews JG, et al. Lebrikizumab treatment in adults with asthma. N Engl J Med 2011; 365: 1088–98.

[31]  Ficha Técnica autorizada de Omalizumab. Available at www.aemps.gob.es.

[32]  Holgate S, Buhl R, Bousquet J, Smith N, Panahloo Z, Jimenez P. The use of omalizumab in the treatment of severe allergic asthma: a clinical experience update. Respir Med 2009; 103: 1098–113.

[33]  Molimard M, de Blay F, Didier A, Le Gros V. Effectiveness of omalizumab (Xolair) in the first patients treated in real-life practice in France. Respir Med 2008; 102: 71–6.

[34]  Korn S, Thielen A, Seyfried S, Taube C, Kornmann O, Buhl R. Omalizumab in patients with severe persistent allergic asthma in a real-life setting in Germany. Respir Med 2009; 103: 1725–31.

[35]  Brusselle G, Michils A, Louis R, Dupont L, Van de Maele B, Delobbe A, et al. Real life effectiveness of omalizumab in patients with severe persistent allergic asthma: the PERSIST study. Respir Med 2009; 103: 1633–42.

[36]  Cazzola M, Camiciottoli G, Bonavia M, Gulotta C, Ravazzi A, Alessandrini A, et al. Italian real-life experience of omalizumab. Respir Med 2010; 104: 1410–6.

[37]  Schatz M, Eisner MD, Zazzali J, Bradley MS, Miller MK. Longitudinal impact of omalizumab on asthma control over two years. Am J Resp Crit Care Med 2011; 183: A4495.

[38]  Vennera MC, Pérez De Llano L, Bardagí S, Ausin P, Sanjuas C, González H, et al.; On Behalf of the Spanish Registry. Omalizumab therapy in severe asthma: experience from the Spanish registry – some new approaches. J Asthma 2012; 49(4): 416–22.

[39]  Barnes P. Intrinsic asthma: not so different from allergic asthma but driven by super-antigens? Clin Exp Allergy 2009; 39: 1145–51.

[40]  Verbruggen K, van Cauwenberge P, Bachert C. Anti-IgE for the treatment of allergic rhinitis – and eventually nasal polyps? Int Arch Allergy Immunol 2009; 148: 87–98.

[41]  Vennera MC, Picado C, Mullol J, Alobid I, Bernal-Sprekelsen M. Efficacy of omalizumab in the treatment of nasal polyps. Thorax 2011; 66: 824–5.

[42]  Gevaert P, Calus L, Van Zele T, Blomme K, De Ruyck N, Bauters W, et al. Omalizumab is effective in allergic and nonallergic patients with nasal polyps and asthma. J Allergy Clin Immunol 2013; 131: 110–6.

[43]  de Llano LP, Vennera MC, Álvarez FJ, Medina JF, Borderías L, Pellicer C, et al.; Spanish Registry. Effects of omalizumab in non-atopic asthma: results from a Spanish multi-center registry. J Asthma 2013; 50: 296–301.

[44] Garcia G, Magnan A, Chiron R, Contin-Bordes C, Berger P, Taillé C, et al. A proof-of-concept, randomized, controlled trial of omalizumab in patients with severe, difficult-to-control, nonatopic asthma. Chest 2013; 144: 411–9.

[45] Pérez-de-Llano LA, Vennera MC, Parra A, Guallar J, Marin M, Asensio O, et al. Effects of omalizumab in Aspergillus-associated airway disease. Thorax 2011; 66(6): 539–40.

[46] Lowe PJ, Tannenbaum S, Gautier A, Jimenez P. Relationship between omalizumab pharmacokinetics, IgE pharmacodynamics and symptoms in patients with severe persistent allergic (IgE-mediated) asthma. Br J Clin Pharmacol 2009; 68: 61–76.

[47] Arm JP, Bottoli I, Skerjanec A, Floch D, Groenewegen A, Maahs S, Owen CE, et al. Pharmacokinetics, pharmacodynamics and safety of QGE031 (ligelizumab), a novel high-affinity anti-IgE antibody, in atopic subjects. Clin Exp Allerg 2014; 44: 1371–85.

[48] Gauvreau GM, Harris JM, Boulet LP, Scheerens H, Fitzgerald JM, Putnam WS. Targeting membrane-expressed IgE B cell receptor with an antibody to the M1 prime epitope reduces IgE production. Sci Transl Med 2014; 6(243): 243ra85.

[49] Berair R, Pavord ID. Rationale and clinical results of inhibiting interleukin-5 for the treatment of severe asthma. Curr Allergy Asthma Resp 2013; 13: 469–76.

[50] Quirce S, Bobolea I, Barranco P. Emerging drugs for asthma. Expert Opin Emerg Drugs 2012; 17: 219–37.

[51] Leckie MJ, ten Brinke A, Khan J, Diamant Z, O'Connor BJ, Walls CM, et al. Effects of an interleukin-5 blocking monoclonal antibody on eosinophils, airway hyper-responsiveness, and the late asthmatic response. Lancet 2000; 356: 2144–8.

[52] Flood-Page PT, Menzies-Grow AN, Kay AB, Robinson DS. Eosinophil's role remains uncertain as anti-interleukin-5 only partially depletes numbers in asthmatic airway. Am J Respir Crit Care Med 2003; 167: 199–204.

[53] Flood-Page P, Swenson C, Faiferman I, Matthews J, Williams M, Brannick L, et al.; International Mepolizumab Study Group. A study to evaluate safety and efficacy of mepolizumab in patients with moderate persistent asthma. Am J Respir Crit Care Med 2007; 176: 1062–71.

[54] Nair P, Pizzichini MM, Kjarsgaard M, Inman MD, Efthimiadis A, Pizzichini E, et al. Mepolizumab for prednisone-dependent asthma with sputum eosinophilia. N Eng J Med 2009; 360: 985–93.

[55] Haldar P, Brightling CE, Hargadon B, Gupta S, Monteiro W, Sousa A, et al. Mepolizumab and exacerbations of refractory eosinophilic asthma. N Eng J Med 2009; 360: 973–84.

[56] Pavord ID, Korn S, Howarth P, Bleecker ER, Buhl R, Keene ON, et al. Mepolizumab for severe eosinophilic asthma (DREAM): a multicentre, double-blind, placebo-controlled trial. Lancet 2012; 380: 651–99.

[57] Liu Y, Zhang S, Li DW, Jiang SJ. Efficacy of anti-interleukin-5 therapy with mepolizu-mab in patients with asthma: a meta-analysis of randomized placebo-controlled trials. PLoS One 2013; 8: e59872.

[58] Castro M, Mathur S, Hargreave F, Boulet LP, Xie F, Young J, et al.; Res-5-0010 Study Group. Reslizumab for poorly controlled, eosinophilic asthma: a randomized, placebo-controlled study. Am J Respir Crit Care Med 2011; 184: 1125–32.

[59] Busse WW, Katial R, Gossage D, Sari S, Wang B, Kolbeck R, et al. Safety profile, pharmacokinetics, and biologic activity of MEDI-563, an anti-IL-5 receptor alpha antibody, in a phase I study of subjects with mild asthma. J Allergy Clin Immunol 2010; 125: 1237–44.

[60] Laviolette M, Gossage DL, Gauvreau G, Leigh R, Olivenstein R, Katial R, et al. Effects of benralizumab on airway eosinophils in asthmatic patients with sputum eosinophilia. J Allergy Clin Immunol 2013; 132: 1086–96.

[61] Oh CK, Geba GP, Molfino N. Investigational therapeutics targeting the IL-4/IL-13/STAT-6 pathway for the treatment of asthma. Eur Respir Rev 2010; 19: 46–54.

[62] Quirce S, Bobolea I, Domínguez-Ortega J, Barranco P. Future biologic therapies in asthma. Arch Bronconeumol 2014; 50(8): 355–61.

[63] Wenzel S, Ford L, Pearlman D, Spector S, Sher L, Skobieranda F, et al. Dupilumab in persistent asthma with elevated eosinophil levels. N Engl J Med 2013; 368: 2455–66.

[64] Wenzel SE, Barnes PJ, Bleecker ER, Bousquet J, Busse W, Dahlén SE, et al. A random-ized, double-blind, placebo-controlled study of tumor necrosis factor alpha blockade in severe persistent asthma. Am J Respir Crit Care Med 2009; 179: 549–58.

[65] Thomson NC, Rubin AS, Niven RM, Corris PA, Siersted HC, Olivenstein R, et al.; AIR Trial StudyGroup. Long-term (5 year) safety of bronchial thermoplasty: asthma Intervention Research (AIR) trial. BMC Pulm Med 2011; 11(8): 581.

[66] Wechsler ME, Laviolette M, Rubin AS, Fiterman J, Lapa e Silva JR, Shah PL, et al.; Asthma Intervention Research (AIR) 2 Trial Study Group. Bronchial thermoplasty: long-term safety and effectiveness in patients with severe persistent asthma. J Allergy Clin Immunol 2013; 132(6): 1295–302.

[67] Torrego A, Solà I, Munoz AM, Roqué i Figuls M, Yepes-Nuñez JJ, Alonso-Coello P, et al. Bronchial thermoplasty for moderate or severe persistent asthma in adults. Co-chrane Database System Rev 2014; (3): CD009910.

# 3

# Asthma-COPD Overlap Syndrome (ACOS): Current Understanding and Future Perspectives

Irina Bobolea and Luis Alejandro Pérez de Llano

## Abstract

This chapter resumes our current understanding of asthma–chronic obstructive pulmonary disease (COPD) overlap syndrome (ACOS), pretending to offer a comprehensive approach for the practicing physician, and provides some future perspectives on this entity.

Although different studies recognize the presence of ACOS, the detection, diagnosis, and treatment of these patients in clinical practice are not always simple and are subject to different interpretations. These patients are of special interest, because they are usually excluded from clinical trials with new medications, and also represent a clinically very important and quite prevalent population, with particular characteristics: more respiratory symptoms, frequent exacerbations, and worse health-related quality of life. They are also characterized by an increase in comorbidity and a greater consumption of health care resources compared to patients with only asthma or COPD alone.

There are currently no universally accepted, validated criteria for the diagnosis of ACOS. The differences between clinical guidelines are discussed here (GINA 2014, GEMA 2015, and GOLD 2014). However, to obtain clear and validated criteria, we think that further research about the underlying mechanisms is needed.

Several potential pathways that might lead to the adult presentation of ACOS are revised. The therapeutic recommendations of the Spanish consensus guideline for patients with overlap phenotype COPD–asthma are provided, and other possible future therapies are discussed in this chapter.

**Keywords:** ACOS, ACOS criteria, ACOS treatment, asthma, COPD

# 1. Introduction

Although different studies recognize the presence of asthma–chronic obstructive pulmonary disease (COPD) overlap syndrome (ACOS), the detection, diagnosis, and treatment of these patients in clinical practice are not always simple and are subject to different interpretations and controversies. These patients are of special interest, because they are usually excluded from clinical trials with new medications for asthma and also represent a clinically very important and quite prevalent population, apparently with particular characteristics: more respiratory symptoms, frequent exacerbations, and worse health-related quality of life [1–5]. They are also characterized by an increase in comorbidity and a greater consumption of health care resources compared to patients with only asthma or COPD alone. There are currently no universally accepted, validated criteria for the diagnosis of ACOS. Also, clinical trials are necessary to verify the response to treatments of this group of patients.

# 2. Definition of ACOS

ACOS is the coexistence of two distinct diseases in the same individual: asthma and COPD. Whether this concept is clinically relevant or not depends on its capacity to describe an entity with differentiated pathogenic mechanisms, prognostic particularities, and potentially specific treatment options. The recently updated Spanish COPD guidelines [6] acknowledge the existence of a syndrome that overlaps characteristics of COPD and asthma, and it proposes a differential treatment.

When considering how to define this entity, existing definitions of asthma and COPD should be taken into account. The new definition of COPD according to GOLD 2014 includes subtle changes regarding the previous definitions, integrating the findings of recent evidence [7]. For instance, there is no longer mention of reversibility, and it emphasizes the role of exacerbations and comorbidities. Thus, COPD is a common, preventable and treatable disorder, defined by persistent airflow obstruction that is mostly progressive, characterized by a chronic inflammatory response in the airways and lungs to noxious particles and gases; exacerbations and comorbidities generally contribute to the severity of the disease in individual patients.

On the other hand, in 2014, GINA [8] defined asthma as "a heterogeneous disease, usually characterized by chronic airway inflammation. It is defined by the history of respiratory symptoms such as wheeze, shortness of breath, chest tightness and cough that vary over time and in intensity, together with variable expiratory airflow limitation". The similarities between asthma and COPD definitions are obvious, but none of their features are pathognomonic, and all of them might be present in individual patients.

For operative purposes, in 2014, GINA and GOLD published a joint document on ACOS [9]. ACOS was defined as the presence of persistent airflow limitation with several features usually associated with asthma and others usually associated with COPD. The document presents the characteristics of asthma and COPD listed separately and suggests that ACOS may be the diagnosis when a similar number of characteristics of both asthma and COPD are identified in a given patient. The joint task force also recommends a stepwise approach to the diagnosis. It uses clinical, spirometric and radiographic findings to help delineate if an adult patient is most likely suffering from asthma or COPD or fulfills enough shared features to be considered within ACOS. This definition and the diagnostic criteria differ from other guidelines, for instance, the Spanish expert report from 2012 [10].

The different diagnostic criteria proposed so far are discussed in Section 5. However, to obtain any clearer and validated criteria, further research about underlying mechanisms is needed.

# 3. Prevalence of ACOS

The exact prevalence of ACOS is unknown. In general, the literature on ACOS has been mostly retrospective and observational, and the studies focused on asthma or COPD populations. It is well known that studies on asthma are usually performed in populations of children or young adults, where the prevalence of COPD is negligible, whereas studies on COPD are usually performed in elderly populations, where the prevalence of asthma is low. The COPDGene study found a prevalence of 13% of ACOS [2]. These patients may have a different clinical natural history, with more frequent and severe exacerbations (odds ratio [OR] 3.55), and different treatment response, which led to recommend early introduction of inhaled corticosteroids (ICS) in these patients. These figures are similar to those reported in the PLATINO study [11]: 12% prevalence for the ACOS phenotype and more risk of exacerbations in these patients (OR 3.01). The inconsistencies and discrepancies that exist upon reported data on prevalence can be in part explained by the absence of a consistent definition and diagnostic standards. In comparison to previous studies that have considered selected groups of patients, such as COPD patients, the study published by de Marco et al [12] assessed the prevalence of ACOS in the general population. They found that this prevalence ranged from a minimum of 1.6% (95% confidence interval (CI): 1.3%–2.0%) in the 20–44 years old age group to 4.5% (95% CI: 3.2%–5.9) in the 60–84 years old age group.

# 4. Pathogenic mechanisms

Several potential pathways might lead to the presentation of ACOS in adults. One such pathway begins in early-onset asthma. Smoking habit later in life might lead to development of fixed airflow limitation and COPD in many of these patients. A second potential pathway recognizes patients with a lifetime smoking history, subsequent COPD, and late-onset features of asthma (adult-onset eosinophilic asthma and aspirin-exacerbated respiratory disease) (see also Figure 1).

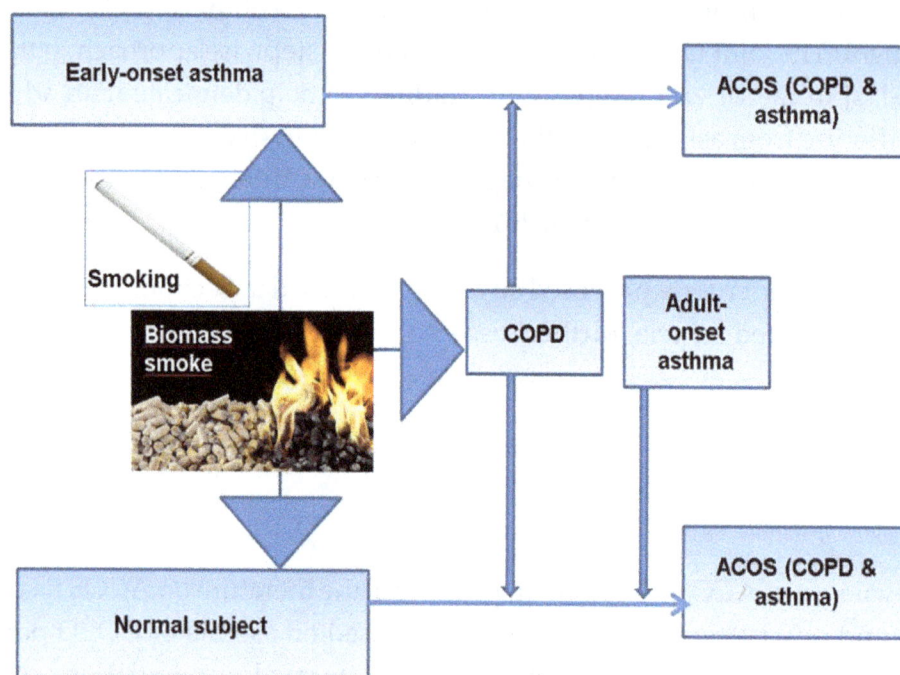

**Figure 1.** Pathogenic pathways leading to ACOS development.

Although no previous studies have addressed the underlying mechanisms of inflammation in ACOS, there is convincing evidence that eosinophils play a pivotal role, similar to what it is found in asthma with a Th2-high profile. Different studies have demonstrated that the presence of significant eosinophilia in an induced sputum sample predicts a good response to ICS, both in patients with COPD and ACOS [13–15]. On the other hand, the presence of more number of neutrophils in sputum has been recently associated with a worse prognosis in asthmatics [16]. Since both asthma and COPD are inflammatory diseases that affect the bronchial tree, it is to be expected to find, in patients with ACOS, some evidence of the Th-1 pattern (characteristic of COPD) and some evidence of Th-2 pattern (characteristic of asthma). The current search for reliable biomarkers of Th1 and Th2 inflammation hopefully will provide additional information in the upcoming years.

Previous studies defined two new asthma molecular phenotypes, namely Th2 high and Th2 low [17]. The Th2–high gene signature includes chloride channel accessory protein 1 (CLCA1), SERPINB2, and periostin (encoded by POSTN), a secreted 90-kDa extracellular matrix protein that is induced by interleukin (IL)-4 and IL-13 in airway epithelial cells and lung fibroblasts. All three genes are induced in bronchial epithelial cells by recombinant IL-13 treatment in vitro, and the expression of these genes correlates with IL-13 and IL-5 expression in the bronchial mucosa, airway and peripheral eosinophilia, airway remodeling, and clinical responsiveness to ICS treatment, but not with atopy. Even more so, periostin seems to become an emerging noninvasive biomarker associated with eosinophilic inflammation, Th2-high molecular phenotype, and airway remodeling, and has potential utility in patient selection for emerging asthma therapeutics targeting Th2 inflammation. A study by Jia et al. [18] identified serum periostin as a systemic biomarker of airway eosinophilia in severe, uncontrolled asthmatics belonging to the BOBCAT cohort (Bronchoscopic Exploratory Research Study of Biomarkers in Corticosteroid-refractory Asthma). In a logistic regression model, serum periostin was the single best predictor of sputum and tissue eosinophilia, showing superiority to blood eosinophils, IgE, and FeNO. Mean periostin levels were significantly higher in "eosinophil-high" when compared with "eosinophil-low" patients, as defined by sputum or tissue eosinophil measurements. Using 25 ng/mL serum periostin as an arbitrary cutoff, eosinophil-low and eosinophil-high patients from the BOBCAT study were effectively differentiated, with a positive predictive value of 93% [18]. Moreover, in 62 patients diagnosed with severe asthma, Bobolea et al. [19] found that periostin levels were higher in patients with fixed airflow limitation than in patients with variable airflow limitation (69.76 vs 43.84 ng/ml, $p < 0.05$) and in patients with eosinophilic phenotype than in patients with mixed granulocytic phenotype (61.58 vs 37.31 ng/ml, $P < 0.05$). However, in a cohort of patients with a broad spectrum of asthma severities, Wagener et al. [20] found that blood eosinophils had the highest accuracy in the identification of sputum eosinophilia. In this study, serum periostin was not able to distinguish eosinophilic from noneosinophilic airway inflammation. Therefore, in view of the differing positions, the exact role of periostin in the diagnosis of Th2 bronchial inflammation remains to be determined.

## 5. Diagnosis of ACOS

The specific criteria for diagnosis of this special syndrome had never been established until 2012, when an expert panel meeting of Spanish key opinion leaders agreed unanimously to confirm the existence of this patient profile and to establish a set of criteria for its diagnosis [10], which has been posteriorly adapted within the Spanish COPD Guideline, although not yet validated. The initial definition of ACOS proposed by the Spanish consensus group is as follows: the diagnosis of ACOS is made when two major criteria or one major and two minor criteria are met. The major criteria include a very positive bronchodilator (BD) test (increase in forced expiratory volume in 1 second [FEV1] >15% and >400 mL), eosinophilia in sputum, and personal history of asthma. Minor criteria include high total IgE, personal history of atopy, and positive BD test (increase in FEV1 >12% and >200 mL) on two or more occasions.

The new Finnish guidelines for the treatment of COPD proposed the same criteria for the diagnosis of ACOS as the Spanish guidelines, with the addition of an elevated FeNO higher than 50 parts per billion as a major criterion and a peak flow follow-up typical for asthma as an additional minor criterion [21]. The latest Czech Republic guidelines, published in 2013, also include ACOS with its own diagnostic criteria, similar to the Spanish recommendations [22]. These are, however, quite restrictive criteria and represent a very conservative approach until more evidence about the characterization of ACOS becomes available from large clinical trials or prospective studies. In fact, two recent studies in Spain, using the previous criteria, identified that only between 5% and 6% of the patients fulfilled the criteria for ACOS, in patients with smoking-related COPD [23, 24]. This percentage is clearly below the expected number of individuals sharing the characteristics of asthma and COPD, according to epidemiological data.

In fact, in a Spanish survey performed among pulmonology specialists, selected as experts in asthma and COPD, aimed at collecting their opinions about ACOS and their attitudes in regard to some case scenarios of ACOS patients, only 34.6% of the specialists surveyed were in agreement with the Spanish criteria, and 30.8% were in an intermediate position between agreement and disagreement. The main aspect highlighted by 76.9% of the specialists was that these criteria had to be validated in prospective studies [25].

On the other hand, the GINA–GOLD approach to diagnosis of ACOS [9] is deliberately descriptive and perhaps not very suitable for clinical applications, but recognizes that this entity, just like asthma and COPD, comprises a heterogeneous group of disorders.

The characteristics that might support the diagnosis of ACOS according to GINA–GOLD are as follows:

1. – Usually age 40 years or older, but may report symptoms in childhood or early adulthood.

2. – Respiratory symptoms, including exertional dyspnea, are persistent, but variability may be prominent.

3. – Airflow limitation that is not fully reversible, but often with evidence of significant current or historical variability.

4. – Persistent airflow limitation.

5. – Frequently, a history of doctor-diagnosed asthma (current or previous), allergies and a family history of asthma, and/or a history of noxious exposures, as seen in COPD.

6. – Symptoms are partly but significantly reduced by treatment. Progression is usual, and treatment needs are high.

7. – Exacerbations may be more common than in COPD, but are reduced by treatment.

8. – Comorbidities can contribute to clinical and functional impairment.

9. – COPD-like findings on the chest X-ray.

10. – Typically eosinophilia (with or without associated neutrophilia) in sputum.

Taking into consideration all these previously proposed criteria, the most recent Spanish guideline on the management of asthma (GEMA 2015) [26] proposes an algorithm designed to guide physicians in their routine clinical practice. The existence of patients who fulfill the criteria for COPD – adult smokers with respiratory symptoms and post-BD FEV1/FVC <0.7 – and who present characteristics of asthma, such as high reversibility of airflow, signs of bronchial and systemic eosinophilic inflammation, history of atopy, or even a previous diagnosis of asthma before the age of 40 years, has been definitely recognized. This approach also includes, as a novelty when compared with all the others, an oral corticosteroid test with prednisone to assess reversibility of the bronchial obstruction. If FEV1/FVC remains below 70% after a BD test, a methacholine test and the presence or absence of biomarkers of Th2 inflammatory response should help the clinician to distinguish between COPD and ACOS [17]. The algorithm is summarized in Figure 2.

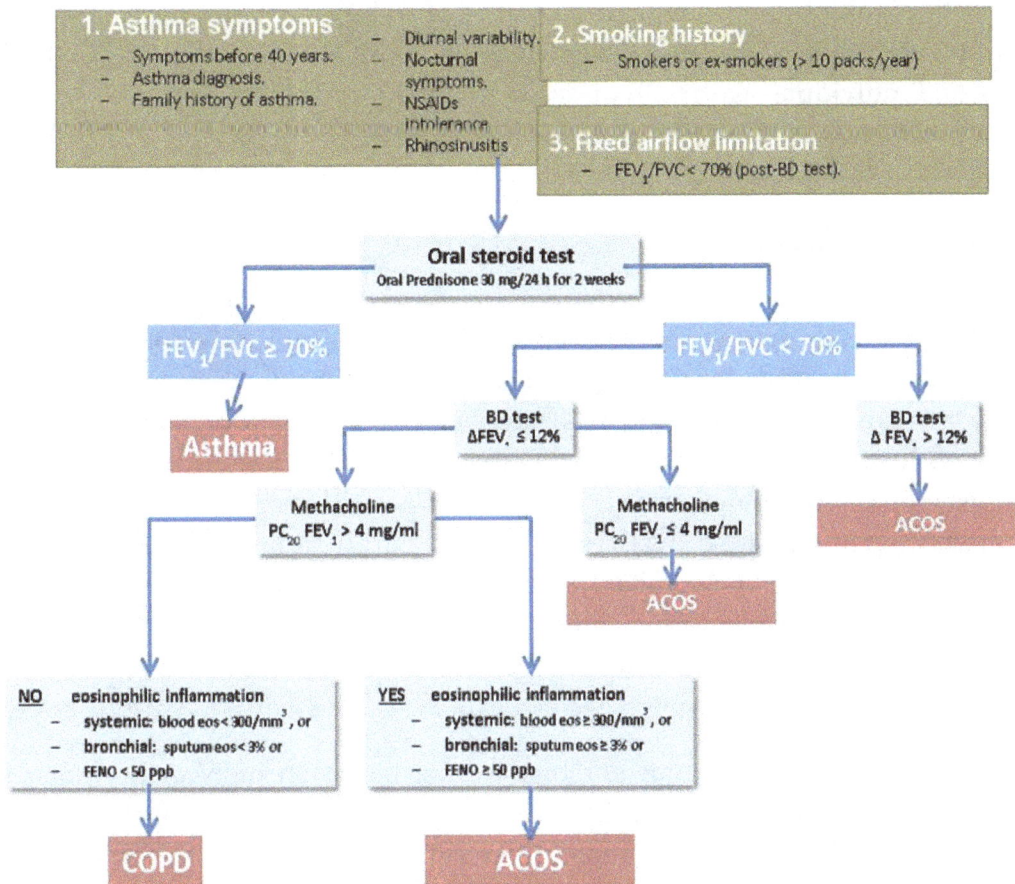

**Figure 2.** Diagnostic algorithm for ACOS according to GEMA 2015 [26].

*BD-test: bronchodilator test; eos: eosinophils.*

# 6. Prognostic implications

It has been reported that patients with ACOS have more frequent exacerbations, are more likely to have a severe exacerbation requiring hospitalization, use more respiratory medications, and have the highest reported pulmonary symptoms. More importantly, patients with ACOS also report worse quality of life than those with either disease alone [27, 28].

However, other authors found that the ACOS phenotype was not clinically different at baseline, in other than the specific criteria used to define it, than patients with no criteria for ACOS. Interestingly, survival after 1 year of follow-up was significantly better in patients with ACOS [29]. To explain such a discrepancy, it should be mentioned that this population included 72% of patients with mild-to-moderate disease, which differs from previous publications with more severe COPD, and of note, 63% of patients with ACOS were receiving ICS, which likely contributed to ameliorate the clinical differences, when compared to the non-ACOS group.

The prognostic significance of having a diagnosis of ACOS must be further assessed in the light of a prospective cohort study, designed to compare the outcomes of COPD patients, asthmatics, and individuals with both diseases.

## 7. Treatment of ACOS

The present approach to pharmacotherapy for ACOS includes trial and error and extrapolation from results of investigations, in particular subpopulations of asthma or COPD patients. The first option recommended by the Spanish consensus guideline for patients with overlap phenotype COPD-asthma is to add ICS to the treatment for COPD [10], as it is also indicated in the Finnish and Czech guidelines [21, 22]. The GINA–GOLD document also indicates that the default position in the case of ACOS should be to start treatment accordingly for asthma, and recommends the LABA/ICS combination, with special attention to avoid the use of LABAs in monotherapy. In the Spanish survey among expert pulmonologists mentioned before [25], 88.5% of the participants agreed that ACOS requires a different treatment compared to COPD, starting with LABA/ICS and stepping up to triple therapy (LABA/ICS+LAMA) in severe cases.

However, these and other recommendations are not based on high-quality data, because patients with ACOS have been classically excluded from pharmacological clinical trials both in asthma and in COPD. As a consequence, there is no clear information about the response of these patients to most of the current pharmacological therapies. The only clinical trial performed to date in patients with ACOS studied the spirometric effects of tiotropium in individuals with concomitant COPD and asthma. Improvement in lung function and a reduction in rescue medication were observed with tiotropium [30].

However, the main interest in differentiating ACOS from COPD lies in the different response to ICS.

Kitaguchi et al. [15], in a retrospective study with a small sample size, found that COPD patients with asthmatic symptoms had high peripheral and sputum eosinophil counts and better reversibility response to treatment with ICS. These findings reproduce those of other studies, in which COPD patients with a positive BD test, or with a positive hyperreactivity test, or with sputum eosinophilia, have been shown to be more responsive to ICS than those without these features [31–36]. Therefore, it seems logical to consider ICSs as the cornerstone of treatment in ACOS with the addition of long-acting β-agonists in those patients who remain symptomatic or suffer recurrent exacerbations.

In addition to the only clinical trial of Magnussen et al., more recent literature has demonstrated the efficacy of long-acting muscarinic antagonists (LAMA), such as tiotropium, in people with asthma with persistent bronchial obstruction [37, 38]. With all these recent data in mind, the Spanish guideline GEMA 2015 recommends the combination of an ICS with a long-acting β-agonist as the first therapeutic choice in patients with ACOS, leaving open the option to add a LAMA if the patients remain uncontrolled [26].

Biological treatments that target Th2-related pathways (omalizumab, anti–IL-5, and perhaps anti–IL-4/-13) might also be effective in ACOS, and they warrant further investigation. This is also the case for drugs that target predominantly neutrophil-driven mechanisms, such as roflumilast.

## 8. Discussion: ACOS as a phenotype or endotype of obstructive airway disease.

Asthma and COPD are themselves heterogeneous disorders that comprise several phenotypes and endotypes. If we admit that ACOS should be characterized by the presence of inflammatory features of both COPD (mainly Th1) and asthma (mainly Th2), we could argue that COPD patients with sputum eosinophilia and with asthma, with a mixed neutrophilic–eosinophilic pattern are, in fact, patients with ACOS, regardless of their clinical presentation. So changing our point of view, from an initial clinically based classification of obstructive airways diseases to another centered on inflammatory underlying mechanisms (endotypes), would allow us to tailor and optimize treatments, leaving behind the rigid categorization of patients into existing diagnostic labels of either asthma or COPD, which do not fully recognize the molecular and clinical heterogeneity of chronic obstructive airway diseases [39].

We need to move toward a new taxonomy of airway diseases that takes into account the underlying pathogenic mechanisms. In this new scenario, ACOS would be an endotype, like early-onset allergic asthma or emphysema. However, things are not so straightforward, and there are several important issues that complicate the settling-in of this new approach:

- Sputum cell count, the method of reference to measure and identify bronchial inflammation, is technically complex and time consuming. At this moment, we do not have substitute reliable biomarkers to identify the bronchial underlying inflammatory mechanisms in a particular patient.

- There is not a complete identification between a particular and well-recognized clinical phenotype (e.g. late-onset eosinophilic asthma) and an exclusive inflammatory pattern (e.g. eosinophilic). In a large cross-sectional study of patients with airway disease, D'Silva et al. [40] reported the cellular profile of over 4,000 induced or spontaneous sputum samples. In the ACOS group, eosinophilic bronchitis was seen in 35%, neutrophilic bronchitis in 19%, and a mixed inflammatory pattern in 10%. In COPD, the phenotypes were respectively 18%, 34%, and 7% and, in asthma alone, 26%, 14%, and 6%. These data bring to the table the heterogeneous nature of airway inflammation in asthma and COPD.

- The inflammatory pattern can vary over time, either spontaneously or as a result of treatment.

It is to be expected that in a near future, advances in the identification of inflammatory patterns can help us to adequately classify patients with chronic obstructive airway disease and offer them the best therapeutic option in each case.

## 9. Conclusions

ACOS is the coincidence of asthma and COPD in the same individual. Prospective studies are required to analyze the underlying inflammatory mechanisms in this entity. So we think that longitudinal studies are required to validate the diagnostic criteria and identify biomarkers of the disease. It also remains to be determined if it has different prognostic and therapeutic implications. If so, perhaps in the future, ACOS will be considered a distinct endotype of chronic obstructive airway disease. There is also a lack of studies to further clarify the best therapeutic options for patients with ACOS. At this moment, it seems reasonable to consider the combination of an ICS and a long-acting β-agonist as the first-choice therapy for these patients.

## Author details

Irina Bobolea[1*] and Luis Alejandro Pérez de Llano[2]

*Address all correspondence to: ibobolea@gmail.com

1 Allergy Department, Hospital 12 de octubre Institute for Health Research (i+12), Madrid, Spain

2 Head of the Pulmonology Department, Hospital Lucus Augusti, Lugo, Spain

## References

[1] Gibson PG, Simpson JL. The overlap syndrome of asthma and COPD: what are its features and how important is it? *Thorax* 2009; 64:728–735.

[2] Hardin M, Silverman EK, Barr RG, et al. The clinical features of overlap between COPD and asthma. *Respir Res* 2011; 12:127.

[3] Miravitlles M, Soriano JB, Ancochea J, et al. Characterisation of the overlap COPD-asthma phenotype. Focus on physical activity and health status. *Respir Med* 2013; 07:1053–1060.

[4] Pleasants RA, Ohar JA, Croft JB, et al. Chronic obstructive pulmonary disease and asthma – patient characteristics and health impairment. *COPD* 2014; 11:256–266.

[5] Rhee CK, Yoon HK, Yoo KH, et al. Medical utilization and cost in patients with overlap syndrome of chronic obstructive pulmonary disease and asthma. *COPD* 2014; 11:163–170.

[6] Miravitlles M, Soler-Cataluna JJ, Calle M, Molina J, Almagro P, Quintano JA et al. Spanish COPD Guidelines (GesEPOC): pharmacological treatment of stable COPD. *Arch Bronconeumol* 2012; 48(7): 247–257.

[7] Global initiative for chronic obstructive lung disease. Global strategy for the diagnosis, management, and prevention of chronic obstructive pulmonary disease. Update 2014. www.goldcopd.com.

[8] GINA. Global strategy for asthma management and prevention. 2014. http://www.ginasthma.org.

[9] Diagnosis of Diseases of Chronic Airflow Limitation: Asthma, COPD and Asthma-COPD Overlap Syndrome (ACOS). GINA 2014 reports are available at http://www.ginasthma.org.

[10] Soler-Cataluna JJ, Cosio B, Izquierdo JL, Lopez-Campos JL, Marin JM, Aguero R et al. Consensus document on the mixed asthma-COPD phenotype in COPD. *Arch Bronconeumol* 2012; 48:331–337.

[11] Menezes AM, Montes de Oca M, Pérez-Padilla R, et al; PLATINO team. Increased risk of exacerbation and hospitalization in subjects with an overlap phenotype: COPD-Asthma. *Chest* 2014; 145 (2):297–304.

[12] de Marco R, Pesce G, Marcon A, et al. The coexistence of asthma and chronic obstructive pulmonary disease (COPD): prevalence and risk factors in young, middle-aged and elderly people from the general population. *PLoS One* 2013; 10; 8 (5):e62985.

[13] Brightling CE, McKenna S, Hargadon B, et al. Sputum eosinophilia and the short term response to inhaled mometasone in chronic obstructive pulmonary disease *Thorax* 2005; 60:193–198.

[14] Fujimoto K, Kubo K, Yamamoto H, et al. Eosinophilic inflammation in the airway is related to glucocorticoid reversibility in patients with pulmonary emphysema. *Chest* 1999; 115:697–702.

[15] Kitaguchi Y, Konatsu Y, Fujimoto K, et al. Sputum eosinophilia can predict responsiveness to inhaled corticosteroid treatment in patients with overlap syndrome of COPD and asthma. *Intern J COPD* 2012; 7:283–289.

[16] Moore WC, Hastie AT, Li X, et al; National Heart, Lung, and Blood Institute's Severe Asthma Research Program. Sputum neutrophil counts are associated with more severe asthma phenotypes using cluster analysis. *J Allergy Clin Immunol* 2014; 133 (6):1557–1563.

[17] Woodruff PG, Modrek B, Choy DF, Jia G, et al. T-helper type 2-driven inflammation defines major subphenotypes of asthma. *Am J Respir Crit Care Med.* 2009; 180:388–395.

[18] Jia G, Erickson RW, Choy DF, et al. Periostin is a systemic biomarker of eosinophilic airway inflammation in asthmatic patients. *J Allergy Clin Immunol* 2012; 130(3):647–654.

[19] Bobolea I, Barranco P, Del Pozo V, et al. Sputum periostin in patients with different severe asthma phenotypes. *Allergy* 2015; 70(5):540–546.

[20] Wagener AH, de Nijs SB, Lutter R, et al. External validation of blood eosinophils, FE(NO) and serum periostin as surrogates for sputum eosinophils in asthma. *Thorax* 2015; 70(2): 115–120.

[21] Kankaanranta H, Harju T, Kilpeläinen M, et al. Diagnosis and pharmacotherapy of stable chronic obstructive pulmonary disease: the Finish guidelines. *Basic Clin Pharmacol Toxicol* 2015; 116:291–307.

[22] Kovlizek V, Chlumsky J, Zindr V, et al. Chronic obstructive pulmonary disease: official diagnosis and treatment guidelines of the Czech Pneumological and Phthisiological Society; a novel phenotypic approach to COPD with patient-oriented care. *Biomed Pap Med Fac Univ Palacky Olomouc Czech Repub.* 2013; 157:189–201.

[23] Golpe R, Sanjuán López P, Cano Jiménez E, et al. Distribution of clinical phenotypes in patients with chronic obstructive pulmonary disease caused by biomass and tobacco smoke. *Arch Bronconeumol.* 2014; 50:318–324.

[24] Miravitlles M, Huerta A, Fernández-Villar JA, et al. Generic utilities in chronic obstructive pulmonary disease patients stratified according to different staging systems. *Health Qual Life Outcomes.* 2014; 12:120.

[25] Miravitlles M, Alcázar B, Alvarez FJ, Bazús T, Calle M, Casanova C, et al. What pulmonologists think about the asthma-COPD overlap syndrome. *Int J Chron Obstruct Pulmon Dis* 2015; 10:1321–1330.

[26] GEMA 4.0. Guía Española para el manejo del asma. 2015. Available at http://www.gemasma.com.

[27] Andersen H, Lampela P, Nevanlinna A, et al. High hospital burden in overlap syndrome of asthma and COPD. *Clin Respir J* 2013; 7(4):342–346.

[28] Kauppi P, Kupiainen H, Lindqvist A, et al. Overlap syndrome of asthma and COPD predicts low quality of life. *J Asthma* 2011; 48(3):279–285.

[29] Cosio BG, Soriano JB, López-Campos JL, et al. Defining the asthma-COPD overlap syndrome in a COPD cohort. *Chest* 2016; 149(1): 45–52.

[30] Magnussen H, Bugnas B, van Noord J, Schmidt P, Gerken F, Kesten S. Improvements with tiotropium in COPD patients with concomitant asthma. *Respir Med* 2008; 102:50–56.

[31] Kerstjens HA, Overbeek SE, Schouten JP, et al. Airways hyperresponsiveness, bronchodilator response, allergy and smoking predict improvement in FEV1 during long-term inhaled corticosteroid treatment. Dutch CNSLD Stud Group. *Eur Respir J* 1993; 6(6):868–876.

[32] Weiner P, Weiner M, Azgad Y, et al. Inhaled budesonide therapy for patients with stable COPD. *Chest* 1995; 108(6):1568–1571.

[33] Leigh R, Pizzichini MM, Morris MM, et al. Stable COPD: predicting benefit from high-dose inhaled corticosteroid treatment. *Eur Respir J* 2006; 27(5):964–971.

[34] Bleecker ER, Emmett A, Crater G, et al. Lung function and symptom improvement with fluticasone propionate/salmeterol and ipratropium bromide/albuterol in COPD: response by beta-agonist reversibility. *Pulm Pharmacol Ther* 2008; 21(4): 682–688.

[35] Leuppi JD, Tandjung R, Anderson SD, et al. Prediction of treatment-response to inhaled corticosteroids by mannitol-challenge test in COPD. A Proof Concept. *Pulm Pharmacol Therap* 2005; 18(2): 83–88.

[36] Kunisaki KM, Rice KL, Janoff EN, et al. Exhaled nitric oxide, systemic inflammation, and the spirometric response to inhaled fluticasone propionate in severe chronic obstructive pulmonary disease: a prospective study. *Ther Adv Respir Dis* 2008; 2(2): 55–64.

[37] Peters SP, Bleecker ER, Kunselman SJ, et al. Predictors of response to tiotropium versus salmeterol in asthmatic adults. *J Allergy Clin Immunol* 2013; 132(5):1068–1074.

[38] Peters SP, Kunselman SJ, Icitovic N, et al. Tiotropium bromide step-up therapy for adults with uncontrolled asthma. *N Engl J Med* 2010; 363(18):1715–1726.

[39] Vanfleteren LE1, Kocks JW, Stone IS, et al. Moving from the Oslerian paradigm to the post-genomic era: Are asthma and COPD outdated terms? *Thorax* 2014; 69(1):72-79.

[40] D'Silva L, Hassan N, Wang HY, et al. Heterogeneity of bronchitis in airway diseases in tertiary care clinical practice. *Can Respir J* 2011; 18(3):144–148.

# 4

# Matrix Metalloproteinases in Asthma-Associated Airway Remodeling

Katarzyna Grzela, Agnieszka Strzelak,
Wioletta Zagórska and Tomasz Grzela

## Abstract

Matrix metalloproteinases (MMPs) are $Zn^{2+}$-dependent endoproteases, which digest extracellular matrix (ECM) components and various non-ECM molecules. Main physiological role of MMPs concerns regulation of tissue remodeling and regeneration. The production and activity of MMPs are tightly supervised by multistage control mechanisms. These mechanisms include regulation of gene expression, and various post-transcriptional/post-translational modifications. However, without proper control MMPs reveal dual nature, similarly to character from the novella by R.L. Stevenson, "Strange Case of Dr Jekyll and Mr Hyde". They become dangerous molecules, involved in cancer metastasis, or cardiovascular diseases.

Recent studies revealed that MMPs are also engaged in asthma. Despite extensive research, exact role of MMPs in this process remains unclear and there is no agreement among scientists, regarding two opposite concepts. The followers of "destructive hypothesis" postulate detrimental effect of MMPs on mucosa. Accordingly, MMPs-mediated damage stimulates chaotic regeneration, and progressive remodeling. Oppositely, enthusiasts of "protective hypothesis" postulate that MMPs actually do not allow formation of excessive collagen deposits, and thus they protect from tissue fibrosis.

The better understanding of "MMPs — Jekyll or Hyde ?" story may be clinically relevant, especially while considering therapies focused on modulation of MMPs activity. Therefore, this issue requires instant elucidation.

**Keywords:** airway remodeling, asthma, extracellular matrix, matrix metalloproteinase, destructive hypothesis and protective hypothesis

# 1. Introduction

Matrix metalloproteinases (MMPs) represent group of 25 endoproteases, which require a presence of zinc ions to reveal their proteolytic activity. According to worldwide accepted nomenclature, MMPs have assigned numbers from 1 to 28. However, till now no respective molecules have been ascribed for numbers 4, 5 and 6, whereas MMP-18 was identified only in *Xenopus* frogs. [1, 2] Apart from regulation of extracellular matrix (ECM) turnover, MMPs are also involved in controlling of numerous non-ECM molecules, including cytokines and growth factors. Thus, MMPs are key molecules in embryo- and organogenesis, angiogenesis and tissue regeneration. However, they are also main destructive factors, responsible for cancer progression, aortic aneurysm rupture or delayed healing of chronic wounds. [3, 4] Recently, their involvement was postulated also in some inflammatory diseases affecting respiratory tract, among them chronic obstructive pulmonary disease and asthma. [5] In this chapter authors will focus especially on possible role of MMPs in asthma and asthma-associated alterations in architecture and function of respiratory tract mucosa, which are better known as airway remodeling.

# 2. MMPs — portrait of the family

## 2.1. MMP structure

Based on molecular structure, substrate specificity and mechanism of activation, MMPs are classified into four groups: gelatinases, matrilysins, archetypal MMPs and furin-activated MMPs (Fig. 1.). Formerly, MMPs were divided into six types – collagenases, gelatinases, stromelysins, matrilysins, membrane-type MMPs and others. However, nowadays this classification possesses rather historical meaning. The overall structure of MMPs reveals some common features, which are similar in all members of the family. [2, 3] One of these features is the presence of signaling peptide, located on the N-terminus of newly synthesized proteins. This leader sequence is necessary for the insertion of maturating MMP molecule into cistern of endoplasmic reticulum, and then it is removed. Unlike to other family members, in MMP-23 the N-terminal signaling sequence is substituted by a type II transmembrane domain, which allows anchorage of these molecules in cell membrane.

The next part common in MMP structure is approximately 80 amino acid-long prodomain. It contains conserved "cysteine switch" motif, responsible for maintaining the latent form of enzyme by the blockade of its catalytic site. The main constant segment present in all family members is their catalytic domain. This sphere-like domain is composed of 160-170 amino acids. It contains shallow slot with two zinc ions inside, which constitutes an active site of MMP molecule. Exclusively, catalytic domains in both gelatinases, MMP-2 and -9, contain unique fibronectin II-like inserts. Most MMPs (except for MMP-7, -23 and -26) have short hinge segment of approximately 10-30 amino acids, which connects the catalytic domain with hemopexin-like domain. Exceptionally, MMP-9 molecule has the longest hinge region, composed of 64 strongly O-glycosylated amino acids. The C-terminal hemopexin-like domain,

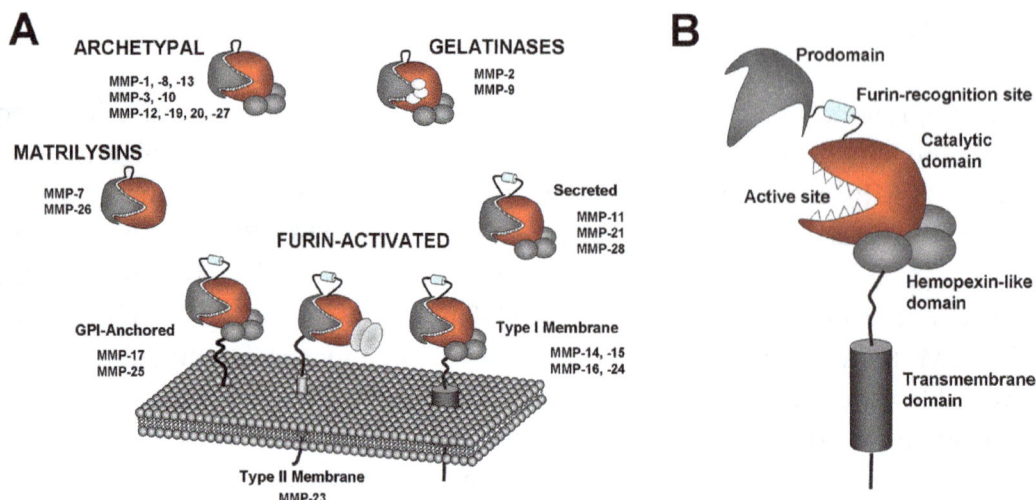

**Fig. 1.** Schematic representation of MMPs family. (A). Main groups of the family and their structure. (B). An example of schematic structure of MMP. Detailed description in text.

not present in MMP-7, -23 and -26, is composed of approximately 200 amino acids and is considered as docking spot for tissue inhibitors of MMPs (TIMPs). In MMP-23 molecule the hemopexin-like domain was replaced by a cysteine-rich immunoglobulin-like domain.

The representatives of membrane-type (MT) subgroup of MMPs (except of already mentioned MMP-23) have hemopexin-like domain connected to a type I transmembrane domain with a short intracellular tail (MMP-14, -15, -16 and -24, also known as MT1, -2, -3 and -5-MMP, respectively), or a cell membrane-anchoring glycosylphosphatidylinositol (GPI) moiety (MMP-17 and -25, known as MT4- and MT6-MMP) (Fig. 1).

Finally, three of secreted MMPs (MMP-11, -21 and -28), all the membrane-type MMPs and MMP-23 have a specific sequence between their prodomain and the catalytic domain, which is recognized by furin. This subtilisin-like serine proteinase from trans-Golgi apparatus and the endoplasmic reticulum removes the prodomain from the catalytic domain and thus may lead to intracellular activation of MMP molecule. [1–6]

## 2.2. Substrate specificity

MMPs are able to digest main components of extracellular matrix (ECM), including high molecular weight polymers of native and denatured collagens and elastin, as well as small ECM molecules, like fibronectin, laminin and aggrecan. Moreover, MMPs may process numerous non-ECM molecules, among them various adhesion molecules, dystroglycan, syndecans, growth factors, pro-cytokines, and their receptors. MMPs were shown to activate via proteolysis pro-forms of interleukin (IL)-1β, IL-8, tumor necrosis factor (TNF), Fas ligand, transforming growth factor (TGF)-β, but also other members of MMPs family (Table 1). [1, 3, 7–9] Noteworthy, some of these cytokines, including vascular endothelial growth factor (VEGF) and TGF-β, may be further entrapped in three-dimensional net of extracellular matrix components or by their binding proteins. Therefore, MMPs may be necessary to reveal biological activity of these factors, through their enzymatic discharge from ECM.

| Group | Representatives | Main ECM substrates | Non-ECM substrates |
|---|---|---|---|
| **ARCHETYPAL MMPs** | **Collagenases**<br>MMP-1, -8- 13 | collagens, gelatin, fibronectin, aggrecan... | pro-IL-1β, pro-IL-8, pro-TNF, other MMPs, PAI, IGFBM |
| | **Stromelysins**<br>MMP-3, -10 | collagens, gelatin, elastin, fibronectin, laminin, aggrecan | pro-IL-1β, other MMPs, IGFBP, MMP/TIMP complex, fibrinogen, plasminogen, antitrombin III |
| | **Others**<br>MMP-12, -19, -20, -27 | collagen IV, gelatin, elastin, fibronectin, laminin | fibrin, plasminogen, myelin basic protein |
| **MATRILYSINS**<br>MMP-7, -26 | | collagen IV, gelatin, elastin, fibronectin, laminin, integrins... | other MMPs, MMP/TIMP complex, fibrinogen, plasminogen |
| **GELATINASES**<br>MMP-2, -9 | | collagens, gelatin, elastin, fibronectin... | pro-IL-1β, plasminogen, other MMPs |
| **FURIN-ACTIVATED MMPs** | **Secreted**<br>MMP-11,-21,-28 | collagen IV, gelatin, laminin, fibronectin | casein, IGFBP |
| | **Type 1 transmembrane**<br>MMP-14,-15,-16,-24 | collagens, gelatin, elastin, laminin, vitronectin | other MMPs |
| | **GPI-anchored**<br>MMP-17,-25 | UNK | |
| | **Type II transmembrane**<br>MMP-23A,-23B | UNK | |

**Table. 1.** Representatives of MMPs family with their main substrates (detailed description in text). ECM – extracellular matrix, Non-ECM- other substrates, PAI – plasminogen activator inhibitor, IGFBP – insulin-like growth factor-binding protein, TIMP – tissue inhibitor of MMPs, UNK – unknown.

## 2.3. MMP expression

Due to a high proteolytic activity and broad substrate specificity, MMPs are recognized as key molecules, engaged in cell proliferation and migration, tissue growth, remodeling, and regeneration. For this reason their expression and activation has to be maintained under precise multistage control. These controlling mechanisms include regulation of gene expression, post-transcriptional and post-translational modifications, but also several ways of pro-enzyme activation or inhibition of active MMP. [3, 4] Nevertheless, if these mechanisms fail, similarly to the well known character from the famous novella by R.L. Stevenson, "Strange Case of Dr. Jekyll and Mr. Hyde", MMPs may also reveal their dual nature. Without sufficient supervision, these endoproteases may become highly dangerous effector molecules, engaged in various pathologies. These conditions include cancer metastasis, formation and rupture of aortic aneurysm, delayed healing of chronic wounds and many others. [1, 3, 10, 11] Recent studies have provided evidence that MMPs may also be involved in pathogenesis of asthma, mainly asthma-associated airway remodeling. [5]

Among all MMPs, only MMP-2 and MMP-9 are produced constitutively, whereas the expression of majority of MMP genes requires some trigger, e.g. tissue damage, or inflammatory reaction. It was found that the promoter region of genes encoding for MMPs comprises sequences recognized by two main specific transcription factors, AP-1 and NF-κB. Both transcription factors merge expression of many inflammatory response-engaged molecules, including MMPs with several intracellular signaling pathways, induced by cytokines and growth factors. Indeed, it was proved that MMPs expression may be controlled by variety of growth factors, including TGF-β, platelet-derived growth factor (PDGF), epidermal growth factor (EGF), and pro-inflammatory cytokines (e.g. IL-1β, IL-6, TNF, etc.). Moreover, the promoter activity of MMPs may also be supervised by family of Ets transcription factors. Since their conserved binding site is located close to target sequence for AP-1, they may interact each other and thus modulate promoter response to various stimuli. [3, 4, 10, 12–14]

The rigid control of MMP genes expression may also be granted by their epigenetic modification. This mechanism is based on alteration in chromatin conformation, which is mediated by differential acetylation-deacetylation of nucleosomal units, due to activity of an enzyme – histone deacetylase (HDAC). Noteworthy, it has been shown that such regulation may result in various responses of particular MMP genes. *In vitro* stimulation with TNF or IL-1β, with simultaneous suppression of HDAC activity resulted in decreased expression of MMP-1 and MMP-9, but increased production of MMP-3. [14, 15] Finally, the expression of MMPs may also be modified on the post-transcriptional level, by the influence on stability or degradation of their transcripts. Recently, it has been proven that the expression of several MMPs may be negatively regulated by the small molecules of non-coding RNA, known as microRNAs (miRs), in mechanism of RNA interference. It has been demonstrated that miR-9, miR-24 and miR-133a may bind to the 3′-UTR of mRNA for MMP-14 (MT1-MMP) and they directly block its translation. On the other hand, down-regulation of miR-199a-5p in murine model induced MMP-1, possibly via Ets-1 derepression. [16–19]

## 2.4. MMP activity

All members of MMPs family are expressed as inactive pro-enzymes. This condition is assured by previously mentioned "cysteine switch", a specific interaction between zinc cations from the active site of the catalytic domain, and a cysteine thiol group from the prodomain. The renouncement of inhibitory influence of the prodomain on the catalytic domain is critical for activation of pro-enzyme and may take place in two concurrent ways (Fig. 2). [3, 14, 20]

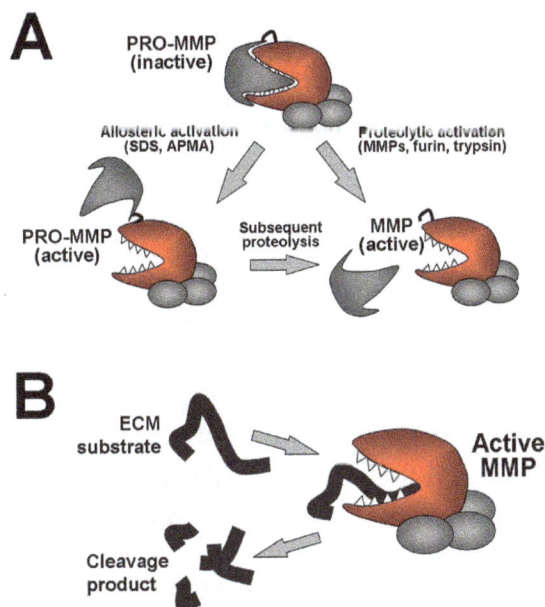

**Fig. 2.** MMPs activation. (A) Two pathways of MMPs activation. (B) Schematic representation of substrate cleavage. Detailed description in text.

### 2.4.1. Activation

The first pathway of MMPs activation is based on direct cleavage of their prodomain. It may be carried by several extracellular proteolytic enzymes, including other MMPs, as well as cysteine, serine and aspartate proteases. This pathway also involves already mentioned intracellular processing and activation by furin. Due to removal of prodomain, molecular weight of pro-enzyme activated in this pathway is significantly reduced, as compared to its initial size. Thus, in zymograms of substrate-specific zymography with SDS-polyacrylamide gel electrophoresis (PAGE) the activated MMP appears as the lower band, below that, corresponding to latent form of enzyme. [21–23]

The second pathway depends on interaction of cysteine thiol groups from prodomain with various compounds, including free radical, disulfides, some detergents with sodium dodecyl sulphate (SDS), alkylating agents, heavy metal ions and organomercurials, with 4-aminophenylmercuric acetate (APMA). This interaction may induce allosteric conversion in MMP structure, which leads to an exposure of the active site in the catalytic domain. Therefore, although the prodomain still remains attached to the entire molecule, such MMP may reveal its proteolytic activity. On the other hand, that MMP, despite being activated, has the same molecular weight, as its inactive pro-form. That explains, why such full length-MMP may be visualized in zymograms on the same level as latent pro-MMP. Noteworthy, the prodomain may be further removed by auto-cleavage, that results in decrease of MMP molecular size and, similarly to the first pathway, an appearance of the lower band in zymograms. [3]

Results of recent studies suggest that *in vitro* proteolysis requires only a substrate and respective MMP, whereas *in vivo* systems usually involve some additional component. These accessory factors may include membrane-, or ECM-associated peptides and glycosaminoglycans, which may determine specificity, as possibly, catalytic rate of MMPs. Accordingly, such accessory molecules may work as a kind of adapters, which bind a substrate and MMP and thus enable their close interaction with an effective concentration. [21–23]

### 2.4.2. Inhibition

As was already noticed, the precise control of MMPs expression and activity is essential for homeostasis of the entire body. Therefore, to counterbalance the mentioned stimulators and activators of MMPs, some agents revealing inhibitory properties are also required. Apart from best known family of specific tissue inhibitors of metalloproteinases (TIMPs), there are also less specific endogenous inhibitors, among them $\alpha$2-macroglobulin, family of serine proteinase inhibitors (serpins), thrombospondin-1 (TSP-1), tissue factor-pathway inhibitor (TFPI)-2, reversion-inducing cysteine-rich protein with Kazal motifs (RECK), etc. [3, 10, 21, 24]

Members of TIMPs family (numbered from 1 to 4) are the best identified specific endogenous inhibitors of MMPs. They are expressed and released by various cell populations, including macrophages, platelets, smooth muscle cells, etc. The mechanism of their action depends on reversible chelating of $Zn^{2+}$ cations from active center of MMP's catalytic domain and, thus, abolishes its proteolytic properties. Since MMP – TIMP interaction occurs in a stoichiometric ratio 1:1, the MMP/TIMP ratio seems to better reflect presumable biological impact of both agents, instead of absolute amount of each of both proteins. Moreover, it is noteworthy that studies concerning *in vivo* interactions between MMPs and TIMPs are also interfered by the highly effective serum antiprotease – $\alpha$2-macroglobulin. [3, 6, 14]

Although all TIMPs may interact with various MMPs, they differ in their specificity, e.g. TIMP-1 preferentially binds to membrane type-MMPs, whereas TIMP-2 is considered as important regulator of MMP-2 activity. Interestingly, the latter regulation actually involves TIMP-2-dependent activation of MMP-2. In this unique mechanism TIMP-2 works as bridging molecule between hemopexin domain of MMP-2 and MT1-MMP (MMP-14), which mediates cleavage of prodomain in "immobilized" MMP-2.

Apart from mentioned above endogenous MMPs inhibitors, there is also an increasing number of exogenous compounds, which reveal direct and/or indirect modulatory properties towards the activity of MMPs. [3, 4] Since they have potential clinical relevance in a treatment of asthma and asthma-associated remodeling, they will be further described in next paragraph (see 2.7).

## 2.5. Methods of MMP measurement

Increasing interest in the role of MMPs in asthma and, especially, asthma-associated remodeling encouraged scientists to develop more specific and sensitive methods to detect MMPs in analyzed samples. However, main obstacle in MMPs research is that most commonly used methods, i.e. enzyme-linked immunosorbent assay (ELISA) and zymography, do not allow simultaneous assessment of amount and activity of MMPs. [3]

## 2.5.1. ELISA

Standard ELISA is a routine laboratory technique, which allows a quantitative detection of minute amounts of MMPs in solution (picograms per ml) using specific antibodies, usually conjugated with peroxidase-based detection system. Noteworthy, standard method provides data concerning specific protein concentration, without any information regarding actual activity of MMPs. Nevertheelss, such activity could be roughly estimated using specially designed ELISA sets, which enable differentiation between truncated forms of activated MMPs and prodomain-containing latent MMPs. However, as mentioned above, allosteric activation not necessarily leads to prodomain removal. Therefore, data provided by ELISA alone are not fully conclusive, and should be verified by some activity assay. [3]

## 2.5.2. Zymography

The substrate-specific zymography is the most commonly used method to evaluate MMPs activity in tested samples. This assay is based on initial separation of samples using electrophoresis in modified polyacrylamide gel, followed by its incubation in reaction buffer and subsequent staining. The key component of such modified gel is substrate, specific for enzyme being analyzed (e.g. collagen for MMP-1 and -13, gelatin for MMP-2 and -9, casein for MMP-1, -3, -7, -10, -12, -13), which is homogenously distributed in whole gel volume. Since polyacrylamide gel contains sodium dodecyl sulphate (SDS), the speed of migration in electrophoresis is determined by molecular weight of separated proteins, resulting in shifted local condensation of full length pro-enzyme and truncated forms of MMPs. During incubation in calcium- and zinc-rich reaction buffer, MMP molecules become reactivated and digest own specific substrate only in place of their condensation. After wash in the staining solution, e.g. Coomassie Brilliant Blue, the entire gel becomes stained, with except of unstained area corresponding to digested substrate. Noteworthy, when compared to respective molecular weight standard, the localization of unstained area enables better identification of analyzed MMP, whereas the size of digested / unstained bands well correlates with amounts of detected enzyme. This amounts may be further determined by comparison to reference sample, e.g. known amounts of recombinant MMP. [3, 25]

Although substrate-specific zymography is sensitive (picograms per sample), and relatively cheap method, it has some weak points. The first issue is long and time-consuming protocol. The next, more important concern, is uncontrolled allosteric activation of MMP mediated by SDS. Since it may strongly affect results of assessment, in current research standard zymography is often replaced by other, faster and more reliable activity assays.

## 2.5.3. Fluorescent activity assay

The unintended interaction with SDS may be avoided, when instead of polyacrylamide gel, MMPs activity is assessed in SDS-free reaction mixture. The measurement of substrate proteolysis in solution implements technology of fluorescence resonance energy transfer (FRET) using substrate (e.g. casein or gelatin) tagged with fluorochrome and quencher. Until labeled substrate stays untouched, the entire energy from fluorochrome is absorbed by quencher, with no fluorescence detectable. When the substrate is cleaved, the fluorochrome-quencher interaction becomes disrupted, that is associated with increased emission of fluorescence under UV light. Since the increase of fluorescence is proportional to enzyme activity, with known quantities of MMP as reference, and with fluorescence reader, this method allows very fast (within few minutes) measurement of proteolytic activity revealed by small amounts (nanograms per ml) of MMP in tested samples. [3, 26]

Noteworthy, in contrast to standard zymography, the fluorescence assay enables studies on proteolytic activity of MMPs, and analysis of modulation of this activity by various agents, e.g. natural and synthetic inhibitors. However, the method is very sensitive to reaction conditions, which may vary depending on protocol of sample preparation. The key factors are concentration of non-ionic detergents, and presence of exogenous protease inhibitors (frequently used to prevent proteolysis in biological material) or metal ion chelators (e.g. EDTA). On the other hand, the tissue sample preparation itself may lead to artificial activation of MMPs or release of their natural inhibitors. [3]

The main disadvantage of the basic variant of mentioned fluorescent method is its non-specificity. Therefore, when analyzing biological samples, to determine, which MMP contributes to the degradation of labeled substrate, it is necessary to use a panel of MMP-specific antibodies, to inhibit proteolytic activity of selected enzyme. Although a such approach enables precise identification of all contributors of observed proteolytic activity, it also significantly increases the cost of that analysis.

### 2.5.4. Immunozymography assay

Recently, a modification of mentioned above fluorescent method was introduced into market. The method combines specificity of standard ELISA and functionality of fluorescent activity assay. In a first step the sample is applied onto test plate, coated by antibody specific for MMP of interest. Then MMP molecules, which are captured by antibody, convert a latent detection reagent into its active form. The activated detection reagent catalyzes enzymatic conversion of colorless substrate into color product. Since the amount of product directly correlates with number of active MMPs, the use of standard calibration curve allows precise measurement of active MMP molecules concentration in tested samples. Furthermore, when using organo-mercurials (e.g. APMA) to activate pro-MMPs in tested material, it also allows an assessment of latent form of MMPs. Thus, the assay incorporates advantages of standard zymography (the assessment of MMP activity and discrimination between pro- and active forms of these enzymes), specificity of ELISA and exceptional sensitivity, reaching 0.1 pg/ml. Therefore, it may be the best choice for research concerning MMPs activity in samples, where the minute amounts of MMPs are expected, e.g. condensates of exhaled air. [27]

### 2.5.5. In situ zymography

The distribution of MMPs in tissue specimens may be studied using immunohistochemistry. However, to assess the local activity of these enzymes, directly on the place of their production, the *in situ* zymography may be used. Similarly to mentioned above fluorescent activity assay, this method also utilizes FRET technology. The tested specimen is incubated with substrate labeled with fluorochrome-quencher complex and then analyzed using fluorescent microscope, or confocal laser scanning microscope. Similarly to fluorescent activity assay, *in situ* zymography does not identify particular MMPs, unless used with specific neutralizing antibodies. Furthermore, it does not provide information concerning quantities of active MMP. Nevertheless, it is still valuable supplement to other methods in MMPs research. [3]

### 2.5.6. Reverse zymography

As previously mentioned, various factors which affect MMPs activity, may be analyzed using fluorescent activity assay, western blot or respective ELISA. However, to detect natural tissue inhibitors of MMP (TIMPs) some functional assay, better known as reverse zymography, has been developed. The method is based on specific interaction between TIMPs from analyzed sample and MMP of interest. Similarly to standard zymography, samples are separated in polyacrylamide gel, which is supplemented with homogenously distributed substrate (e.g. gelatin), but also selected MMP. After electrophoresis the gel is incubated in reaction buffer. Since both, MMP and substrate, are present in the entire gel volume, MMP cleaves the whole substrate, except of places corresponding to the TIMPs condensation after electrophoresis. In these places TIMPs protect substrate from digestion, therefore, after Coomassie staining they appear as blue bands, whereas the remaining gel volume stays unstained. [3]

## 2.6. MMPs in patients with asthma

### 2.6.1. Mr. Hyde...?

Extensive studies, focused on asthma and asthma-associated airway remodeling, have revealed clear involvement of MMPs in pathogenesis of that disease. [5] However, the exact role of MMPs in this process remains vague. The postulated link between metalloproteinases and asthma was based mainly on observations concerning increased amounts and/or activities of various MMPs in samples collected in patients with asthma. The samples were obtained using various methods of collection and/or various material, among them serum or plasma, mucosal biopsies, induced sputum, broncho-alveolar lavage (BAL) fluid and, most recently, exhaled breath condensates (EBC). [27–31] Majority of studies concerned MMP-9, however, other MMPs, including MMP-1, -2, -3, or -12 were also studied. It is noteworthy that substrate specificity of mentioned MMPs entirely enables their self-sufficient work with full repertoire of ECM components. Collagen IV, and laminin, two main components of basement membranes, are cleaved by MMP-9 and MMP-12. Native molecules of collagen I, main fibrillar ECM component of mucosal connective tissue, are initially digested by MMP-1, whereas their further degradation may be continued by all mentioned MMPs (MMP-2, -3, -9, and -12). Elastin molecules are degraded mainly by MMP-12, but also MMP-2 and -9. [3] Although nominal values of MMPs (especially MMP-9) concentrations differed between various studies, in vast majority of mentioned reports similar regularity was observed. MMPs levels and /or activity in individuals with asthma were several fold higher than in control subjects. [28, 29, 32] The number of MMPs-positive cells in sputum or BAL inversely correlated with values of forced expiratory volume in 1 second (FEV1), whereas MMPs amounts in sputum, BAL and EBC positively correlated with severity of disease. They were significantly higher in severe asthma or in asthma exacerbation, and lower in mild asthma or in remission. [31, 33] Also bronchial smooth myocytes/myofibroblasts (BSM) from mucosal biopsies of patients with fatal asthma produced increased levels of MMP-9 and -12, whereas BSM from non-asthmatics expressed only small quantities of MMP-2,-3 and -9. [34]

These observations could support concept of "destructive hypothesis", which emphasizes detrimental effect of metalloproteinases on disease progression. In this scenario, similarly to Mr. Hyde from previously mentioned novella by R.L. Stevenson, MMPs reveal their dark nature. The overexpression and hyperactivation of these enzymes may result in progressive damage of epithelium, basement membrane and subepithelial connective tissue. These events may endorse local inflammatory reaction, and thus further increase the damage zone. [5, 35] On the other hand, they may induce excessive and poorly controlled tissue repair, with increased deposition of ECM components, proliferation and hypertrophy of myofibroblasts, as well as goblet cells hyperplasia with mucus hypersecretion. These changes result in structural and functional changes in bronchial tree mucosa, which is known as airway remodeling (Fig. 3). [5, 34] In fact, in animal model of asthma it was found that an increase in MMP-9 activity in the airway mucosa was associated with epithelial damage, alteration of subepithelial basement membrane, but also increased levels of TGF-β and subepithelial collagen deposition. [36, 37] In patients with asthma Vignola and coauthors have observed positive correlation between sputum levels of MMP-9 and the intensity of functional and structural abnormalities, which may be easily visualized using air flow measurement and high resolution computed tomography, respectively. [38, 39]

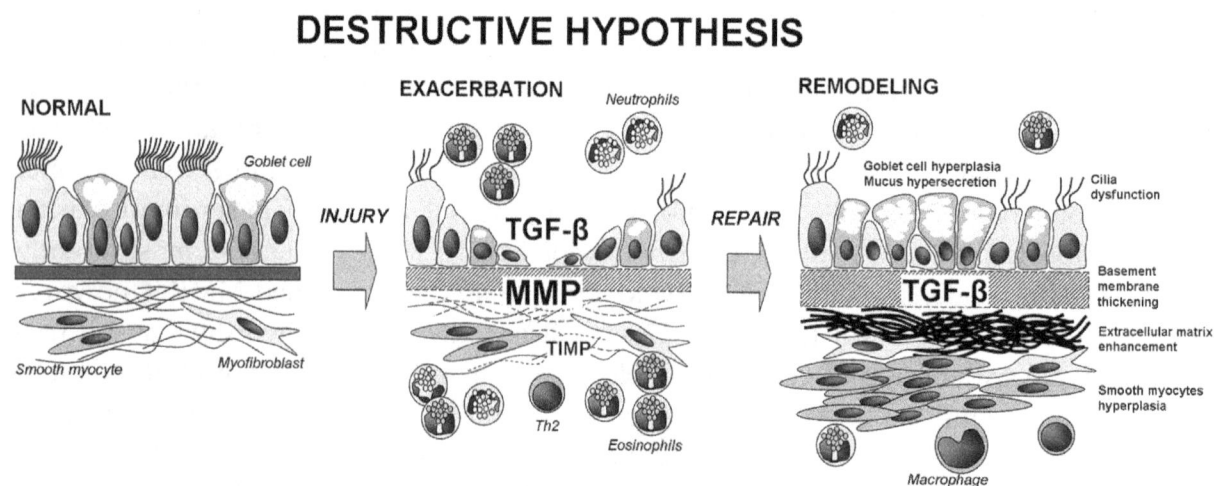

Fig. 3. Schematic representation of the "destructive hypothesis". Detailed description in text.

Interestingly, some authors did not confirm direct correlation of MMPs levels with symptoms severity, especially when using serum or plasma samples for the analysis. [30] The last finding may suggest that a main source of MMPs overproduction in asthma is located in airway system, with limited systemic influence. This assumption may be supported by association between MMP-9 level measured in breath condensates and predominant population of inflammatory cells in induced sputum or BAL. Barbaro and coauthors have shown that patients with neutrophilic airway inflammation revealed MMP-9 concentrations significantly higher than individuals with severe eosinophilic asthma. [40] Thus, one could conclude that, essentially, neutrophils and, to a lesser extent, eosinophils would be main sources of MMPs in mild and severe asthma. Nevertheless, there is strong evidence that functional and structural changes in bronchial wall are also contributed by other producers of MMPs – epithelial cells, bronchial smooth myocytes, fibroblasts and mast cells. [5, 27] In fact, recent studies have shown that epithelium- and myocytes-derived metalloproteinases may be involved in pathogenesis of asthma and asthma-associated remodeling much earlier, even before clinical manifestation of first symptoms. That hypothesis emerged as an ancillary result of embryological studies, focused on development of bronchial tree. It has been proposed that pouches of epithelium, submerged in mesenchyma, work together during organogenesis as an functional entity, which was named the epithelial-mesenchymal trophic unit (EMTU). [41] Apart from large variety of cytokines and growth factors, produced by EMTU during embryogenesis, the important role in regulation of bronchial growth play metalloproteinases. Their list is still expanding and includes several soluble MMPs, mainly MMP-3, -9 and -12 [34, 42], as well as membrane-type 1 MMP (MT1-MMP/MMP-14). [43] The latter is involved in regulation of cell proliferation, migration and differentiation, since all these events are in some extent associated with pericellular proteolytic activity of this membrane-bound MMP.

Recently, another membrane-bound metallopeptidase, member of distinct class of disintegrin and metalloproteinases (ADAM), denoted as ADAM33, has been added to this list. [44] Similarly to MT-MMPs, function of these metalloproteinases relies on degradation of ECM components located in the close proximity to the cell, that enables further growth and branching of respiratory tree. However, this involvement also comprises processing of cytokines and their receptors. Therefore, although they remain under strict control, including methylation-dependent epigenetic regulation of promoter activity [45], even small abnormality in that system may be responsible for aberrant function of EMTU. This may lead to enhanced response to some stimuli, e.g. oxidative stress or viral infection. [46] Such triggers may result in reactivation of EMTU in adulthood, excessive stimulation of epithelial cells and bronchial myofibroblasts. They start again to express large quantities of metalloproteinases and cytokines, among them TGF-β. Both mentioned enzymes, ADAM33 and MT1-MMP/MMP-14, are supposed to trigger TGF-β-dependent stimulation of BSM and subepithelial fibroblasts, which, in response, start with excessive production and deposition of ECM components. Hereby EMTU reactivation may be associated with an increased risk of airway malfunction. Interestingly, in some individuals the initial ultrastructural changes in basement membrane, a characteristic feature of asthma-associated remodeling, were observed long before the onset of clinical symptoms of disease. [47, 48] Accordingly, one could expect, that EMTU hypothesis should be supported by some genetic background. Indeed, analysis of genome-wide association has indicated the possible role of nucleotide polymorphisms of metalloproteinases in increased susceptibility to asthma. [49] Among them, a significant association with early onset of bronchial hyperresponsiveness and asthma was noted in case of several polymorphic variants of ADAM33. [50] However, due to ethnic variability, the significance level of this association differs between analyzed populations. Noteworthy, among analyzed polymorphisms of ADAM33, only T1, V4, T+1 and F+1 variants were found to correlate with asthma in the general population [51], whereas other, including ST+7 or haplotype H4, were characteristic solely for certain populations. [52, 53]

Furthermore, several groups have suggested correlation between increased risk of asthma development and occurrence of some nucleotide polymorphisms in genes encoding for "classic" matrix metalloproteinases, mainly MMP-9. The postulated associations concerned single nucleotide polymorphisms (SNPs) of MMP-9 gene, located in promoter region (-1562C/T), the substrate binding site in catalytic domain (279Q/R) and TIMP docking region of hemopexin domain (574P/R and 668R/Q). [5, 54] However, majority of mentioned studies were conducted in rather small groups, with various ethnic origins. Therefore, results of these studies, although relevant, should be considered with some caution. Till now, based on studies involving group of 4,000 children, only allele R of 279 SNP was confirmed as being associated with significant increase of asthma risk. [54] On the other hand, some SNPs in MMP genes may also be associated with eventual benefit for a patient. Recently, the mutant T allele of MMP-2 promoter (-1306C/T) SNP, supposed to decrease MMP-2 production, has been described as conferring significant protection against asthma in North Indian population. [55]

### 2.6.2. ... or Dr. Jekyll ?

As already mentioned, research involving asthma patients, animal models and *in vitro* studies provide strong support for "destructive hypothesis". [56] MMPs are abundantly produced and activated during acute and chronic asthma, and their level negatively correlates with lung function. However, those observations should be interpreted with some caution, especially since recent studies yielded some contradicting data. [57, 58] Based on these data an opposite, or "protective hypothesis" has been formulated. According to this concept, MMPs are responsible for cleavage of excessive amounts of ECM components, which are secreted in response to inflammation-mediated damage of mucosa. [59] Therefore, MMPs are supposed to protect mucosa from uncontrolled fibrosis, whereas their natural inhibitors – TIMPs (especially TIMP-1), since they prevent cleavage of abnormal ECM deposits, would, paradoxically, appear as key detrimental molecules in that system (Fig. 4). In fact, increased TIMP-1 concentrations in BAL were related to persistent wheezing in preschool children. [31] However, an attribution of altered ECM turnover solely to MMPs activity or TIMPs concentration seems to be unfounded simplification. Presumably, enhanced accumulation of matrix components results rather from imbalance between proteolytic activity of MMPs and anti-proteolytic properties of TIMPs. Consequently, instead of absolute levels of MMPs or TIMPs, their relative amounts, expressed as respective MMP/TIMP ratios, may be more relevant for course of disease. Indeed, in several studies decreased MMP-9/TIMP-1 ratio was observed in sputum, BAL and mucosal biopsies of adults and children with asthma. [60, 61] Moreover, it was associated with the airflow aggravation and reduced airway lumen, observed in computed tomography of asthmatic patients. [62] The low MMP-9/TIMP-1 ratio was also reported in asthmatic smokers with persisted airflow obstruction and thickening of bronchial mucosa. [63]

## PROTECTIVE HYPOTHESIS

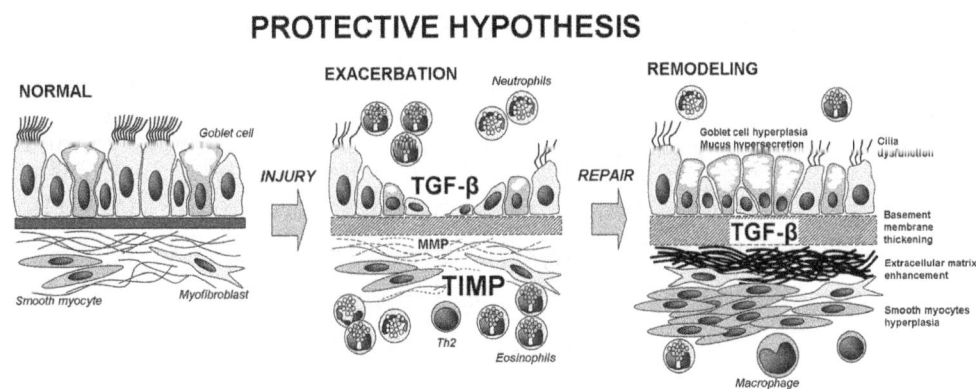

**Fig. 4.** Schematic representation of the "protective hypothesis". Detailed description in text.

When considering protective role of MMPs in asthma and asthma-associated remodeling, their main function concerns normalization of ECM turnover. However, one has to mention MMP-mediated regulation of cell-to-cell and cell-to-ECM interactions, as well as their involvement in cytokines/growth factors network. [56] As previously described, MMPs have been shown to process some cytokines, including TGF-β and VEGF, but also cleave several cell surface receptors, among them fibroblast growth factor (FGF) receptor 1 (FGFR1), CD44, or alpha subunits of receptors for IL-2, -5 and -13. [56, 64–67] Possibly, MMPs could also reveal their protective effect on asthma progression by interference with trafficking of immune cells and/or shedding key receptors engaged in Th2 signaling, thus attenuating allergic inflammation. This hypothesis was confirmed in murine models with MMP-deficient animals. Indeed, in mice lacking MMP-2, -8, -9 or -19 an allergen challenge resulted in increased allergic inflammation and airway hyperresponsiveness with augmented release of Th2 cytokines – IL-4, -5 and -13. [65, 68–74] Interestingly, MMPs deficiency was also associated with delayed clearance of immune cells from the airway. [68, 69, 71] This finding could be explained by involvement of MMPs in conditioning of leukocytes. [71] The possible mechanism of that phenomenon may exploit MMP-9-mediated cleavage of IL-2Rα subunit on the surface of T lymphocytes, which results in down-regulation of their proliferative capacity and subsequent apoptosis. [75] Apart from mentioned Th2 cytokines, MMPs may modulate inflammatory and immune response via processing of CC and CXC chemokines. Metalloproteinases have been shown to cleave macrophage inflammatory protein (MIP)-2 and monocyte chemoattractant proteins (MCPs) – MCP-2, -3, and -4. [76, 77]

The data mentioned above imply, that allergic inflammation and airway remodeling seem to be intricately related to MMPs activity, since MMPs may represent key mediators, or rather modulators, involved in vigorous crosstalk between airway constituent cells, invading inflammatory cells, and the extracellular matrix. [78] From that point of view the idea concerning protective role of MMPs in asthma and asthma-associated remodeling seems to be convincing. However, the issue becomes more complicated, when analyzing involvement of MMPs in processing of ECM components and their direct input in airway destruction and remodeling. Noteworthy, both concepts, "destructive" and "protective", may be supported by some clinical data. In fact, there is still reasonable doubt, whether MMPs reveal some similarity to Dr. Jekyll, or they are recognized rather unfriendly, like Mr. Hyde. However, in addition to some philosophical background, this issue has also an outstanding practical meaning, especially in context of possible pharmacological interventions in asthma-associated remodeling, which may be addressed to modulate MMPs activity. Obviously, when favoring "protective" role of MMPs, they would require some support to increase MMP/TIMP ratio. In contrast, if considering the "destructive hypothesis" as more likely, an opposite action should be undertaken. According to that concept, actually the inhibition of MMPs should provide some benefit for patient. Therefore, univocal clarification of that issue is of great clinical relevance.

### 2.7. MMP modulation — pharmacological interventions

Apart from previously mentioned (see chapter 2.4.2) endogenous or "physiological" inhibitors, several exogenous MMP modulators are also available. Noteworthy, in addition to few agents originally designed as MMP inhibitors (e.g. batimastat or marimatsat), nowadays in clinical practice are used many drugs, originally not intended to modulate MMPs activity. [3, 4, 10] The list of these agents is still expanding and includes tetracyclines, inhibitors of angiotensin converting enzyme (ACE), inhibitors of cholesterol synthesis (better known as statins), corticosteroids, etc. Some of them display direct inhibitory influence on MMPs activity (tetracyclines, ACE inhibitors), whereas in others mechanism of their action is indirect and more complex. Moreover, modulation of MMPs expression has been related to the use of clarithromycin, imatinib, inhibitors of Rho-kinase, antagonists of VEGF receptors, as well as inhibitors of some signaling pathways, including NF-κB, MAPK, and others (Fig. 5). [79–81]

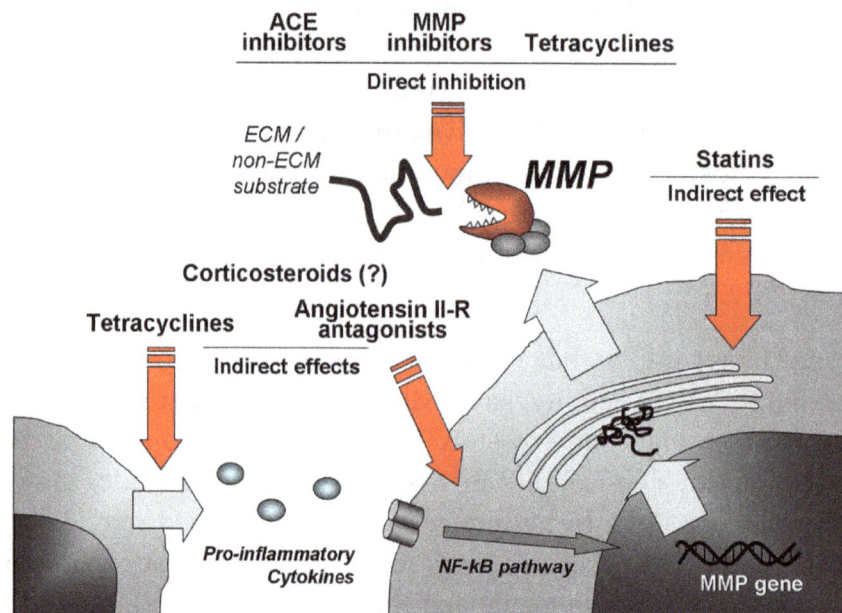

**Fig. 5.** Schematic representation of main strategies for MMPs modulation. Detailed description in text.

## 2.7.1. MMP inhibitors

The first group of broad-spectrum MMP inhibitors (batimastat, marimastat, ilomastat, etc.) is based on hydroxamate derivatives. These small zinc ion chelators were originally developed as anti-cancer drugs, and were expected to protect from cancer metastasis and tumor-related angiogenesis. [82] In murine asthma model a treatment with these compounds (marimastat, neovastat, GM6001, and others) was associated with reduced development of allergic inflammation, whereas in patients with atopic asthma these agents decreased bronchial hyperresponsiveness after allergen challenge. [68, 83, 84] However, due to low specificity, nearly all first generation synthetic MMP inhibitors may reveal inhibitory activity against various zinc-containing metalloproteins, including numerous non-MMP enzymes and transcription factors. Therefore, due to reported severe adverse effects, including so-called musculo-skeletal syndrome, mentioned compounds are currently withdrawn from the clinical practice. Regrettably, also novel MMP inhibitors, designed to specifically target particular MMPs, although encouraging in animal studies, did not ensure better safety and, most importantly, satisfactory clinical efficacy in humans. [85–90] The possible explanation of unexpectedly low clinical effectiveness of specific MMP inhibitors concerned compensatory induction of other MMPs after specific down-regulation of the target one.

Noteworthy, some other strategies of MMPs inhibition include use of monoclonal antibodies or anti-sense technologies. [3, 91] However, relatively high cost due to sophisticated technological process, and parenteral route for administration are enumerated as main limitations for development and broad use of these solutions.

## 2.7.2. Tetracyclines

Tetracyclines are natural antibiotics discovered in *Streptomyces*, which, apart from well defined anti-microbial properties, may also reveal some other, non-antibiotic activities. Tetracyclines may stabilize ECM turnover, presumably by direct inhibition of catalytic site of MMPs, but also indirectly, by suppression of inflammatory cascade and modulation of MMPs expression. [92] Indeed, anti-MMP properties of semi-synthetic tetracycline — doxycycline have been reported in various clinical conditions, including adult periodontitis, abdominal aortic aneurysm, atherosclerosis, autoimmune diseases and in cancer research. [93–96] Thus, doxycycline has received a Food and Drug Administration approval as potent MMP inhibitor, nevertheless its effect on asthma and asthma-associated remodeling still requires extensive studies. Data available from animal studies are promising in terms of attenuated airway hyperresponsiveness after allergen challenge and decreased airway inflammation. [97–99] Moreover, it was observed that long-term administration of doxycycline together with standard therapy was associated with significant improvement in lung function parameters and possible reversal of remodeling in patients with chronic asthma. [100]

## 2.7.3. Statins

The inhibitors of 3-hydroxy-3-methylglutaryl-coenzyme A (HMG-CoA) reductase, better know as statins, are potent inhibitors of cholesterol biosynthesis. Due to their mechanism of action statins are currently used as standard constituent of primary and secondary prevention of atherosclerosis and arterial insufficiency. In addition to decreasing serum cholesterol levels, statins are know to exert various pleiotropic, cholesterol-independent effects. [3, 101] The latter are mediated by inhibition of isoprenoids, which modulate the function of intracellular signaling molecules. Thus, statins, among them lovastatin, cerivastatin, simvastatin, rosuvastatin, or pitavastatin, may reveal some anti-inflammatory activities, including inhibition of MMPs. Therefore, they have been extensively studied mainly in cancer and cardiovascular diseases. [102, 103] Recently, in a randomized controlled study atorvastatin has been shown to significantly reduce sputum concentrations of acute inflammatory mediators, including MMP-8 and -9, in smoking asthmatic patients. [104] Thus, statins, especially when combined with standard therapy, may offer some protection from exacerbation and, possibly, airway remodeling. Noteworthy, simvastatin was found to modulate TGF-β-induced mesenchymal-epithelial transition of alveolar epithelial cells *in vitro*. Interestingly, simvastatin sufficiently suppressed TGF-β to induce expression of connective tissue growth factor (CTGF) and MMP-2 and -9, but it failed to reverse TGF-β-induced morphological changes in epithelial cells. [105] Therefore, although that observation could be a rationale behind the use of statins in prevention of subepithelial fibrosis and airway remodeling, this issue still requires further research.

### 2.7.4. Renin-Angiotensin System modulators

Another group of potential MMP modulators comprises several compounds designed to control the function of the renin-angiotensin system (RAS). These agents, although originally designed to manage arterial hypertension through the inhibition of angiotensin-converting enzyme, appeared to be effective also against MMPs. The mechanism of their action is based on dose-dependent, direct blockage of active site in catalytic domain of the enzyme. [3] Interestingly, also antagonists of angiotensin II receptor were found to modulate MMPs expression, possibly by inhibition of NF-κB pathway. [106] Since early clinical experience with modulators of RAS may suggest their great potential in novel therapy of respiratory diseases, these compounds are recently in focus of interest of several groups. [5, 107, 108]

### 2.7.5. Inhaled corticosteroids

Inhaled corticosteroids (ICS) are currently used as a standard treatment to control asthma symptoms. However, it has to be determined, whether they can block or even reverse epithelial–mesenchymal transition and subepithelial fibrosis in the respiratory tract of asthmatic patients. Noteworthy, decreased amounts of MMP-9 in reticular lamina of basement membrane have been recently shown to contribute to the beneficial effect of ICSs on epithelial–mesenchymal transition in chronic obstructive pulmonary disease. [109] Unexpectedly, data from clinical studies in asthmatic patients are limited and disappointing. [27, 110] In particular, no significant decrease in levels and/or activity of MMP-9 was observed after prolonged therapy with ICS in patients with asthma. [27, 111] This finding may suggest that inhaled corticosteroids alone could not be as effective in preventing asthma-associated airway remodeling, as postulated previously. [27, 110]

In contrast to ICS alone, the improved control of asthma severity, possibly due to better modulation of MMPs system, may be achieved by introducing a combination therapy, which comprises ICS and long acting β-agonists (LABA). Although both, *in vitro* and *in vivo* studies, confirmed superiority of combination therapy over ICS or LABA alone in this regard, they did not determine exactly, how this combination may affect MMP levels. [112–114] Possibly, the augmented effect of ICS-LABA combination can be, at least partially, explained by LABA ability to modulate NF-κB signaling pathway. Thus, inhibition of NF-κB will result in decreased expression of MMP-9 gene, as has been recently shown for ultra-LABA – indacaterol. [115] Indeed, combination of ICS with LABA as both, maintenance and reliever therapy, significantly reduced MMP-9 levels in induced sputum of asthmatic patients. [116, 117] Remarkably, MMP-9 levels, observed in patients with asthma before and after combined treatment with ICS and LABA, seem to reflect the intensity of airways remodeling, as they revealed good correlation with bronchial wall thickening, visualized using high-resolution computed tomography. [116]

### 2.7.6. Leukotriene-receptor antagonists

Leukotriene-receptor antagonists (LTRA) may be considered as an alternative to ICS as "first-line asthma-controller therapy" or as "add-on therapy" in patients already receiving ICS. Montelukast, most commonly used LTRA, was found to decrease the expression of MMP-9 in activated eosinophils *in vitro*. [118] In children with asthma a treatment with LTRA resulted in clinical improvement –reduction of symptoms and increase of peak expiratory flow, which were associated with significant decrease of MMP-9 levels in plasma. [119] In experimental asthma model in mice LTRA treatment was shown to reverse airway remodeling and decreased airway hyperresponsiveness after allergen challenge. Again, mentioned improvement correlated with decrease of MMP-2 and -9 levels in BAL fluid. [120]

## 3. Conclusions

Despite extensive studies focused on role of MMPs in asthma and asthma-associated remodeling, our knowledge regarding this issue is still far from a satisfactory level. Since there is no agreement among scientists regarding superiority of "destructive" or "protective" concept, the clarification of "Dr. Jekyll or Mr. Hyde ?" issue seems to have outstanding clinical relevance, especially when considering possible pharmacological interventions. Regrettably, the interpretation of results concerning exact place of MMPs in asthma pathogenesis may be impeded by different methodology and various populations analyzed in these studies. Such differences may certainly affect result of MMPs assessment across the studies. [57, 121] On the other hand, these discrepancies can be ascribed to real differences in MMPs amount and/or activity, depending on sample type and disease severity. Furthermore, local expression and activity of individual MMPs may vary in different airway compartments, thus adding complexity to the network of allergic inflammatory response. [61, 78, 122] Accordingly, the distribution of MMP-2, MMP-9 and MMP-12 in bronchial wall was shown to differ between large and small airways. Moreover, it varied between healthy controls and patients with asthma, and further changed depending on severity of disease. [61, 78]

Noteworthy, mentioned compartmental differences may be easily averaged for the entire bronchial tree, especially when using site-unspecific samples, like induced sputum, BAL, breath condensate and, obviously, serum or plasma. On the other hand, due to such averaging, small local changes, although clinically relevant, may be disregarded. Therefore, further research should focus on more precise assessment of distribution and activity of MMPs, the balance between MMPs and their natural inhibitors, as well as association of those findings with alterations in architecture and function of respiratory tract mucosa.

# Author details

Katarzyna Grzela, Agnieszka Strzelak, Wioletta Zagórska and Tomasz Grzela[*]

*Address all correspondence to: tomekgrzela@gmail.com

The Medical University of Warsaw, Department of Paediatrics, Pneumonology and Allergology (KG, AS, WZ), and Department of Histology and Embryology (TG), Poland

# References

[1] Amălinei C, Căruntu ID, Bălan RA. Biology of metalloproteinases. Rom J Morphol Embryol. 2007;48:323–334.

[2] Fanjul-Fernández M, Folgueras AR, Cabrera S, López-Otín C. Matrix metalloproteinases: evolution, gene regulation and functional analysis in mouse model. Biochim Biophys Acta. 2010;1803:3–19. DOI: 10.1016/j.bbamcr.2009.07.004.

[3] Grzela T, Bikowska B, Litwiniuk M. Matrix metalloproteinases in aortic aneurysm — executors or executioners? In: Grundmann RT, editors. Etiology, pathogenesis and pathophysiology of aortic aneurysms and aneurysm rupture. Rijeka: Intech Publ; 2011:25–54. DOI: 10.5772/17861.

[4] Krejner A, Litwinuk M, Grzela T. Matrix metalloproteinases in the wound microenvironment: therapeutic perspectives. Chronic Wound Care Management and Research 2016 (accepted for publication)

[5] Grzela K, Litwiniuk M, Zagorska W, Grzela T. Airway remodeling in chronic obstructive pulmonary disease and asthma: the role of matrix metalloproteinase-9. Arch Immunol Ther Exp 2016;64:47–55. DOI: 10.1007/s00005-015-0345-y.

[6] Nagase H, Visse R, Murphy G. Structure and function of matrix metalloproteinases and TIMPs. Cardiovasc Res. 2006;69:562–573. DOI: 10.1016/j.cardiores.2005.12.002.

[7] Endo K, Takino T, Miyamori H, et al. Cleavage of syndecan-1 by membrane type matrix metalloproteinase-1 stimulates cell migration. J Biol Chem. 2003;278:40764–40770. DOI: 10.1074/jbc.M306736200.

[8] Mott JD, Werb Z. Regulation of matrix biology by matrix metalloproteinases. Curr Opin Cell Biol. 2004;16:558–564. DOI:10.1016/j.ceb.2004.07.010.

[9] Yamada H, Saito F, Fukuta-Ohi H, et al. Processing of beta-dystroglycan by matrix metalloproteinase disrupts the link between the extracellular matrix and cell membrane via the dystroglycan complex. Hum Mol Genet. 2001;10:1563–159. DOI: 10.1093/hmg/10.15.1563.

[10] Hadler-Olsen E, Fadnes B, Sylte I, Uhlin-Hansen L, Winberg JO. Regulation of matrix metalloproteinase activity in health and disease. FEBS J. 2011;278:28–45. DOI: 10.1111/j.1742-4658.2010.07920.x.

[11] Ravanti L, Kahari VM. Matrix metalloproteinases in wound repair. Int J Mol Med. 2000;6:391–407. DOI: 10.3892/ijmm.6.4.391

[12] Yan C, Boyd DD. Regulation of matrix metalloproteinase gene expression. J Cell Physiol. 2007;211:19–26. DOI: 10.1002/jcp.20948.

[13] Kapila S, Xie Y, Wang W. Induction of MMP-1 (collagenase-1) by relaxin in fibrocartilaginous cells requires both the AP-1 and PEA-3 promoter sites. Orthod Craniofac Res. 2009;12:178–186. DOI: 10.1111/j.1601-6343.2009.01451.x.

[14] Clark IM, Swingler TE, Sampieri CL, Edwards DR. The regulation of matrix metalloproteinases and their inhibitors. Int J Biochem Cell Biol. 2008;40:1362–1378. DOI: 10.1016/j.biocel.2007.12.006.

[15] Clark IM, Swingler TE, Young DA. Acetylation in the regulation of metalloproteinase and tissue inhibitor of metalloproteinases gene expression. Front Biosci. 2007;12:528–535. DOI: 10.2741/2079.

[16] Di Gregoli K, Jenkins N, Salter R, White S, Newby AC, Johnson JL. MicroRNA-24 regulates macrophage behavior and retards atherosclerosis. Arterioscler Thromb Vasc Biol. 2014;34:1990–2000. DOI: 10.1161/ATVBAHA.114.304088.

[17] Zhang H, Qi M, Li S, et al. microRNA-9 targets matrix metalloproteinase-14 to inhibit invasion, metastasis, and angiogenesis of neuroblastoma cells. Mol Cancer Ther. 2012;11:1454–1466. DOI: 10.1158/1535-7163.MCT-12-0001.

[18] Xu M, Wang YZ. miR-133a suppresses cell proliferation, migration and invasion in human lung cancer by targeting MMP-14. Oncol Rep. 2013;30:1398–1404. DOI: 10.3892/or.2013.2548.

[19] Chan YC, Roy S, Huang Y, Khanna S, Sen CK. The microRNA miR-199a-5p down-regulation switches on wound angiogenesis by derepressing the v-ets erythroblastosis

virus E26 oncogene homolog 1-matrix metalloproteinase-1 pathway. J Biol Chem. 2012;287:41032–41043. DOI: 10.1074/jbc.M112.413294.

[20] Chakraborti S, Mandal M, Das S, Mandal A, Chakraborti T. Regulation of matrix metalloproteinases: an overview. Mol Cell Biochem. 2003;253:269–285.

[21] Klein T, Bischoff R. Physiology and pathophysiology of matrix metalloproteases. Amino Acids. 2011;41:271–290. DOI: 10.1007/s00726-010-0689-x.

[22] Pei D, Weiss SJ. Furin-dependent intracellular activation of the human stromelysin-3 zymogen. Nature. 1995;375:244–247. DOI: 10.1038/375244a0.

[23] Ra HJ, Parks WC. Control of matrix metalloproteinase catalytic activity. Matrix Biol. 2007;26:587–596. DOI: 10.1016/j.matbio.2007.07.001.

[24] Litwiniuk M, Bikowska B, Niderla-Bielinska J, et al. Potential role of metalloproteinase inhibitors from radiation-sterilized amnion dressings in the healing of venous leg ulcers. Mol Med Rep. 2012;6:723–728. DOI: 10.3892/mmr.2012.983.

[25] Grzela T, Brawura-Biskupski-Samaha R, Jelenska MM, Szmidt J. Low molecular weight heparin treatment decreases MMP-9 plasma activity in patients with abdominal aortic aneurysm. Eur J Vasc Endovasc Surg. 2008;35:159–161.

[26] Grzela T, Niderla-Bielinska J, Litwiniuk M, White R. The direct inhibition of MMP-2 and MMP-9 by an enzyme alginogel: a possible mechanism of healing support for venous leg ulcers. J Wound Care. 2014;23:278-285. DOI: 10.12968/jowc.2014.23.5.278.

[27] Grzela K, Zagorska W, Krejner A, et al. Prolonged treatment with inhaled corticosteroids dose not normalize high activity of matrix metallopreoteinase-9 in exhaled breath condensates of children with asthma. Arch Immunol Ther Exp. 2015;63:231–237. DOI: 10.1007/s00005-015-0328-z.

[28] Suzuki R, Kato T, Miyazaki Y, et al. Matrix metalloproteinases and tissue inhibitors of matrix metalloproteinases in sputum from patients with bronchial asthma. J Asthma. 2001;38:477–484.

[29] Belleguic C, Corbel M, Germain N, et al. Increased release of matrix metalloproteinase-9 in the plasma of acute severe asthmatic patients. Clin Exp Allergy. 2002;31:217–223. DOI: 10.1046/j.1365-2222.2002.01219.x.

[30] Ko FW, Diba C, Roth M, et al. A comparison of airway and serum matrix metalloproteinase-9 activity among normal subjects, asthmatic patients, and patients with asthmatic mucus hypersecretion. Chest. 2005;127:1919–1927. DOI: 10.1378/chest.127.6.1919.

[31] Erlewyn-Lajeunesse M, Hunt L, Pohunek P, et al. Bronchoalveolar lavage MMP-9 and TIMP-1 in preschool wheezers and their relationship to persistent wheeze. Pediatr Res 2008;64:194–199. DOI: 10.1203/PDR.0b013e318175dd2d.

[32] Lee Y, Lee B, Rhee Y, Song C. The involvement of matrix metalloproteinase-9 in airway inflammation of patients with acute asthma. Clin Exp Allergy. 2001;31:1623–1630. DOI: 10.1046/j.1365-2222.2001.01211.x.

[33] Karakoc G, Yukselen A, Yilmaz M, Altintas D, Kendirli G. Exhaled breath condensate MMP-9 level and its relationships with asthma severity and interleukin-4/10 levels in children. Ann Allergy Asthma Immunol. 2012;108:300–304. DOI: 10.1016/j.anai.2012.02.019.

[34] Bara I, Ozier A, Tunon de Lara JM, Marthan R, Berger P. Pathophysiology of bronchial smooth muscle remodeling in asthma. Eur Respir J. 2010;36:1174–1184. DOI: 10.1183/09031936.00019810.

[35] Grzela K, Zagorska W, Jankowska-Steifer E, Grzela T. Chronic inflammation in the respiratory tract and ciliary dyskinesia. Centr Eur J Immunol. 2013;38:122–128. DOI: 10.5114/ceji.2013.34369.

[36] Royce SG, Shen M, Patel KP, Huuskes BM, Ricardo SD, Samuel CS. Mesenchymal stem cells and serelaxin synergistically abrogate established airway fibrosis in an experimental model of chronic allergic airways disease. Stem Cell Res. 2015;15:495–505. DOI: 10.1016/j.scr.2015.09.007.

[37] Wenzel SE, Balzar S, Cundall M, Chu HW. Subepithelial basement membrane immunoreactivity for matrix metalloproteinase 9: association with asthma severity, neutrophilic inflammation, and wound repair. J Allergy Clin Immunol. 2003;111:1345–1352. DOI: 10.1067/mai.2003.1464.

[38] Vignola AM, Riccobono L, Mirabella A, et al. Sputum metalloproteinase-9/tissue inhibitor of metalloproteinase-1 ratio correlates with airflow obstruction in asthma and chronic bronchitis. Am J Respir Crit Care Med. 1998;158:1945–1950. DOI: 10.1164/ajrccm.158.6.9803014.

[39] Vignola AM, Paganin F, Capieu L, et al. Airway remodelling assessed by sputum and high-resolution computed tomography in asthma and COPD. Eur Respir J. 2004;24:910–917. DOI: 10.1183/09031936.04.00032603.

[40] Barbaro M, Spanevello A, Palladino G, Salerno F, Lacedonia D, Carpagnano G. Exhaled matrix metalloproteinase-9 (MMP-9) in different biological phenotypes of asthma. Eur J Int Med. 2014;25:92–96. DOI: 10.1016/j.ejim.2013.08.705.

[41] Holgate S. A brief history of asthma and its mechanisms to modern concepts of disease pathogenesis. Allergy Asthma Immunol Res. 2010;2:165–171. DOI: 10.4168/aair.2010.2.3.165.

[42] Lavigne MC, Thakker P, Gunn J, et al. Human bronchial epithelial cells express and secrete MMP-12. Biochem Biophys Res Commun. 2004;324:534–546. DOI: 10.1016/j.bbrc.2004.09.080.

[43] Araya J, Cambier S, Morris A, Finkbeiner W, Nishimura SL. Integrin-mediated transforming growth factor- activation regulates homeostasis of the pulmonary

epithelial-mesenchymal trophic unit. Am J Pathol. 2006;169:405–415. DOI: 10.2353/ajpath.2006.060049.

[44] Davies DE. The Role of the epithelium in airway remodeling in asthma. Proc Am Thorac Soc. 2009;6:678–682. DOI: 10.1513/pats.200907-067DP.

[45] Yang Y, Haitchi HM, Cakebread J, et al. Epigenetic mechanisms silence a disintegrin and metalloprotease 33 expression in bronchial epithelial cells. J Allergy Clin Immunol. 2008;121:1393-1399,1399.e1-14. DOI: 10.1016/j.jaci.2008.02.031.

[46] Tacon CE, Wiehler S, Holden NS, Newton R, Proud D, Leigh R. Human rhinovirus infection up-regulates MMP-9 production in airway epithelial cells via NF-κB. Am J Respir Cell Mol Biol. 2010;43:201–209. DOI: 10.1165/rcmb.2009-0216OC.

[47] Barbato A, Turato G, Baraldo S, et al. Airway inflammation in childhood asthma. Am J Respir Crit Care Med. 2003;168:798–803. DOI: 10.1164/rccm.200305-650OC.

[48] Saglani S, Payne DN, Zhu J, et al. Early detection of airway wall remodeling and eosinophilic inflammation in preschool wheezers. Am J Respir Crit Care Med. 2007;176:858–864. DOI: 10.1164/rccm.200702-212OC.

[49] Madore AM, Laprise C. Immunological and genetic aspects of asthma and allergy. J Asthma Allergy. 2010;3:107–121. DOI: 10.2147/JAA.S8970.

[50] Holgate ST, Yang Y, Haitchi HM, et al. The genetics of asthma: ADAM33 as an example of a susceptibility gene. Proc Am Thorac Soc. 2006;3:440–443. DOI: 10.1513/pats.200603-026AW.

[51] Liang S, Wei X, Gong C, Wei J, Chen Z, Deng J. A disintegrin and metalloprotease 33 (ADAM33) gene polymorphisms and the risk of asthma: a meta-analysis. Hum Immunol. 2013;74:648–657. doi: 10.1016/j.humimm.2013.01.025.

[52] Werner M, Herbon N, Gohlke H, et al. Asthma is associated with single-nucleotide polymorphisms in ADAM33. Clin Exp Allergy. 2004;34:26–31. DOI: 10.1111/j.1365-2222.2004.01846.x.

[53] Schedel M, Depner M, Schoen C, et al. The role of polymorphisms in ADAM33, a disintegrin and metalloprotease 33, in childhood asthma and lung function in two German populations. Respir Res. 2006;7:91. DOI: 10.1186/1465-9921-7-91.

[54] Pinto LA, Depner M, Klopp N, et al. MMP-9 gene variants increase the risk for non-atopic asthma in children. Respir Res. 2010;11:23. DOI: 10.1186/1465-9921-11-23.

[55] Birbian N, Singh J, Jindal SK. Highly protective association of MMP-2 -1306C/T promoter polymorphism with wsthma in a North Indian population: a pilot study. Allergy Asthma Immunol Res. 2014;6:234–241. DOI: 10.4168/aair.2014.6.3.234.

[56] Gueders MM, Foidart JM, Noel A, Cataldo DD. Matrix metalloproteinases (MMPs) and tissue inhibitors of MMPs in the respiratory tract: potential implications in asthma and

other lung diseases. Eur J Pharmacol. 2006;533:133–144. DOI: 10.1016/j.ejphar. 2005.12.082.

[57] Bissonnette ÉY, Madore AM, Chakir J, et al. Fibroblast growth factor-2 is a sputum remodeling biomarker of severe asthma. J Asthma. 2014;51:119–126. DOI: 10.3109/02770903.2013.860164.

[58] McDougall CM, Helms PJ, Walsh GM. Airway epithelial cytokine responses in childhood wheeze are independent of atopic status. Respir Med. 2015;109:689–700. DOI: 10.1016/j.rmed.2015.04.001.

[59] Roberts ME, Magowan L, Hall IP, Johnson SR. Discoidin domain receptor 1 regulates bronchial epithelial repair and matrix metalloproteinase production. Eur Respir J. 2011;37:1482–1493. DOI: 10.1183/09031936.00039710.

[60] Doherty GM, Kamath SV, de Courcey F, et al. Children with stable asthma have reduced airway matrix metalloproteinase-9 and matrix metalloproteinase-9/tissue inhibitor of metalloproteinase-1 ratio. Clin Exp Allergy. 2005;35:1168–1174. DOI: 10.1111/j. 1365-2222.2005.02326.x.

[61] Weitoft M, Andersson C, Andersson-Sjöland A, et al.Controlled and uncontrolled asthma display distinct alveolar tissue matrix compositions. Respir Res. 2014;15:67. DOI: 10.1186/1465-9921-15-67.

[62] Matsumoto H, Niimi A, Takemura M, et al. Relationship of airway wall thickening to an imbalance between matrix metalloproteinase-9 and its inhibitor in asthma. Thorax. 2005;60:277–281. DOI: 10.1136/thx.2004.028936.

[63] Chaudhuri R, McSharry C, Brady J, et al. Low sputum MMP-9/TIMP ratio is associated with airway narrowing in smokers with asthma. Eur Respir J. 2014;44:895–904. DOI: 10.1183/09031936.00047014.

[64] Atkinson JJ, Senior RM. Matrix metalloproteinase-9 in lung remodeling. Am J Respir Cell Mol Biol. 2003;28:12–24. DOI: 10.1165/rcmb.2002-0166TR.

[65] Chen W, Tabata Y, Gibson AM, et al. Matrix metalloproteinase 8 contributes to solubilization of IL-13 receptor alpha2 in vivo. J Allergy Clin Immunol. 2008;122:625–632. DOI: 10.1016/j.jaci.2008.06.022.

[66] Cook-Mills JM. Hydrogen peroxide activation of endothelial cell-associated MMPs during VCAM-1-dependent leukocyte migration. Cell Mol Biol (Noisy-le-grand). 2006;52:8-16.

[67] Matsumura M, Inoue H, Matsumoto T, et al. Endogenous metalloprotease solubilizes IL-13 receptor $\alpha$2 in airway epithelial cells. Biochem Biophys Res Commun. 2007;360:464–469. DOI: 10.1016/j.bbrc.2007.06.076.

[68]  Corry DB, Rishi K, Kanellis J, et al. Decreased allergic lung inflammatory cell egression and increased susceptibility to asphyxiation in MMP2-deficiency. Nat Immunol. 2002;3:347–353. DOI: 10.1038/ni773.

[69]  McMillan SJ, Kearley J, Campbell JD, et al. Matrix metalloproteinase-9 deficiency results in enhanced allergen-induced airway inflammation. J Immunol 2004;172:2586–2594. DOI: 10.4049/jimmunol.172.4.2586.

[70]  Owen CA, Hu Z, Lopez-Otin C, Shapiro SD. Membrane-bound matrix metalloproteinase-8 on activated polymorphonuclear cells is a potent, tissue inhibitor of metalloproteinase-resistant collagenase and serpinase. J Immunol. 2004;172:7791–7803. DOI: 10.4049/jimmunol.172.12.7791.

[71]  Gueders MM, Balbin M, Rocks N, et al. Matrix metalloproteinase-8 deficiency promotes granulocytic allergen-induced airway inflammation. J Immunol. 2005;175:2589–2597. DOI: 10.4049/jimmunol.175.4.2589.

[72]  Page K, Ledford JR, Zhou P, Wills-Karp M. A TLR2 agonist in German cockroach frass activates MMP-9 release and is protective against allergic inflammation in mice. J Immunol. 2009;183:3400–3408. DOI: 10.4049/jimmunol.0900838.

[73]  Gueders MM, Hirst SJ, Quesada-Calvo F, et al. Matrix metalloproteinase-19 deficiency promotes tenascin-C accumulation and allergen-induced airway inflammation. Am J Respir Cell Mol Biol. 2010;43:286–295. DOI: 10.1165/rcmb.2008-0426OC.

[74]  Mehra D, Sternberg DI, Jia Y, et al. Altered lymphocyte trafficking and diminished airway reactivity in transgenic mice expressing human MMP-9 in a mouse model of asthma. Am J Physiol Lung Cell Mol Physiol. 2010;298:L189–96. DOI: 10.1152/ajplung.00042.2009.

[75]  Sheu BC, Hsu SM, Ho HN et al. A novel role of metalloproteinase in cancer-mediated immunosuppression. Cancer Res. 2001;61:237–242.

[76]  Yoon HK, Cho HY, Kleeberger SR. Protective role of matrix metalloproteinase-9 in ozone-induced airway inflammation. Environ Health Perspect. 2007;115:1557–1563. DOI: 10.1289/ehp.10289.

[77]  McQuibban GA, Gong JH, Wong JP, et al. Matrix metalloproteinase processing of monocyte chemoattractant proteins generates CC chemokine receptor antagonists with anti-inflammatory properties in vivo. Blood. 2002;100:1160–1167.

[78]  Araujo BB, Dolhnikoff M, Silva LF, et al. Extracellular matrix components and regulators in the airway smooth muscle in asthma. Eur Respir J. 2008;32:61–69. DOI: 10.1183/09031936.00147807.

[79]  Simpson JL, Powell H, Boyle MJ, et al. Clarithromycin targets neutrophilic airway inflammation in refractory asthma. Am J Respir Crit Care Med. 2008;177:148–155. DOI: 10.1164/rccm.200707-1134OC.

[80] Righetti RF, Pigati PA, Possa SS, et al. Effects of Rho-kinase inhibition in lung tissue with chronic inflammation. Respir Physiol Neurobiol. 2014;192:134–146. DOI: 10.1016/j.resp.2013.12.012.

[81] Azizi G, Haidari MR, Khorramizadeh M, et al. Effects of imatinib mesylate in mouse models of multiple sclerosis and in vitro determinants. Iran J Allergy Asthma Immunol. 2014;13:198–206.

[82] Shono T, Motoyama M, Tatsumi K, et al. A new synthetic matrix metalloproteinase inhibitor modulates both angiogenesis and urokinase type plasminogen activator activity. Angiogenesis. 1998;2:319–329.

[83] Bruce C, Thomas PS. The effect of marimastat, a metalloprotease inhibitor, on allergen-induced asthmatic hyper-reactivity. Toxicol Appl Pharmacol. 2005;205:126–132. DOI: 10.1016/j.taap.2004.10.005.

[84] Lee SY, Paik SY, Chung SM. Neovastat (AE-941) inhibits the airway inflammation and hyperresponsiveness in a murine model of asthma. J Microbiol. 2005;43:11–16.

[85] Jung YW, Zindl CL, Lai JF, Weaver CT, Chaplin DD. MMP induced by Gr-1+ cells are crucial for recruitment of Th cells into the airways. Eur J Immunol. 2009;39:2281–2292. DOI: 10.1002/eji.200838985.

[86] Mukhopadhyay S, Sypek J, Tavendale R, et al. Matrix metalloproteinase-12 is a therapeutic target for asthma in children and young adults. J Allergy Clin Immunol. 2010;126:70–76. DOI: 10.1016/j.jaci.2010.03.027.

[87] Li W, Li J, Wu Y, et al. Identification of an orally efficacious matrix metalloprotease 12 inhibitor for potential treatment of asthma. J Med Chem. 2009;52:5408–5419. DOI: 10.1021/jm900809r.

[88] Yu Y, Chiba Y, Sakai H, Misawa M. Effect of a matrix metalloproteinase-12 inhibitor, S-1, on allergic airway disease phenotypes in mice. Inflamm Res. 2010;59:419–428. DOI: 10.1007/s00011-009-0153-0.

[89] Lagente V, Le Quement C, Boichot E. Macrophage metalloelastase (MMP-12) as a target for inflammatory respiratory diseases. Expert Opin Ther Targets. 2009;13:287–295. DOI: 10.1517/14728220902751632.

[90] Dahl R, Titlestad I, Lindqvist A, et al. Effects of an oral MMP-9 and -12 inhibitor, AZD1236, on biomarkers in moderate/severe COPD: a randomised controlled trial. Pulm Pharmacol Ther. 2012;25:169–177. DOI: 10.1016/j.pupt.2011.12.011.

[91] Vandenbroucke RE, Dejonckheere E, Libert C. A therapeutic role for matrix metalloproteinase inhibitors in lung diseases? Eur Respir J. 2011;38:1200–1214. DOI: 10.1183/09031936.00027411.

[92] Hu J, Van den Steen PE, Sang QX, Opdenakker G. Matrix metalloproteinase inhibitors as therapy for inflammatory and vascular diseases. Nat Rev Drug Discov. 2007;6:480–498. DOI: 10.1038/nrd2308

[93] Cerisano G, Buonamici P, Valenti R, et al. Effects of a timely therapy with doxycycline on the left ventricular remodeling according to the pre-procedural TIMI flow grade in patients with ST-elevation acute myocardial infarction. Basic Res Cardiol. 2014;109:412. DOI: 10.1007/s00395-014-0412-2.

[94] Fiotti N, Altamura N, Moretti M, et al. Short term effects of doxycycline on matrix metalloproteinases 2 and 9. Cardiovasc Drugs Ther. 2009;23:153–159. DOI: 10.1007/s10557-008-6150-7.

[95] Prins HJ, Daniels JM, Lindeman JH, et al. Effects of doxycycline on local and systemic inflammation in stable COPD patients, a randomized clinical trial. Respir Med. 2016;110:46–52. DOI: 10.1016/j.rmed.2015.10.009.

[96] Nukarinen E, Tervahartiala T, Valkonen M, et al. Targeting matrix metalloproteinases with intravenous doxycycline in severe sepsis — A randomised placebo-controlled pilot trial. Pharmacol Res. 2015;99:44–51. DOI: 10.1016/j.phrs.2015.05.005.

[97] Lee KS, Jin SM, Kim SS, at al. Doxycycline reduces airway inflammation and hyper-responsiveness in a murine model of toluene diisocyanate-induced asthma. J Allergy Clin Immunol. 2004;113:902–909. DOI: 10.1016/j.jaci.2004.03.008.

[98] Gueders MM, Bertholet P, Perin F et al. A novel formulation of inhaled doxycycline reduces allergen-induced inflammation, hyperresponsiveness and remodeling by matrix metalloproteinases and cytokines modulation in a mouse model of asthma. Biochem Pharmacol. 2008;75:514–526. DOI: 10.1016/j.bcp.2007.09.012.

[99] Avincsal MO, Ozbal S, Ikiz AO, Pekcetin C, Güneri EA. Effects of topical intranasal doxycycline treatment in the rat allergic rhinitis model. Clin Exp Otorhinolaryngol. 2014;7:106–111. DOI: 10.3342/ceo.2014.7.2.106.

[100] Bhattacharyya P, Paul R, Bhattacharjee P, et al. Long-term use of doxycycline can improve chronic asthma and possibly remodeling: the result of a pilot observation. J Asthma Allergy. 2012;5:33–37. DOI: 10.2147/JAA.S31402.

[101] Feleszko W, Młynarczuk I, Olszewska D, et al. Lovastatin potentiates antitumor activity of doxorubicin in murine melanoma via an apoptosis-dependent mechanism. Int J Cancer. 2002;100:111–118. DOI: 10.1002/ijc.10440.

[102] Yoshimura K, Nagasawa A, Kudo J, et al. Inhibitory effect of statins on inflammation-related pathways in human abdominal aortic aneurysm tissue. Int J Mol Sci. 2015;16:11213–11228. DOI: 10.3390/ijms160511213.

[103] Shen YY, Yuan Y, Du YY, Pan YY. Molecular mechanism underlying the anticancer effect of simvastatin on MDA-MB-231 human breast cancer cells. Mol Med Rep. 2015;12:623–630. DOI: 10.3892/mmr.2015.3411.

[104] Thomson NC, Charron CE, Chaudhuri R, Spears M, Ito K, McSharry C. Atorvastatin in combination with inhaled beclometasone modulates inflammatory sputum mediators in smokers with asthma. Pulm Pharmacol Ther. 2015;31:1–8. DOI: 10.1016/j.pupt.2015.01.001.

[105] Yang T, Chen M, Sun T. Simvastatin attenuates TGF-β1-induced epithelial-mesenchymal transition in human alveolar epithelial cells. Cell Physiol Biochem. 2013;31:863–874. DOI: 10.1159/000350104.

[106] Fujiwara Y, Shiraya S, Miyake T, et al. Inhibition of experimental abdominal aortic aneurysm in a rat model by the angiotensin receptor blocker valsartan. Int J Mol Med. 2008;22:703–708. DOI: 10.3892/ijmm_00000075.

[107] Kaparianos A, Argyropoulou E. Local renin-angiotensin II systems, angiotensin-converting enzyme and its homologue ACE2: their potential role in the pathogenesis of chronic obstructive pulmonary diseases, pulmonary hypertension and acute respiratory distress syndrome. Curr Med Chem. 2011;18:3506–3515. DOI: 10.2174/092986711796642562.

[108] Shrikrishna D, Astin R, Kemp PR, Hopkinson NS. Renin-angiotensin system blockade: a novel therapeutic approach in chronic obstructive pulmonary disease. Clin Sci. 2012;123:487–498. DOI: 10.1042/CS20120081.

[109] Sohal SS, Soltani A, Reid D, et al. A randomized controlled trial of inhaled corticosteroids (ICS) on markers of epithelial-mesenchymal transition (EMT) in large airway samples in COPD: an exploratory proof of concept study. Int J Chron Obstruct Pulmon Dis. 2014;9:533–542. DOI: 10.2147/COPD.S63911.

[110] Obase Y, Rytilä P, Metso T, et al. Effects of inhaled corticosteroids on metalloproteinase-8 and tissue inhibitor of metalloproteinase-1 in the airways of asthmatic children. Int Arch Allergy Immunol. 2010;151:247–254. DOI: 10.1159/000242362.

[111] Mattos W, Lim S, Russell R, Jatakanon A, Chung KF, Barnes PJ. Matrix metalloproteinase-9 expression in asthma: effect of asthma severity, allergen challenge, and inhaled corticosteroids. Chest. 2002;122:1543–1552. DOI: 10.1378/chest.122.5.1543.

[112] Todorova L, Gürcan E, Westergren-Thorsson G, Miller-Larsson A. Budesonide/formoterol effects on metalloproteolytic balance in TGFbeta-activated human lung fibroblasts. Respir Med. 2009;103:1755–1763. DOI: 10.1016/j.rmed.2009.03.018.

[113] Todorova L, Bjermer L, Westergren-Thorsson G, Miller-Larsson A. TGFβ-induced matrix production by bronchial fibroblasts in asthma: budesonide and formoterol effects. Respir Med. 2011;105:1296–1307. DOI: 10.1016/j.rmed.2011.03.020.

[114] Perng DW, Su KC, Chou KT, et al. Long-acting β2 agonists and corticosteroids restore the reduction of histone deacetylase activity and inhibit H2O2-induced mediator release from alveolar macrophages. Pulm Pharmacol Ther. 2012;25:312–318. DOI: 10.1016/j.pupt.2012.04.001.

[115] Lee SU, Ahn KS, Sung MH, et al. Indacaterol inhibits tumor cell invasiveness and MMP-9 expression by suppressing IKK/NF-κB activation. Mol Cells. 2014;37:585-591. DOI: 10.14348/molcells.2014.0076.

[116] Wang K, Liu CT, Wu YH, et al. Effects of formoterol-budesonide on airway remodeling in patients with moderate asthma. Acta Pharmacol Sin. 2011;32:126–132. DOI: 10.1038/aps.2010.170.

[117] Lin CH, Hsu JY, Hsiao YH, et al. Budesonide/formoterol maintenance and reliever therapy in asthma control: acute, dose-related effects and real-life effectiveness. Respirology. 2015;20:264–272. DOI: 10.1111/resp.12425.

[118] Langlois A, Ferland C, Tremblay GM, Laviolette M. Montelukast regulates eosinophil protease activity through a leukotriene-independent mechanism. J Allergy Clin Immunol. 2006;118:113–119. DOI: 10.1016/j.jaci.2006.03.010.

[119] Chuang SS, Hung CH, Hua YM et al. Suppression of plasma matrix metalloproteinase-9 following montelukast treatment in childhood asthma. Pediatr Int. 2007;49:918–922. DOI: 10.1111/j.1442-200X.2007.02497.x.

[120] Hsu CH, Hu CM, Lu KH, et al. Effect of selective cysteinyl leukotriene receptor antagonists on airway inflammation and matrix metalloproteinase expression in a mouse asthma model. Pediatr Neonatol. 2012;53:235–244. DOI: 10.1016/j.pedneo.2012.06.004.

[121] Todorova L, Bjermer L, Miller-Larsson A, Westergren-Thorsson G. Relationship between matrix production by bronchial fibroblasts and lung function and AHR in asthma. Respir Med. 2010;104:1799–1808. DOI: 10.1016/j.rmed.2010.06.015.

[122] Katainen E, Kostamo K, Virkkula P, et al. Local and systemic proteolytic responses in chronic rhinosinusitis with nasal polyposis and asthma. Int Forum Allergy Rhinol. 2015;5:294–302. DOI: 10.1002/alr.21486.

# 5

# Managing Bronchial Asthma in Underprivileged Communities

Yousser Mohammad and Basim Dubaybo

## Abstract

The definition of a primary care facility is the site where the first patient contact occurs. In developing countries, primary healthcare (PHC) facilities are officially healthcare centers, hosting World Health Organization (WHO) programs for tuberculosis and chronic respiratory diseases. In addition, there are many other providers of PHC services, which include emergency departments, general outpatient clinics in public hospitals. Asthma patients may present for treatment in any of these primary care facilities. An international study achieved by the Union showed that 51% of asthma patients in Syria are treated in emergency departments only, many developing countries like Sudan, Algeria, and some African countries had the same use of ER. There are questions about the quality of care provided in these clinics with regard to their adherence to Global Initiatives for Asthma (GINA) guidelines. Evidence suggests that there may be over prescribing of oral corticosteroids and antibiotics and under-prescription of inhaled corticosteroids, so there is a need to improve practice bringing it more into alignment to international guidelines. It may be considered by many that it is not possible to follow guidelines in developing countries and those that have economic and political pressures. However, a pilot program to test the feasibility of a providing systematic follow-up of uncontrolled asthma patients in a general free of charge hospital in Syria showed that it is possible to achieve asthma control following to GINA guidelines even in very deprived community. The same was mentioned by the Union in an international survey for other developing African and Mediterranean countries. WHO launched programs for non-communicable disease including chronic respiratory disease: Practical Approach to lung Health (PAL) and Package of essential no communicable (PEN) disease interventions for primary health care in low-resource settings. The IPCRG also worked on how to improve implementation of guidelines. We will provide the results and following evidence-based recommendations from our field surveys in developing countries, as well comment on international programs. Although much progress has been realized in the diagnosis and management of asthma in developed nations, progress in one variant of asthma, inner city asthma, has been slow. Inner city asthma is that variant of the disease which afflicts residents of urban environments with low socioeconomic conditions, poor housing, and rampant environmental risks. This variant of asthma appears to be more severe, associated with increased psychological burden as well as morbidity and mortality, has a diverse array of predisposing factors, and poses significant challenges in management and treatment. One important aspect of treatment is education which leads to the participation of the patient and the families in the care resulting in a more favorable outcome.

**Keywords:** asthma, primary care, WHO, chronic respiratory diseases, essential drugs for asthma, inner city, developed nations

---

## Background

This chapter deals with asthma in developing nations and touches on one variant of asthma in the developed world which has significant resemblance to its counterpart in developing nations. The first section is derived from studies in Syria, while the second from the United States.

## 1. Introduction - Managing bronchial asthma in primary health care

According to the International Study for Asthma and Allergies in Childhood (ISAAC), comparing phase one in 1994 to three in 2000–2003, asthma prevalence expressed by wheezing the last 12 months in 13–14 years old is increasing in developing countries. Asthma prevalence is higher in developed countries, but asthma is more severe in developing countries [1].

The definition of a primary care facility is the site where the first patient contact occurs [2]. If we take Syria as an example of developing county, primary healthcare (PHC) facilities are officially healthcare centers under the control of the Ministry of Health, which among other services provided, host World Health Organization (WHO) programs for tuberculosis and chronic respiratory diseases [3, 4]. In addition, there are many other providers of PHC services which include emergency departments(ED), general outpatient clinics in public hospitals, school health clinics, clinics in workplace settings, and internal and general clinics within the private sector.

Asthma patients may present for treatment in any of these primary care facilities in Syria. A multicenter survey of primary care clinics revealed that 13% of patients aged over 6 years attended with asthma [5]. Another study showed that 51% of asthma patients are treated in ED only, and only 9% are treated in primary care centers [6]. Many developing countries like Sudan, Algeria and some African countries had the same use of ED [6]. The same under-utilization of community primary healthcare services has also been observed in China in 2014 [7].

There are questions about the quality of care provided in these clinics with regard to their adherence to Global Initiatives for Asthma (GINA) guidelines. Evidence suggests that there may be over prescribing of oral corticosteroids and antibiotics and under-prescription of inhaled corticosteroids [5, 6], so there is a need to improve practice bringing it more into alignment to international guidelines.

It may be considered by many that it is not possible to follow guidelines in developing countries and those that have economic and political pressures. However, a pilot program to test the feasibility of a providing systematic follow-up of uncontrolled asthma patients in a general free of charge hospital in Syria showed that it is possible to achieve asthma control following to GINA guidelines even in very poor community [8]. The same was mentioned by the Union in an international survey for other developing African and Mediterranean countries [9], the same in a recent study in Sudan [10].

A Ministry of Health—WHO program for non-communicable diseases in Syria including an intensive courses for asthma and COPD for GPs in health centers has been launched since the beginning of 2015 in a pilot site from Syria. However, unlike developed countries, in Syria, presentations are very personalized, there are no established accredited modules or curriculum for continuing medical education for primary care physicians and nurses. In order to make optimum improvements in care across the country, we need to ensure that high-quality training interventions are made available for healthcare providers who are working in a primary care setting, aiming to increase both their competence and confidence in the essentials of asthma management. This program needs to incorporate accredited educational materials, a process for monitoring and continuous evaluation, and collaborative efforts with an international agency such as the Global Alliance against Chronic Respiratory Diseases (WHO–GARD www.who.int/gard ) [8]. A survey conducted by the International COPD Coalition gave the same conclusions about absence of curriculum for education for asthma and COPD [11].

Primary healthcare services are free of charge in Syria, and other developing countries hosting WHO programs, and are staffed by full-time qualified nurses who are supported by part-time physicians, who also provide services in the private sector. In addition, some patients who are able to pay for healthcare may refer themselves directly to private pulmonologists, without being referred from primary care. Since 2006, WHO launched programs for asthma and COPD at primary care level in Syria and other developing countries, and training was undertaken on site [3–5, 8].

In this paper, we share our experience in developing countries and will present first field surveys in developing countries. Second, we will comment on the international programs of WHO and International Primary Care Respiratory Group (IPCRG). And third, we will give our evidence-based recommendations.

## 2. Discussion

### 2.1. Field surveys and what we learned

Asthma is under-diagnosed in primary care [5, 6, 8, 12–14]. The Global Alliance against chronic respiratory disease (GARD–WHO: www.who.int/gard ) survey on chronic respiratory diseases prevalence and risk factors in Syria revealed that although 27% of the 1599 patients surveyed had evidence of reactive airway disease and reversible obstruction by spirometry, but only 13% had been diagnosed as asthma by the primary care practitioners. Indicating that 50% were under-diagnosed [4]. This finding is not unique to Syria. Under-diagnosis has also been reported in the same GARD survey in Cape Verde [12]. There are several hypotheses for these high rates of under-diagnosis. The condition's variability of symptoms, misdiagnosis such as an infection, some may be mislabeling of patients as COPD when in fact, they may have uncontrolled asthma [5, 15], increasing workload, and demand on services and limited experienced doctors. It is important for practitioners to follow standard diagnostic procedures and good history taking such as recurrent symptoms (wheezing, cough, difficult breathing, and chest tightness) and the presence of triggers. In addition, practitioners should obtain objective tests and look for reversibility of peak expiratory flow rate (PEFR) expressed as increase of 20% and 60 l/min, or 12% increase in forced expiratory volume in one second (FEV1) and 200 ml after short-acting beta agonists (SABA), or a decrease in these measurements after exercise testing. Practitioners could also rely on variability of PEFR or FEV1 between two visits. In situations where spirometry or peak flow meter results are not available, or patients are under 5 years of age, practitioners should rely on clinical history and treatment trials [16]. WHO recommend peak flow meter to be available in the most remote healthcare centers, and referral for spirometry in healthcare centers or hospitals at central level is available [3, 4].

Asthma is under-treated and under-controlled: The GARD–WHO multicentre national survey 2010 for chronic respiratory diseases [5] revealed that only 25% of inhaled corticosteroid (ICS) prescriptions included adequate doses according to the GINA guidelines. In addition, 46% of patients received oral corticosteroids which could be avoided if ICS were prescribed in PHC according to the guidelines. Similarly, 56% of asthma patients received oral antibiotics without a clinical indication. Another important issue is that 56% of asthma patients surveyed have FEV1 < 80% after bronchodilators, which points to poor control [5, 16].

Despite asthma being poorly diagnosed and treated, it is possible to observe improvements in asthma control to the level of published guidelines in underserved areas. In a pilot study conducted on economically deprived patients in an underserved area, we systematically followed up patients with uncontrolled asthma in a general free of charge outpatient clinic in a public hospital 2006–2007 [8]. A trained postgraduate medical student asked every patient questions about the parameters of asthma control, measured PEFR, and ensured prescription of ICS at their first presentation. The student also taught patients proper inhaler technique and educated them about how to avoid risk factors. Weekly follow-up data were collected by the GP. After 3 months, 44 of 66 patients who had not been followed up previously were properly controlled. We conclude that GINA guidelines could be realistic even in underserved areas. In 2006, an international multicenter survey of the Union showed that implementation of asthma guidelines was possible in primary care in developing countries [13]. The same recently in Sudan (2014): In a new model specialized center for asthma, a survey aiming at describing the epidemiological and clinical characteristics of asthma patients concluded that most patients had abnormal spirometry with more than half having an FEV1 that is 60% or less of their predicted normal reading. The majority improved with combined treatment (Formoterol, budesonide) with 60% normalizing their spirometry highlighting the feasibility and applicability of specialized asthma care centers in resource-poor countries [10].

The global initiative for asthma guidelines are based on the level of control [16] such that for each asthmatic presenting to a primary healthcare facility, the general practitioner (GP) should ask standard questions about the clinical control of asthma including:

- Frequency of symptoms
- Need for inhaled bronchodilators
- Frequency of night awakening
- Exercise limitation
- Number of exacerbations.
- values of PEFR or FEV1

To improve care, training should emphasize that: Patients with uncontrolled asthma need to be prescribed low-dose or medium-dose inhaled corticosteroids, educated on inhaler technique, and referred to higher level of care for further assessment if not controlled after follow-up visits [3–5, 16], and referred back to primary care for long-term follow-up and education.

### 2.1.1. Review of international WHO programs and other programs

*WHO–MOH programs*: Three programs have been introduced for chronic respiratory diseases (CRD) in Syria since 2006 [3, 4, 11, 16]:

1. Practical Approach to Lung Health (PAL) program, integrating asthma, and COPD care in the National Tuberculosis program, adopting for the first time a referral policy and initiating a respiratory disease dispensary at central level equipped with peak flow, oximetry, and spirometry.

2. The Package for the essential needs for non-communicable diseases (NCD) at primary care level in low resources settings: WHO–PEN program. Integrating all major NCD including CRD at primary care level.

3. GARD program www.who.int/gard Survey on CRD risk factors and prevalence. And the resulting evidence based guidelines, and training. WHO country office is involved.

### 2.1.2. Other programs

1. The GINA world Asthma day program: Conferences in World Asthma Days are improving asthma care: Make health workers in PHC familiar with asthma symptoms, asthma control, peak flow meter, and corticoid inhalers.

2. Civil societies, in collaborating with the International COPD Coalition www.internationalcopd.org, are helping patients with CRD and allergy is wide-spreading patient education for asthma and COPD, and health education.

3.  Educational Program for nurses about asthma and COPD: Two national workshops were run for this purpose in 2004 and 2007 by the Education for health center of Excellence— UK in Syria www.educationforhealth.org, but also in Bangladesh, and many other developing countries, aiming to introduce the role of nurses in national programs.

4.  The new intensive course of WHO–MOH mentioned above for non-communicable diseases in Syria and other EMRO countries.

*2.1.3. International Primary Care Respiratory Group (IPCRG)*

The IPCRG tried to resolve the question on how to deal with asthma and COPD in primary care in developing countries, elaborating a symptomatic approach and algorithms, but they recommend providing primary care in developing countries with PEF and Inhalers [17]. While PAL–WHO went further (Spirometry and referral) [4].

Research priority to improve asthma management in primary care have been investigated by the IPCRG, 2009: Conclusion, primary care research should include awareness about local asthma triggers like biomass fuel, early diagnosis, and management in remote areas where there are no tools for diagnosis, the reliability of medication trial, how to overcome taboos about cultural misbelieves and inhalers, how to make essential drugs available, and how to adapt and evaluate guidelines implementation [18].

PEN–WHO opted for an integrated approach with other NCD; the approach was symptoms and PEAK flow measurements; primary care physician prescribes ICS if asthma; and treat acute attacks with oral corticosteroids and inhaled bronchodilators; referral rules to confirm diagnosis or help for better long-term treatment are stated if failure of control at follow-up visit. Necessary tools are PEF, oximetry, oxygen, and nebulisers or inhalers via spacer [3]

PAL–WHO, integrating CRD with tuberculosis program was very ambitious, referral and spirometry were recommended [4], but unfortunately, there were discontinuity and no evaluation process for the implementation of these programs, in conflict zones.

GARD–WHO was a success with the survey, and following publications and guidelines [5]

## 2.2. The core messages from the field surveys and international national programs

To empower the role of PHC in controlling asthma and lessen related mortality. Core messages are as follows:

1.  The first consultation with the uncontrolled patient is crucial. It is vital that the correct diagnosis is made and good education is delivered. The correct treatment should be initiated at this time which will be an appropriate dose of inhaled corticosteroid and a short-acting reliever inhaler (Bronchodilator). Inhaler technique needs to be taught and the initiation of a self-management plan including what to do in an emergency and whom to contact. A follow-up appointment is important, and the PHC should consider a referral if not controlled during a follow-up visit [19]

2.  Prescription of oral corticosteroids on discharge from emergency room, if not hospitalized, is recommended. By contrast, expectorants and antibiotics are often unnecessarily prescribed [5, 13, 19].

3.  Methodical follow-up leads to control and is feasible even in poor settings by using standard guideline-based protocols and follow-up records. [8, 13]

4.  The core equipment and medicines that health facilities should have include peak flow meter, pulse oximetry, bronchodilator inhalers, spacers (which could be built up in very poor settings/plastic bottle), [20–22], nebulizers and solution of short acting beta agonists (SABA) and if possible anticholinergics, oxygen extractor or oxygen bottle, and systemic corticosteroids.

5.  Short-acting beta-agonists (via spacer, which can be built in poor settings using a plastic bottle) is as effective as nebulizer to relieve symptoms, except for very severe attacks [21–23]. The asthma-trained nurses or community healthcare workers key role is to educate patients, particularly in inhaler technique and self-management [23]. This is common practice in many developed countries and the UK and Australia have been leaders in developing nurses to fulfill this role. In the UK, much of the asthma management in primary care is provided by appropriately trained nurses [23].

6.  Every uncontrolled asthma patient in spite prescription of ICS and regular follow-up in Primary care should be referred to a specialist or well-trained physician with an interest in asthma and placed in an asthma management plan and then referred back to the PHC for follow-up.

7.  A toolbox for general practitioners and nurses should consist of the following:

    • Questions related to symptoms suggestive of asthma diagnosis to face under-diagnosis

    • Asthma control test for initial evaluation and follow up

    • Use of peak flow and table of values

    • Educational photos about inhaler and spacer use (Photos of all available inhalers to educate.)

    • What to do in an emergency

    • Education on how inhaled corticosteroids reverse inflammation

    • A patient self-management plan

8.  Every follow-up visit should be the occasion to improve the partnership with patients according to their literacy level of education and cultural believes. A follow-up record to monitor clinical control, PEFR, compliance, and trigger avoidance should be filled at every visit. Education for inhaler technique should be part of every follow-up visit.

9.  Including these core elements on the role of primary care in curriculum of medical schools, nursing schools, and pharmacies is recommended.

10. WHO programs of NCD, PEN, and PAL have been introduces in PHC dispensaries in many developing countries including Syria, and training for those programs was done at pilot sites, but the humanitarian crisis in Syria and other conflict zones discontinued progress. Effort should be done to continue [3, 4].

11. Conferences and World Asthma Days as recommended by GINA are improving asthma care: Make health workers in PHC familiar with asthma control, peak flow meter, and corticoid inhalers, but there is a great need for more education, which can also be provided online.

12. Patient organizations are playing a role on patient education and providing free medications [11].

13. According to the GARD Survey results, training sessions for the essential on asthma and COPD are needed for health workers at primary care level. This needs to adapt educational materials.

14. The list of essential medications for asthma, especially inhaled corticosteroids [24], is not available in all countries; in Sudan, a survey pointed this issue [25]. In a general review, researchers reported [26]: Another issue is in some developing countries, the essential medication as listed by WHO is not available. Health services in low-resource countries are poorly adapted to treating chronic diseases. Designed to respond episodically to acute disease, almost all historical investment has focused on infectious diseases. Crucial to the successful management of chronic diseases is an infrastructure designed to support pro-active management, providing not only an accurate diagnosis, but also a secure supply of cost-effective drugs at an affordable price. When in very poor health systems, ICS are not available, a variety or a phenotype of severe asthma prevails (defined by WHO as the non-treated severe asthma) [27], while the ATS/ERS definition for severe asthma is asthma refractory to ICS.

15. The WHO issued a guide on prevention and control of non-communicable diseases in: Guidelines for primary healthcare in low-resource settings: 2012, and urged developing countries to follow the directives for chronic respiratory disease as well [28].

## 3. Inner city asthma - Introduction

Inner city asthma is a variant of asthma that afflicts patients who reside in some of the poorest neighborhoods of some urban localities [29]. These patients frequently have economic and financial difficulties and reside in housing projects that are environmentally poor with increased likelihood of pollution [30]. Several studies have demonstrated that these factors coupled to barriers to appropriate asthma care, as well as reliance on emergency care, poor medication compliance, limited availability of primary and specialty asthma care and poor communication between patient and physicians are responsible for the unique nature of this entity [31–33]. Because of these factors, the character of inner city asthma may be different from that observed in other localities. Different patterns of prevalence, predisposing factor, severity, morbidity, mortality, and management have been observed.

# 4. Prevalence

Over the past several decades, a gradual increase in the prevalence of asthma has been noted in several industrialized countries [29]. Although some of this increase may be related to changes in health insurance policies resulting in better coverage and increased access to care and improvements in diagnostic testing, other factors may be involved. Some of the increase is attributed, in part, to a gradual increase in prevalence of asthma in individuals of lower socioeconomic status who reside in inner cities [29, 34]. For example, statistical analysis shows that between the years 2001 and 2010, rates of asthma in adolescents in the United States of America have increased at a rate of around 1.4% reaching 9.5% in 2010 [34]. Careful analysis of this phenomenon indicates that this increase was most realized among various minority groups including African-Americans and Hispanics.

African-American children are reported to have a rate of asthma per population that is 1.6 times the level observed in white children [34, 35]. Some Hispanic groups, like children originally from Puerto Ricco, have been reported to have asthma prevalence that is almost 2.4 times that of white children [35, 36]. The prevalence of asthma among children in some Chicago neighborhoods is estimated to be as high as 44%, with the highest rate observed and reported in neighborhoods with a higher proportion of residents of African-American and Hispanic ancestry [37]. In one district of New York City, asthma prevalence was reported 13.2% for Puerto Ricans [38]. Racial background is not the only factor responsible for this disparity. Asthma prevalence varies among various localities with those localities with low income levels manifesting an increase in prevalence irrespective or racial and ethnic mix [29, 33].

# 5. Severity

Numerous studies have shown that inner city asthma, especially among children, is characterized by increased intensity and poor response to therapy [39]. It is not clear why this population of asthmatics is more difficult to control. Some investigators speculate that a myriad of factors may be involved including environmental, socioeconomic, psychosocial, behavioral, or genetic ones [39, 40]. Other authorities believe that the poor control may be related to inappropriate asthma management practices, limited access to care, poor compliance with therapy, and limited communication between physicians and patients [41, 42]. The practical implications of these observations are that these children have a higher rate of hospital admissions [43] and their condition at the time admission is serious and is frequently described as near fatal [44] which refers to a group of individuals predisposed to acute respiratory failure from their disease state with acidosis and altered mental status.

The increased acuity of inner city asthma has several short-term and long-term implications. The collective cost resulting from loss of work and productivity as well as absenteeism from school and work is hard to measure. The added cost of overutilization of healthcare facilities and emergency department adds to the financial implications of this phenomenon. Overconsumption of pharmaceutical agents and other supportive agents and procedures further increases the overall cost. Finally, the impact on the general health of the individuals, stunted growth, and development of long-term respiratory impairment adds to the overall societal impact.

# 6. Predisposing factors

The factors contributing to the high prevalence of asthma among inner city residents are varied. Cohen et al. [45] suggest that a key factor in this regard is the poor access to healthcare that patients in urban environments experience. This may be related to a limited number of physicians and healthcare facilities as well as limited availability of safe transportation. Limited access to care has a negative impact on most clinical conditions including the availability of effective prenatal care. Another major predisposing factor which increases the prevalence of asthma in residents of inner cities is exposure to tobacco smoke [45]. Tobacco smoke is known to affect the rate of lung growth, clearance of secretions, and defense mechanisms against particulate matter and infectious agents.

Studies have shown that children living in urban environments have a higher rate of emergency room visits and lower use of inhaled corticosteroids [46]. This may be related to lower rates of diagnosis as shown by the 1999 National Health Interview Study [34]. Specific factors that have been examined include poverty with reduced access to and quality of care [47]. The resultant additional health issues such as prematurity [48, 49] and obesity [29, 50] further confound the problem. In addition, poor housing [51] with exposure to indoor pollutants and environmental tobacco [52] plays a significant role in aggravating the condition. Finally, the psychological impact of the disease in the setting of poor resources worsens the perception among patients, impacts coping, and results in further deterioration in symptomatology [53, 54].

# 7. Morbidity and mortality

In general, inner city asthma has a higher index of severity, is associated with increased morbidity, and has a higher mortality rate than asthma outside the inner city milieu [29]. Several criteria may be used to evaluate the level of acuity. These include, among others, emergency room visits, hospitalizations, office visits, time lost from work, and absenteeism from school. Research shows that inner city asthma is associated with increased morbidity in each of these criteria. The national database report of 2006 indicated that around 3.5 million visits to physician offices, half a million visits to hospital outpatient departments, an equivalent number of visits to an emergency department, and over 150,000 hospitalizations were related to asthma in this population [55].

Inner city asthma is associated with increased mortality when adjusted for the level of acuity. As far as mortality is concerned, there were 167 deaths from asthma in 2005 among children and adolescents [29, 55]. Interestingly, African-Americans demonstrate a sevenfold increase in mortality, around threefold increase in emergency department visits, threefold increase in hospitalization, but 20% lower nonemergency ambulatory visits than white children. Data on Hispanic children show emergency department visits to be twice that of whites [55].

## 8. Management

Management of inner city asthma places additional demands on patients and healthcare providers alike. Patients need to be maintained on the usual asthma medications including short-acting and long-acting bronchodilators, inhaled corticosteroids, leukotriene antagonists, and possibly methyl xanthines. In addition, one has to focus on eliminating or minimizing the effect of the predisposing factors listed in the previous paragraphs. Specifically, dealing with poor housing, indoor pollutants, and environmental tobacco makes it necessary for patients and their families to invest in home improvement projects that are costly and demanding. Since this may be beyond the capabilities of several patients, this poses a significant burden on the public health and social safety networks in various cities. These services are already oversubscribed and have limited resources.

Several interventions have focused on the fact that patient and family education are critical to the process of managing and controlling inner city asthma. Patients and their families need to learn the components of quality care so that they can participate in their own care. An important component of this strategy is making sure patients, and their families have the requisite knowledge to reach healthcare providers in a timely and structured manner. Therefore, efforts should focus on educating patients to improve their ability to acquire the knowledge needed to navigate the healthcare system. A family-based intervention performed by a trained counselor has been shown to improve care and decrease morbidity [56]. School-based asthma education is also effective [57]. Emphasis should also be placed on reducing environmental triggers such as the use of pest control [58] services and reduction of exposure to tobacco smoke [59] and weatherizing homes to decrease mold and moisture [60, 61] Good management of inner city asthma requires the same kind of proactive care that has been shown to be effective in other situations. These include guidelines-driven care and assured access to the appropriate controller medication [62] and the addition of a biologic such as omalizumab in selected cases [63].

## 9. Summary and conclusions

To the pulmonologist, inner city asthma is a complex and challenging entity that requires consolidated management efforts and a comprehensive approach that includes awareness of the unique predisposing factors, the increased acuity, and the need to focus on improved access to care. A multifaceted approach that targets a wide array of risk factors including allergens, indoor pollution, housing quality, and external sources of pollution, such as neighborhood trash collection receptacles must be utilized. Guidelines-based management that is effective in other types of asthma may not be sufficient to provide adequate control. In addition, the structure of the healthcare system must change to allow the needed access and the recognition and management of social factors which impact on asthma management.

## Author details

Yousser Mohammad[1,2,3*] and Basim Dubaybo[4]

*Address all correspondence to: ccollaborating@gmail.com

1 Department of Pulmonary and Family Medicine, Syrian Private University, Damascus, Syria

2 Department of Pulmonary, Damascus University, Damascus, Syria

3 Center for Research and Training for CRD, Tishreen University, Latakia, Syria

4 Department of Internal Medicine, Wayne State University School of Medicine, Detroit, Michigan, USA

## References

[1] Lai CKW, Beasley R, Crane J, Foliaki S, Shah J, Weiland S, and the ISAAC Phase Three Study Group. Global variation in the prevalence and severity of asthma symptoms: Phase Three of the International Study of Asthma and Allergies in Childhood (ISAAC).Thorax. 2009;64:476–483.

[2] International Classification of Primary Care, Second edition (ICPC-2), available as "print on demand" from OUP website: www.oup.uk

[3] Package of essential noncommunicable (PEN) disease interventions for primary health care in low-resource settings. Geneva, Switzerland: World Health Organization. c2010. Available from: http://whqlibdoc.who.int/ publications/2010/9789241598996_eng.pdf

[4] World Health Organization. Practical approach to lung health. Manual on initiating PAL implementation. Geneva, World Health Organization, 2008. (WHO/HTM/TB/ 2008.410, WHO/NMH/CHP/CPM/08.02).

[5] Mohammad Y, Shaaban R, Yassine F, Allouch J, Daaboul N, Bassam A, Mohammad A, Taha D, Sabba S, Dyban G, Al-Sheih K, Balleh H, Ibrahim M, Al Khaer H, Dayoub M, Halloum R, Fadhil I, Abbas A, KHouri A, Khaltaev N, Bousquet J, Khaddouj M, Suleiman I, Meri M, Bakir M, Naem A, Said H, Al-Dmeirawi F, Myhoub H, Dib G.

Executive summary of the multicenter survey on the prevalence and risk factors of chronic respiratory diseases in patients presenting to primary care centers and emergency rooms in Syria. J Thorac Dis. 2012;4(2):203–205. doi:10.3978/j.issn. 2072-1439.2011.11.07.

[6] Burney P, Potts J, Aït-Khaled N, Sepulveda RM, Zidouni N, Benali R, Jerray M, Musa OA, El-Sony A, Behbehani N, El-Sharif N, Mohammad Y, Khouri A, Paralija B, Eiser N, Fitzgerald M, Abu-Laban R.. A multinational study of treatment failures in asthma management. Int J Tuberc Lung Dis. 2008;12(1):13–18.

[7] Yang H, Huang X, Zhou Z, Wang HH, Tong X, Wang Z, Wang J, Lu Z. Determinants of initial utilization of community healthcare services among patients with major non-communicable chronic diseases in South China. Plos One. 2014;9(12):e116051. doi: 10.1371/journal.pone.0116051. eCollection 2014.

[8] http://www.ginasthma.org/Mediterranean

[9] Bousquet J, Dahl R, Khaltaev N. Global alliance against chronic respiratory diseases. Allergy 2007:62:216–223.

[10] Imad H, Yasir G. Pan African Medical Journal Epidemiological and clinical characteristics, spirometric parameters and response to budesonide/formoterol in patients attending an asthma clinic: an experience in a developing country. Pan Afr Respir Med. Pan Afr Med J. 2015; 21: 154.

[11] Mohammad Y, Fink-Wagner A-H, Nonikov D. Assets and needs of respiratory patient organizations: differences between developed and developing countries. J Thorac Dis 2013; 5(6):914–918. doi:10.3978/j.issn.2072-1439.2013.08.72.

[12] Martins P, Rosado-Pinto J, do Céu Teixeira M, Neuparth N, Silva O, Tavares H, Spencer JL, Mascarenhas D, Papoila AL, Khaltaev N, Annesi-Maesano I. Under-report and underdiagnosis of chronic respiratory diseases in an African country. Allergy 2009;64(7):1061–1067.

[13] Ait-Khaled N, Enarson DA, Bencherif N, Boulhbal F, Camara LM, Dagli E, Jankirie TK, Karadag B, Keita B, Ngoran K, Adhiambo J, Ottmanis SE, Pham N, Sow O, Yousser M, Zaidouni N. Implementation of asthma guidelines in health centers of several developing countries. Int J Tuberc Lung Dis. 2006;10(1):104–109.

[14] Shahror N, Bardan H. Prevalence and risk factors of asthma in Damascus school children aged 10–14. Rev Mal Respir. 2006;23:10S109–10S139.

[15] Mohammad Y, Shaaban R, Al-Zahab BA, Khaltaev N, Bousquet J, Dubaybo B. Impact of active and passive smoking as risk factors for asthma and COPD in women presenting to primary care in Syria: first report by the WHO-GARD survey group. Int J Chronic Obstr Pulm Dis. 2013-11-04.

[16] 16-Global Initiative for Asthma. Global Strategy for Asthma management and prevention on www.ginasthma.org accessed.

[17]  Levy M, Fletcher M. International primary care respiratory group guidelines. Prim Care Respir J. 2006;15:20–34.

[18]  Pinnock H, Thomas M, Tsiligianni I, Lisspers K, Østrem A, Ställberg B, Yusuf O, Ryan D, Buffels J, Cals JW, Chavannes NH, Henrichsen SH, Langhammer A, Latysheva E, Lionis C, Litt J, van der Molen T, Zwar N, Williams S. The International Primary Care Respiratory Group (IPCRG) Research Needs Statement 2010. Prim Care Respir J. 2010;19 Suppl 1:S1–S20.

[19]  AAAAI guidelines 2007: Section 3, component 2, education for a partnership on asthma care, pp. 100–106 on www.aaaai.org.

[20]  Alhaidera SA, Alshehrib HA, and Al-Eid K. Replacing nebulizers by MDI-spacers for bronchodilator and inhaled corticosteroid administration: Impact on the utilization of hospital resources. International Journal of Pediatrics and Adolescent Medicine. 2014; 1(1):26–30.

[21]  Yasmin S, Mollah AH, Basak R, Islam KT, Chowdhury YS. Mymensingh Med J. Efficacy of salbutamol by nebulizer versus metered dose inhaler with home-made non-valved spacer in acute exacerbation of childhood asthma. Mymensingh Med J. 2012;21(1):66–71.

[22]  Zar HJ, Levin ME. Challenges in treating pediatric asthma in developing countries. Paediatr Drugs. 2012;14(6):353–359. doi:10.2165/11597420-

[23]  Charlton I, et al. Audit of the effect of a nurse run asthma clinic on workload and patient morbidity in a general practice. Br J Gen Pract. 1991;41:227–231.

[24]  http://www.who.int/medicines/publications/essentialmedicines/en/index.html: accessed on Juin 2014

[25]  El Sony AI, Chiang C-Y, Malik E, Hassanain SA, Hussien H, Khamis AH, Bassilli AF, Enarson DA. Standard case management of asthma in Sudan: a Pilot Project. Public Health Action. PHA 2013;3(3):247–252.

[26]  Beran D, Zar HJ, Perrin C, Menezes AM, Burney P. Burden of asthma and chronic obstructive pulmonary disease and access to essential medicines in low-income and middle-income countries. Lancet Respir Med. 2015;3(2):159–170. doi:10.1016/S2213-2600(15)00004-1.

[27]  Bousquet J, Baena-Cagnani CE, Mantzouranis E, Bleecker ER, Burney P, et al. Workshop summary. Uniform definition of asthma severity, control, and exacerbations: Document presented for the World Health Organization Consultation on Severe Asthma. J Allergy Clin Immunol 2010;126(5):926–938.

[28]  Prevention and Control of Non communicable Diseases: Guidelines for primary health care in low-resource settings. Geneva: WHO, 2012.

[29]  Gergen PJ, Togias A. Inner city asthma. Immunol Allergy Clin N Am 2015;35:101–114.

[30] Forno E, Celedón JC. Asthma and Ethnic Minorities: Socioeconomic Status and Beyond. Curr Opin Allergy Clin Immunol. 2009;9(2):154–160. PMCID: PMC3920741

[31] Akinbami L. The state of childhood asthma, United States, 1980–2005. Adv Data. 2006; (381):1–24

[32] Sarver N, Murphy K. Management of asthma: new approaches to establishing control. J Am Acad Nurse Pract 2009;21:54–65.

[33] Celano MP, Linzer JF, Demi A, Bakeman R, Smith CO, Croft S, et al. Treatment adherence among low-income, African American children with persistent asthma. J Asthma 2010;47:317–22. NIHMSID: NIHMS94525

[34] Moorman JE, Akinbami LJ, Bailey CM, et al. National surveillance of asthma: United States, 2001–2010. Vital Health Stat 2012;3:1–67.

[35] Akinbami LJ, Moorman JE, Garbe PL, et al. Status of childhood asthma in the United States, 1980–2007. Pediatrics 2009;123(Suppl 3):S131–45.

[36] Carter-Pokras OD, Gergen PJ. Reported asthma among Puerto Rican, Mexican-American, and Cuban children, 1982 through 1984. Am J Public Health 1993;83:580–582.

[37] Gupta RS, Zhang X, Sharp LK, et al. Geographic variability in childhood asthma prevalence in Chicago. J Allergy Clin Immunol 2008;121:639–645.e1.

[38] Ledogar RJ, Penchaszadeh A, Garden CC, et al. Asthma and Latino cultures: different prevalence reported among groups sharing the same environment. Am J Public Health 2000;90:929–935.

[39] Breysse J, Dixon S, Gregory J, et al. Effect of weatherization combined with community health worker in-home education on asthma control. Am J Public Health 2014;104:e57–e64.

[40] Takaro TK, Krieger J, Song L, et al. The breathe-easy home: the impact of asthma-friendly home construction on clinical outcomes and trigger exposure. Am J Public Health 2011;101:55–62.

[41] Szefler SJ, Mitchell H, Sorkness CA, et al. Management of asthma based on exhaled nitric oxide in addition to guideline-based treatment for inner-city adolescents and young adults: a randomised controlled trial. Lancet 2008;372:1065–1072.

[42] Busse WW, Morgan WJ, Gergen PJ, et al. Randomized trial of omalizumab (anti-IgE) for asthma in inner-city children. N Engl J Med 2011;364:1005–1015.

[43] Scott L, Morphew T, Bollinger ME, Samuelson S, Galant S, Clement L, O'Cull K, Jones F, and Jones CA. Achieving and maintaining asthma control in inner-city children. J Allergy Clin Immunol 2011;128:56–63.

[44] Bryant-Stephens T. Asthma disparities in urban environments. J Allergy Clin Immunol 2009;123:1199–1206.

[45] Cohen RT, Canino GJ, Bird HR, et al. Area of residence, birthplace, and asthma in Puerto Rican children. Chest 2007;131:1331–1338.

[46] Esteban CA, Klein RB, McQuaid EL, et al. Conundrums in childhood asthma severity, control, and health care use: Puerto Rico versus Rhode Island. J Allergy Clin Immunol 2009;124:238–244, 244.e1–e5.

[47] Information on poverty and income statistics: a summary of 2013 current population survey data. ASPE Issue Brief: Department of Health and Human Services, Office of the Assistant Secretary for Planning and Evaluation; 2013. Available at: aspe.hhs.gov/hsp/13/PovertyandIncomeEst/ib_poverty2013.pdf.

[48] Gessner BD, Chimonas MA. Asthma is associated with preterm birth but not with small for gestational age status among a population-based cohort of Medicaid-enrolled children <10 years of age. Thorax 2007;62:231–236.

[49] Svanes C, Omenaas E, Heuch JM, et al. Birth characteristics and asthma symptoms in young adults: results from a population-based cohort study in Norway. Eur Respir J 1998;12:1366–1370.

[50] Jensen ME, Gibson PG, Collins CE, et al. Diet-induced weight loss in obese children with asthma: a randomized controlled trial. Clin Exp Allergy 2013;43:775–784.

[51] Northridge J, Ramirez OF, Stingone JA, et al. The role of housing type and housing quality in urban children with asthma. J Urban Health 2010;87:211–224.

[52] Akinbami LJ, Kit BK, Simon AE. Impact of environmental tobacco smoke on children with asthma, United States, 2003–2010. Acad Pediatr 2013;13:508–516.

[53] Weil CM, Wade SL, Bauman LJ, et al. The relationship between psychosocial factors and asthma morbidity in inner-city children with asthma. Pediatrics 1999;104:1274–1280.

[54] Bartlett SJ, Kolodner K, Butz AM, et al. Maternal depressive symptoms and emergency department use among inner-city children with asthma. Arch Pediatr Adolesc Med 2001;155:347–353.

[55] Moorman, J.E. et al. National surveillance for asthma–United States, 1980–2004. MMWR Surveill Summ. 2007;56:1–54.

[56] Flores G, Bridon C, Torres S, et al. Improving asthma outcomes in minority children: a randomized, controlled trial of parent mentors. Pediatrics 2009;124:1522–1532.

[57] Bruzzese JM, Sheares BJ, Vincent EJ, et al. Effects of a school-based intervention for urban adolescents with asthma. A controlled trial. Am J Respir Crit Care Med 2011;183:998–1006.

[58]  Morgan WJ, Crain EF, Gruchalla RS, et al. Results of a home-based environmental intervention among urban children with asthma. N Engl J Med 2004;351:1068–1080.

[59]  Morgan WJ, Crain EF, Gruchalla RS, et al. Results of a home-based environmental intervention among urban children with asthma. N Engl J Med 2004;351:1068–1080.

[60]  Akinbami LJ, Moorman JE, Garbe PL, Sondik EJ. Status of childhood asthma in the United States, 1980–2007. Pediatrics 2009;123(suppl 3):S131–S145.

[61]  Eakin M, Rand C, Bilderback A, Bollinger M, Butz A, Kandasamy V, Riekert K. Asthma in head start children: effects of the breathmobile program and family communication on asthma outcomesJ Allergy Clin Immunol 2012;129:664–670.

[62]  Talreja N, Soubani AO, Sherwin RL, et al. Modifiable factors associated with severe asthma exacerbations in urban patients. Ann Allergy Asthma Immunol. 2012;109:128–132.

[63]  Restrepo RD, Peters J. Near-fatal asthma: recognition and management. Curr Opin Pulm Med. 2008;14:13–23.

**6**

# Non-invasive Biomarkers in Asthma: Promises and Pitfalls

Helena Pite, Mário Morais-Almeida,
Tjeert Mensinga and Zuzana Diamant

### Abstract

The asthma concept has evolved throughout the years: one major step in asthma management is the recognition of the chronic (airway) inflammation; another major step is further understanding of asthma heterogeneity and subsequent development of targeted therapies. While the concept of chronic inflammation, airway structural changes and their variability over time are widely accepted, their measurement and monitoring have gone through many hardships.

In this chapter, we discuss the need for applicable biomarkers in asthma management and focus on the currently available and most promising totally non-invasive samplings and detection techniques, ranging from single biomarkers to biomarker panels and composite signatures, including molecular high-throughput "omics" technologies outcomes. Limitations of these biomarkers are compared with minimal-, semi- and invasive techniques. Additionally, we discuss the benefits of an integrative systems medicine approach, considering asthma phenotypes based on cluster analysis of multidimensional biomarker datasets and its contribution to recent developments towards the promise of better understanding asthma and personalised asthma management.

**Keywords:** asthma, biomarkers, composite signature, phenotype, personalised medicine

## 1. Introduction

According to the concurrent paradigm, asthma should not be regarded as a single disease, but rather as a complex of multiple, overlapping syndromes. The heterogeneity of asthma has been recognised already for over a century, for instance, as intrinsic and extrinsic ("allergic") asthma [1].

The introduction and subsequent validation of hypertonic saline-induced sputum analysis revealed different inflammatory asthma phenotypes: i.e. eosinophilic versus non-eosinophilic [2]. Asthma phenotypes comprise shared similar observable characteristics, produced by the interactions of an individual's genetic make-up and the environment that can be affected by several triggers and respond to treatment. However, phenotypes may vary over time and do not directly link to the underlying pathophysiology. Factor analyses involving various disease characteristics and biomarkers, including fractional exhaled nitric oxide (FeNO) levels and sputum cell differentials, helped to further define asthma (sub)phenotypes [3, 4].

In the 1990s, in analogy with animal models, asthma was thought to be a typical T-helper (Th)2- and immunoglobulin E (IgE)-driven disease, and hence, the proof of clinical effectiveness of potential asthma therapeutics was tested in the allergen challenge model. More recently, genomics and other sophisticated "omics" techniques enabled further characterisation of various inflammatory cells and other biomarkers, and helped to link asthma subphenotypes or endotypes to specific cellular and molecular pathways. For instance, gene expression profiling revealed two major subtypes: i.e. "Th2-high" and "Th2-low" asthma providing evidence for responders and non-responders to Th2-targeted therapies [5, 6]. Apart from the involvement of the adaptive immune responses, pathognomonic for parasites and allergens, more recent insight showed the major involvement of the innate system (ILC2s: innate lymphoid type 2 cells) in some asthma endotypes [7]. Interestingly, both Th2 cells and ILC2s produce type 2 cytokines (i.e. interleukin (IL)-4, IL-5 and IL-13) and these type 2 responses are mainly mediated by eosinophils. However, the underlying "upstream" mechanisms differ: while allergens mainly drive Th2-responses [8], viruses and pollutants are common triggers for ILC2-mediated type 2 responses that involve epithelial cells and IL-25, IL-33 and thymic stromal lymphopoietin [9]. Presently, it is not fully clarified how exactly both type 2 response pathways interrelate.

Apart from disease typing, the discovery of new inflammatory pathways and related bio-markers resulted into the development of endotype-specific, individualised asthma treatment.

In this review, we aim to highlight the key non-invasive and semi-invasive biomarkers currently used in the management of asthma.

## 2. Do we need biomarkers in asthma?

Given the heterogeneity of asthma and the evidence that standard therapy is not (fully) effective in all patients, especially in those with more severe disease and those at risk for frequent exacerbations, the need for appropriate biomarkers allowing the identification and subsequent targeted treatment of these patients has been increasingly recognised. Since asthma is multidimensional and thus presents at several different levels including clinical, physiological, histological, cytological and molecular, various approaches have been developed to identify effective biomarkers (**Table 1**) [10]. In addition, given the complexity of the disease, (unbiased) biomarker clustering within different asthma populations has been performed by several research groups, which revealed different disease subphenotypes with varying disease course and/or response to treatment [3, 4].

| Disease level | Parameters/biomarkers |
| --- | --- |
| Clinical | Age of onset |
| | Frequent exacerbators |
| | Therapy resistance |
| | Cofactors, including allergy, nasal polyps, recurrent viral infections, air pollutants including passive and/or active tobacco smoke, obesity |
| Physiological | Lung function (normal, reversible, fixed obstruction) |
| | Airway hyperresponsiveness |
| Cytological | Inflammatory cells and soluble markers in: |
| | Sputum (central airways); |
| | BAL, bronchial wash/brushings (peripheral airways) |
| Histological | (Trans)bronchial biopsies (inflammatory and structural cells and structures) |
| Exhaled air | FeNO (fractional exhaled nitric oxide) |
| | EBC (exhaled breath condensate) |
| | VOCs (volatile organic compounds: eNose) |
| | EBT (exhaled breath temperature) |
| Systemic biomarkers | Peripheral blood: |
| | eosinophils, CRP, IgE, periostin, cytokines |
| Molecular | Genomic SNP analysis (i.e. the large-scale genotyping of single nucleotide polymorphisms) |
| | Transcriptomic analysis (i.e. the measurement of all gene expression values in a cell or tissue type simultaneously) |
| | Proteomic analysis (i.e. the identification of all proteins present in a cell or tissue type) |
| | Metabolomic analysis (i.e. the identification and quantification of all metabolites present in a cell or tissue type; eNose) |

BAL: bronchoalveolar lavage; CRP: C-reactive protein; eNose: electronic nose; IgE: immunoglobulin E; SNP: single nucleotide polymorphism

**Table 1.** Clinical and biological biomarkers in asthma.

Using a systems biology approach in large cohorts of patients, researchers within the Innovative Medicines Initiative Severe Asthma Project U-Biopred have been collecting data, including molecular analyses, tissue, exhaled air and blood samplings, as well as clinical and lung function data, and patient-reported symptoms [11]. By combining this information, the researchers aimed to generate a "handprint", i.e. a combination of clinical and biological characteristics (biomarkers) indicative of a specific asthma subphenotype/endotype. Subsequent studies are being undertaken to test if one's "handprint" can predict the disease course and can indicate a response to (targeted) asthma treatments. This approach will provide a key step to personalised medicine [12–14].

Generally, an ideal biomarker should possess the following key characteristics: clinical relevance, adequate sensitivity and specificity for (targeted) treatment effects, repeatability, simplicity and cost-effectiveness [10].

# 3. Promising single non-invasive biomarkers of asthma

The concept of asthma has undergone considerable changes throughout the years, from a disease mainly manifesting by variable symptoms and bronchoconstriction to airway inflammation and remodeling. More recently, heterogeneity has gained an outstanding position in asthma definition. So far, one of the most important steps in asthma history, bringing significant reduction in morbidity and mortality, was the recognition of airway inflammation in asthma and the introduction of efficacious and safe anti-inflammatory therapy for asthma control. Despite ongoing developments, current guidelines for both diagnosis and follow-up of patients with asthma are still grounded on clinical and lung function parameters. Thus, functional biomarkers were the first objective measures coming forward into clinical practice and, in general, the promise of delivering valuable molecular, cellular or histological biomarkers to daily clinical practice has not yet been met. However, intense research in asthma has brought together scientists from academia, research institutes, the pharmaceutical industry and patient organisations, with significant progress taking place in the recent years. In this section, we discuss the currently available and more advanced non-invasive biomarkers in asthma.

Clinicians and researchers dedicated to asthma may benefit from a direct analysis of the airways, profiting the patients. In fact, non-invasive airway assessment is possible through lung function tests (LFTs) and airway sampling. Furthermore, other "more distant" to the airway biomarkers (such as blood or urinary biomarkers) can also be regarded as potentially useful, considering the systemic properties of asthma.

## 3.1. Functional biomarkers

LFTs are essential in routine clinical practice. They are non-invasive, well validated and reproducible. At present, LFTs provide the only generally accepted functional biomarkers to objectively aid in the diagnosis, risk assessment and monitoring of asthma. Thus, asthma definition currently implies the objective detection of variable airflow limitation, while the "best personal lung function" is a hallmark of asthma monitoring and future risk assessment.

LFTs provide relative features (phenotypes) that aid in differential diagnosis, namely in the distinction from chronic obstructive pulmonary disease (COPD), but are not diagnostic in its use. For instance, neither post-bronchodilator airway obstruction, lack of bronchodilation response or hyperinflation can be used to rule out asthma.

Presently, LFTs patterns alone are not considered to define disease subsets that respond to particular therapies. However, lung function has been shown to be predictive of clinical outcomes and provide complementary information to subphenotype asthma. For instance, variability measures of lung function can predict the loss of asthma control and response to long-term beta2-agonist treatment [15].

Airway hyperreactivity (AHR) is a basic pathophysiological hallmark of asthma, but remains a complex component of this disease. A growing number of variable airway smooth muscle (ASM) and non-muscle factors contributing to AHR has been recognised. Besides its high negative predictive value in the diagnosis of asthma, AHR has been advocated as a surrogate biomarker related to airway inflammation to guide asthma management. It has been shown that anti-inflammatory therapy directed at reducing AHR may imply higher corticosteroid doses, but leads to improved lung function and better control [16, 17]. AHR evaluation has also been suggested useful in back titration of inhaled corticosteroids. However, the reduction in AHR with higher doses appears targeted to the persistent structural component of AHR (defined as opposed to the variable inflammation component of AHR). Emerging data support that it is the structural changes of the airway that mainly contribute to AHR (i.e. reticular layer thickness and ASM hypertrophy) [16]. This effect also depends on the type of challenge used: assessing AHR to indirect bronchoconstrictor stimuli is superior in the detection of changes associated with airway inflammation, while direct stimuli, mediated through direct interaction with ASM, better reflect the structural changes. Assessment of AHR is a useful non-invasive tool providing complementary information, though its routine feasibility in general practice can be hard to settle.

Summing up, lung function measurements may not, per se, reflect the precise underlying pathological processes responsible for different phenotypes. However, in a multidimensional approach to evaluate asthma as a complex dynamic disease, functional biomarkers and their variability must definitely be part of future composite parameters in asthma.

### 3.2. Exhaled air biomarkers

Exhaled breath can be sampled in a fully non-invasive manner across all age groups. However, exhaled breath analysis is not useful for analysing cellular or histological biomarkers and, in general, the search for useful molecular biomarkers has been hampered by methodologic difficulties mainly dealing with very low molecular concentrations, variability and lack of sampling and analysing methods standardisation [10].

*FeNO* is so far the most commonly used molecular biomarker in exhaled air. Nitric oxide (NO) is a gaseous chemical compound, which can be measured in exhaled breath either by chemiluminescence and electrochemical analysers. The American Thoracic Society and the European Respiratory Society recommendations for standardised procedures for the FeNO measurement have been published [18]. Accordingly, FeNO is measured at a flow rate of 50 mL/s, thus reflecting NO production from the central airways. Currently available devices allow accurate and highly reproducible measurements, through simple, fast and non-invasive methodology. Hand-held devices are now widely available in clinical practice and used in both adults and children (since preschool age, usually above the age of 4 years) [10].

Evidence-based guidelines for adequate interpretation of FeNO measurement have been developed [19]. This biomarker can be affected by several perturbing factors, mainly age, height and recent active or passive smoking. Other variables that have been reported to affect FeNO levels include weight, gender, race, atopic status, diet or alcohol intake [20]. Large variation of normal FeNO values exists, with wide inter-individual differences and significant overlaps between healthy/non-asthmatic and asthmatic populations. Intriguingly, the afore-mentioned confounding factors explain few of the substantial variations within the general population [20]. For these reasons, guideline-recommended cut-points are supported for routine interpretation of FeNO levels [19].

Presently, there is evidence to support the use of FeNO thresholds essentially for assessing the likelihood of Th2-mediated airway inflammation and responsiveness to corticosteroids [19]. Low FeNO levels do not rule out asthma [19].

Persistently high FeNO levels may be attributed to poor adherence to corticosteroid therapy, poor inhaled drug delivery or persistent/high allergen exposure [19]. This has also been suggested to reflect a highly reactive asthma phenotype [21]. Although FeNO may be indicative of loss of disease control or exacerbation, some patients remain with high FeNO despite good clinical asthma control, and clinical trials of FeNO-guided management have yielded conflicting results [22–24]. Increased knowledge on asthma pathophysiology and the source and biochemistry of FeNO may help to further understand these findings. Traditionally, FeNO is known to originate in the airway epithelium as a result of inducible nitric oxide synthase (iNOS) upregulation, which occurs with inflammation [19]. Recent data give further support to this view by showing iNOS overexpression in the airway epithelium of patients with asthma [25]. However, it is interesting to note that despite the strong association between FeNO and Th2-mediated/eosinophilic inflammation and atopy, eosinophils are not the principal cells in the airways that express iNOS and this enzyme is upregulated by Th1 cytokines [26]. Anti-IL-5 and anti-IgE therapy for asthma reduced sputum eosinophilia without affecting FeNO, contrary to IL-13 inhibition that significantly decreased FeNO [27]. Studies have shown that FeNO levels are not elevated in many patients with severe asthma, compared to mild and moderate asthma, despite evidence of airway inflammation [13, 28]. Other sources of FeNO need also to be considered. For instance, as NO is a highly reactive molecule, it can be trapped and directly regenerated by abundant free thiol-containing biomolecules [26]. One of these thiols is S-nitrosoglutathione, which has been shown to be depleted in severe asthma, possibly contributing to comparative lower FeNO levels in these patients. Another important reservoir of nitrogen species is nitrite/nitrous acid. These agents are physiologically recycled in blood and tissues to form NO and other bioactive nitrogen oxides. When airway pH increases, more nitrite is formed and FeNO levels fall. On the other hand, FeNO may be high with acidification [26]. Still, many questions regarding the source of FeNO and its specific role need to be explored. Another area of research that may bring additional knowledge and clinical usefulness is dedicated to partitioning of FeNO. In particular, alveolar FeNO can be obtained by measuring FeNO at multiple flow rates and has been shown to be an independent parameter that is putatively associated with increased distal lung inflammation and more severe disease [29].

In summary, the clinical importance of FeNO as a marker of Th2-mediated airway inflammation that is likely to respond to corticosteroid treatment may be "indirect," but is well established. Further analysis is needed to address the possible need to define FeNO levels cut-points in different situations, according to the presence or absence of pertinent confounders. The application of FeNO measurement to identify particular asthma phenotypes or as part of a more comprehensive panel of biomarkers including also other "Th2 type" biomarkers may allow taking better profit of this readily available biomarker [30]. Partitioning of FeNO is a promising area of research, whose clinical usefulness is yet to be established.

Other biomarkers have been studied in exhaled breath vapor namely *volatile organic compounds* (VOCs). In general, reactive oxygen species result from inflammation and promote polyunsaturated fatty acids degradation, originating volatile hydrocarbons. These VOCs are subsequently excreted in exhaled breath. Thus, exhaled VOCs may originate from systemic metabolism or from local airway inflammation. It is important to consider also that VOCs in exhaled breath may also be originated from pathogenic bacteria or from exogenous sources such as ambient air pollution [31]. Some studies have suggested that single VOCs such as pentane or ethane could be significantly higher in patients with asthma. However, VOCs profiles analyses bring significant additional value [31].

Another potential single biomarker in exhaled air is *exhaled breath temperature* (EBT), which reflects heat, a cardinal sign of inflammation. EBT has been shown to correlate with bronchial blood flow [32], which is advocated as the main mechanism to explain EBT changes in disease status.

Several studies have shown that EBT is higher in patients with asthma [32–34]. Conflicting data have been reported regarding a possible association between EBT and asthma control, with several studies supporting [34, 35], and others rejecting this relation [36, 37]. Correlation between EBT and other biomarkers, such as sputum eosinophils and FeNO, has resulted in inconsistent reports [32, 37]. Furthermore, EBT has been shown to increase after eucapnic voluntary hyperventilation, methacholine challenge test or exercise, but no difference was found between asthmatics and healthy individuals [38], suggesting this increase in EBT to be physiologic.

However, it is important to stress that different methods have been used to measure EBT. Some studies used a flow and pressure-controlled maximal slow continuous exhalation to residual volume to measure EBT, while others measured EBT in tidal volume until a temperature plateau was reached. Different variables have been analysed: plateau EBT, rate of temperature increase, time to achieve plateau EBT. These different methods preclude results comparison and, to our knowledge, no study has analysed both methods simultaneously. The recent development of improved, easier-to-use, portable devices has improved feasibility, including in children and in the elderly [34, 36, 39].

Moreover, further studies are needed when it concerns interpretation of the results. Variables such as room temperature and relative-ambient humidity may influence the results [39]. Some studies point a correlation between gender [37, 39], age [36, 39] and lung volume [36], which needs to be addressed. No significant correlation has been documented between EBT and auricular temperature, suggesting EBT to be a distinct variable and not just another measurement of body temperature [33, 34].

Conclusively, EBT assessment may be an appealing method enabling completely non-invasive and patient-friendly evaluation and deserves further standardisation and validation as a potentially useful biomarker in asthma.

## 3.3. Exhaled breath condensate biomarkers

Exhaled breath has been a source for intense research in the latest years and many other biomarkers have been studied. *Exhaled breath condensate* (EBC) has the advantage of being a more stable matrix than exhaled breath vapor, including volatile and also non-volatile compounds. It is obtained by cooling exhaled air and is thought to reflect the composition of the airway lining fluid. Many molecules have been analysed in EBC, including metabolites and also proteins. Although methodological recommendations for exhaled breath sampling and analysis have been published [40], the procedures for EBC collection and biomarker detection are not fully standardised and there is significant heterogeneity between different working groups yielding (highly) variable data.

Many biomarkers analysed in EBC reflect oxidative stress. Among these, the most extensively studied include $H_2O_2$ and isoprostanes.

$H_2O_2$ is a reactive oxygen species that contributes to oxidative stress within the airways. A meta-analysis has reported that EBC $H_2O_2$ concentrations were significantly higher in adults with asthma, and associated with disease severity and control [41]. This has also been reported in children. Of importance, smoking increases $H_2O_2$ levels. EBC $H_2O_2$ levels were inversely correlated with lung function parameters and improved with inhaled corticosteroids [41]. Thus, EBC $H_2O_2$ has been suggested a promising biomarker for asthma control monitoring.

Oxidative stress can also be assessed through the determination of lipid peroxidation-derived products. *8-isoprostane* derives from arachidonic acid peroxidation. Increased levels of 8-isoprostane have been found in EBC in patients with asthma, correlating with disease severity [42]. EBC 8-isoprostane levels have been shown to be particularly useful to indicate asthma control and severity in childhood when combined with different markers [30]. Increased 8-isoprostane levels in EBC of children with exercise-induced bronchoconstriction (EIB) have been described, suggesting a role for oxidative stress in EIB [43].

Markers of inflammation have also been addressed. *Leukotrienes (LT)* are important mediators of airway inflammation in asthma, and the most extensively studied molecular biomarkers of inflammation in EBC. Increased levels of LTs have been detected in EBC of patients with asthma, correlated with disease severity and were effectively reduced by oral corticosteroids or LT receptor antagonist [44, 45]. However, the reported effect of inhaled corticosteroids on LTB4 EBC levels is controversial [46]. LTs have been suggested as markers of asthma severity [42]. Likewise, LTs have been associated with EIB severity [47].

Various *cytokines* and other molecules have been analysed in EBC. In particular, IL-4 has been found to be higher in EBC of patients with asthma, especially in asthma associated with atopy [30, 42]. Cytokine ratios and biomarker panels in EBC including cytokines have been suggested to be useful to assess asthma control (including IL-4 and interferon-gamma) and to predict asthma exacerbations (e.g. IL-5) [30, 48].

Last but definitely not least, the measurement of *pH* is one of the simplest and most technically validated biomarkers in EBC. EBC pH reflects airway acidification [49]. Several research groups have found higher pH levels in healthy subjects, compared to patients with asthma [10]. Significant decline in EBC pH occurred during asthma exacerbations. EBC pH shows good reproducibility, having low running costs and normal data sets have been published in self-reported healthy subjects [50].

Although some biomarkers may be useful to measure in EBC, samples are highly diluted, biomarker concentrations are difficult to measure, require specialised equipment, laboratory techniques and normalisation standards are lacking. Unfortunately, EBC has been hampered by serious drawbacks in the methodology, detection techniques and result interpretation, all consistent with large intra and intersubject variability, precluding validation for most single biomarkers.

### 3.4. Biomarkers in non-respiratory specimens

Other non-invasive matrices have also been analysed in search for biomarkers in asthma. *Saliva* is a readily available specimen and allows metabolites, proteins and also deoxyribonucleic acid (DNA)/ribonucleic acid (RNA) extracting (although buccal swabs perform better), including also oral microbiota assessment. *Cotinine* in saliva has been one of the most extensively studied biomarkers, with interest in asthma as a measure of tobacco exposure. Salivary *cortisol* has also been used for the evaluation of adrenal function. Morning salivary cortisol was significantly lower in patients with asthma than in healthy individuals, and poor asthma control has recently been associated with lower salivary cortisol levels [51]. Preliminary data have suggested that *inflammatory salivary markers* may also be associated with asthma control, including eosinophil-related (such as eosinophil cationic protein) and myeloid/innate mediators [52]. Additionally, a significant decrease in salivary antioxidant enzyme-peroxidase activity was observed in children during asthma exacerbations [53]. A salivary pH decline has also been associated with asthma and AHR [54]. Another area of research includes the analysis of oral microbiota, which may change in asthma, either through disease status or its pharmacotherapy. The interest in saliva studies in relation to asthma is still preliminary and the role of many possible confounders needs to be considered.

Although *urine* does not directly reflect the airways, samples are easily obtained across the full age spectrum. Several urine molecular biomarkers have been described to be associated with asthma. Here, we focus on four molecules which have been studied in more detail.

Of the potent lipid inflammatory mediators comprising the cysteinyl *LTs*, only LTE4 is stable, making this molecule the dominant LT detectable in biological fluids. Urinary levels of this end product of LT metabolism have been shown to be elevated in asthma, both in children and adults, and in patients with aspirin-exacerbated respiratory disease [55, 56]. It has been associated with the degree of airflow limitation and acute exacerbations [55, 57]. Although inhaled corticosteroids are the most effective treatment for asthma, they do not alter LTE4 excretion. Urinary LTE4 levels have been suggested as potential predictors of better response to anti-LT therapy compared to other therapeutic approaches, though further studies are needed, including other biomarkers, to predict individual responses.

As LTs, *prostaglandins* (PG) are the end products of arachidonic metabolism. PGD2 results from cyclooxygenase pathway and is excreted in urine after being metabolised to $9\alpha,11\beta$-PGF2. Increased urinary excretion occurs in patients with asthma and after challenge tests, and a negative association has been found with lung function [58].

*Bromotyrosine* is another molecule with possible interest in asthma. It is generated from protein oxidation by eosinophils. The oxidised amino acid is stable and excreted in urine. Urinary bromotyrosine levels are higher in patients with asthma and have been associated with asthma control and lung function, predicting exacerbations [59]. Its levels have been shown to reduce during inhaled corticosteroid therapy. High urinary bromotyrosine levels could predict a favorable clinical response to inhaled corticosteroid therapy, especially in combination with high FeNO values [59]. These results warrant further developments.

Though urinary biomarkers may become useful tools, many require specialised equipment and their measurement is not fully validated or standardised. There is a current need for normalisation standards and assessment of intra and inter-individual variation to select the potentially useful biomarkers. It is also important to address urine dilution when reporting quantitative absolute results.

### 3.5. Airway imaging biomarkers

Airway imaging biomarkers are also emerging, offering the potential of adding complementary information, namely on small airways function and remodeling. High-resolution computed tomography (HRCT) images are used to measure airway narrowing, wall thickening, air trapping and ventilation inhomogeneity [27]. The first two measures have been correlated with lung function and asthma severity. Increased parenchymal lucency has also been associated with severe asthma exacerbations, lung function and neutrophilic inflammation. HRCT is easily performed though it requires that lungs are scanned at a standard volume for validity and reproducibility. The risk of exposure to significant ionising radiation needs to be considered and normal ranges have not been established.

## 4. Composite biomarkers in non-invasive sampling: what is known and what could be useful in the future?

The complexity and dynamics of asthma drive the need to establish distinct disease phenotypes and endotypes. There are several different triggers in asthma, with various pathophysiological pathways in parallel resulting in clinical expression that may be rather similar. Therefore, repeated multiscale, multidimensional measurements may be needed to capture this complexity, which may yield more useful information than single or even panels of combined biomarkers [60]. In this view, molecular composite signatures may be obtained by high-throughput "omics" technologies, which are increasingly standardised. Several large-scale studies of the genome, transcriptome, proteome or metabolome have produced an enormous amount of data and it is pivotal to follow the available guidelines in order to avoid false discoveries [60]. The composite high-dimensional signatures or fingerprints are based on pattern recognition underlying complex non-linear biology systems. Some evidence that this approach may be successful in asthma has already emerged concerning differential diagnosis [61]. Regarding non-invasive, direct assessment of exhaled breath, it is interesting to note that while many problems arise in specific molecular biomarkers validation, recent studies have shown encouraging results with the application of metabolomics strategies to study exhaled biomarkers [60, 62, 63].

Among "omics" systems biology, metabolomics is considered the one that comes closest to phenotype expression. It involves the identification and quantification of small molecular weight metabolites. Real-time metabolomics measurements are already feasible for several clinical applications with electronic noses (eNoses). These handheld, portable devices can capture various combinations of VOCs in exhaled breath, with nanosensors arrays. The nanosensors are based on conducting polymers, metal oxide, metal oxide field effect transistors, surface or bulk acoustic waves, optical sensors, colorimetric sensors, ion mobility spectrometry, infrared spectroscopy, gold nanoparticles and gas-chromatography (GC) coupled with mass spectrometry (MS) or flame ionisation detection [60, 64]. The pattern recognition algorithms using various eNose sensor systems indicate fingerprints of exhaled VOCs, called breathprints, which have shown to discriminate patients with asthma from healthy subjects and COPD with accuracies between 80% and 100% [65]. Breathprints have also been studied to phenotype asthma. Recent studies indicate that eosinophilic and non-eosinophilic asthma can be distinguished when using a composite eNose platform. Breath analysis by eNose could also predict the response to corticosteroids with greater accuracy than sputum eosinophils or FeNO [66]. These data suggest that composite signatures of breath analysis could be used for assessment and monitoring of airway inflammation. Important methodologic issues of technique optimisation and standardisation deserve deeper analysis, from breath sampling, to modulating factors including comorbidities and incompatibility between eNoses. These should enable external validation to determine possible disease-specific breathprints with clinical applicability.

Besides the analysis of exhaled breath vapour with GC-MS and eNoses, the novel metabolomics approach has also been applied to EBC. It has been shown to enable characterisation of metabolic compounds in even small EBC volumes, using high-resolution proton nuclear magnetic resonance (NMR) or MS. This has proved capable of discriminating healthy individuals from those with asthma [62, 63, 67, 68]. It could also discriminate between severe and non-severe asthma [63], supporting the hypothesis that severe asthma has specific metabolic features.

Interestingly, the metabolomics analysis of urine also discriminated healthy individuals from those with asthma [69], and could distinguish patients with stable asthma from those with acute exacerbations based on profiles [69, 70]. Metabolomics analysis of urine samples has also been recently suggested as a useful clinical tool to differentiate asthma from COPD [71].

Pinkerton et al. [72] demonstrated for the first time that differences between healthy controls and asthma patients could be detected via micro-RNA (miRNA) expression in EBC, and suggest that different types of inflammation may have unique miRNA signatures. These small non-coding RNAs are known to be important in the post-transcriptional regulation of inflammation, thus opening a new research field using non-invasive direct air sampling.

Proteomics has also recently been applied to EBC. Liquid chromatography (LC)-MS has been used to separate and detect proteolytic peptides present in EBC with differentiating profiles based on asthma status [73]. However, this preliminary study faced several problems such as insufficient sample volume, possible salivary contamination and difficulties in peptides identification due to their low concentration.

Besides allowing an overview of molecular signatures, the "omics" approach may potentially lead to new knowledge regarding asthma pathophysiology, due to its untargeted, hypothesis-generating approach. All biomedical researchers are facing not only the opportunities but also the challenges in accessing, managing, analysing and integrating diverse data sets that are larger, more diverse and more complex than ever before, and that exceed the abilities of current management and analysis approaches [60, 74]. Composite biomarkers research such as that coming from molecular profiling assays including various "omics" is a live example that needs to be critically interpreted and cautiously validated to yield truly significant advances in personalised medicine.

## 5. Non-invasive biomarkers limitations: can more invasive sampling do better?

Asthma syndromes are characterised for being dynamic, with varying changes in symptoms pattern, lung function, inflammation and remodelling throughout time. In this setting, non-invasive direct airway sampling, such as exhaled breath analysis, seems especially appealing, allowing easy and repeatable measures over time. However, low molecular concentrations and variable sample dilution lead to difficulties in methods sensitivity and validation, with consequent issues in replication of biomarker findings (**Table 2**). In comparison, bronchoscopy allows direct visual examination of the airways and direct collection of fluid (bronchoalveolar lavage, bronchial washing) and tissue (brushing, biopsy). These techniques are mostly impractical because they are invasive, require specialised equipment and qualified personnel, have contraindications and carry potential risks / complications. Therefore, ethical issues preclude bronchoscopic sampling broad use in asthma, even less when repeated samplings are needed, thus being mainly reserved for selected severe patients and for research purposes. Apart from practical issues, standard bronchoscopy techniques hold several other limitations, including lack of reproducibility and sample dilution effect, despite recently proposed improvements (Table 2) [75]. In between invasive and non-invasive airway samplings, semi-invasive induced-sputum analysis may also reflect the airways and is easier to perform. Moreover, although indirect, blood sampling is minimally invasive and is a known relevant biomarker source in asthma.

| Biomarker source | Pros | Cons |
| --- | --- | --- |
| Exhaled breath | Totally non-invasive<br>Validated for FeNO measurement<br>Portable (FeNO, eNose, EBT, EBC)<br>Direct results (FeNO, eNose, EBT)<br>Multiple molecular biomarkers<br>May be collected across all ages<br>May be collected in severe patients<br>Allows serial measurements | Validation not complete (except FeNO)<br>Many perturbing factors<br>Upper airways/salivary possible contamination<br>Require expertise, expensive and time-consuming specialised lab assays (EBC)<br>Soluble markers subject to dilution |
| Induced-sputum | Semi-invasive<br>Validated tool<br>Molecular and cellular biomarkers<br>Useful to guide treatments (sputum-eosinophils) | Impossible in young children<br>Contraindicated in severe bronchoconstriction / active cardiovascular disorders<br>Rescue medication / procedures needed<br>Non-repeatable over short time-period (<12 to 18 h)<br>Procedure itself may induce changes in airways/lab results<br>Upper airways/salivary possible contamination<br>Require expertise, expensive and time-consuming specialised lab assays<br>Soluble markers subject to dilution |
| Bronchoscopy | Direct airway assessment | Invasive<br>Several medical contraindications<br>Rescue medication/procedures needed<br>Non-repeatable in many patients<br>Expertise and experience required for procedure<br>Require expertise, expensive and time-consuming specialised lab assays<br>BAL markers subject to dilution<br>Procedure itself may induce changes in airways/lab results (BAL) |
| Blood | Minimally invasive<br>Some biomarkers routinely available (e.g. eosinophil counts)<br>Useful to guide treatments (e.g. eosinophils counts)<br>Molecular and cellular biomarkers<br>May be collected across all ages<br>May be collected in severe patients<br>Allows serial measurements | Not directly reflecting the airways<br>Not patient-friendly in all subjects (e.g. children)<br>Require expertise, expensive and time-consuming specialised lab assays (some biomarkers) |
| Urine | Totally non-invasive<br>May be collected across all ages<br>May be collected in severe patients<br>Allows serial measurements | Not directly reflecting the airways<br>Require expertise, expensive and time-consuming specialised lab assays |

BAL: bronchoalveolar lavage; EBC: exhaled breath condensate; EBT: exhaled breath temperature; eNose: electronic nose; FeNO: fractional exhaled nitric oxide.

Table 2. Pros and cons of main biomarker sample sources in asthma.

In this section, we will discuss these sampling methods and related current main biomarkers for asthma management.

## 5.1. Sputum biomarkers

Induced sputum is a validated sampling method of the more central airways. Sputum is collected after inhalations of hypertonic saline. Although relatively safe, induced-sputum requires specialised training, equipment and laboratory processing. Monitoring lung function during the induction procedure reduces the risk of excessive bronchoconstriction. Patient's active cooperation is needed for collection, making this technique unsuitable for some patients, especially for children below the age of 7 years [76].

Induced-sputum provides a rich source of soluble and cellular biomarkers and has exceptionally allowed a successful single biomarker-based clinical management approach in asthma. This is the case with sputum eosinophil percentage, which identifies patients who have eosinophilic and non-eosinophilic asthma phenotypes and can be predictive of poor asthma outcome and targeted treatment response, with demonstrated treatment-guided superior efficacy in reducing asthma exacerbations in adults [2, 27, 77, 78]. Thus, sputum eosinophil percentage acts as a key marker and correlates with severe exacerbations and AHR. It has also been useful in a panel of biomarkers to select patients who may benefit from IL-5 targeted therapies, including mepolizumab (anti-IL-5), reslizumab (anti-IL-5) and benralizumab (anti-IL-5R). In contrast with adults [77, 78], eosinophil sputum-guided therapy was not associated with decreased asthma exacerbations or improved asthma control in school-aged children and adolescents [79]. Sputum inflammatory phenotype was shown to be unstable in children with asthma, and this was not related to treatment or disease control [80].

Besides eosinophils, other sputum biomarkers are currently in research. Sputum neutrophils are often related to severe non-eosinophilic asthma with fixed airway obstruction. Soluble sputum biomarkers have been associated with asthma severity (e.g. eosinophilic cationic protein, LT, IL-4, IL-5, IL-13, IL-6, IL-12, tumour necrosis factor-$\alpha$, granulocyte-macrophage colony-stimulating factor), exacerbations (e.g. IL-8, neurokinin A) or remodelling (procollagen synthesis peptides, tissue inhibitors of metalloproteinase or transforming growth factor-$\beta$) [10]. Many biomarkers can be measured, but most require highly sensitive detection methods and results may be affected by sputum processing or variable dilutions. These factors need to be taken into account to select and validate useful biomarkers in sputum.

Induced sputum may also be an interesting source for composite biomarkers. Unsupervised clustering of induced-sputum gene expression profiles identified three transcriptional asthma phenotypes that related to clinical and inflammatory parameters (resembling eosinophilic, neutrophilic and paucigranulocytic asthma) [81]. Differentially expressed genes were related to immune and inflammatory responses, proving a framework to investigate asthma endo-types.

In summary, logistic and practical difficulties have precluded the wide use of induced sputum in clinical practice, but sputum eosinophil percentage is recommended as a supplemental measure in future asthma clinical research studies to identify specific cellular profiles and to predict or to monitor a treatment response in adult patients [27]. It is important to highlight that sputum eosinophils and FeNO are not duplicative outcome measures, even though low sputum eosinophil and low FeNO are strongly linked [27].

## 5.2. Blood biomarkers

Peripheral blood can be collected across all age groups, with minimal risk. Some biomarkers are routinely standardised in medical institutions and therefore readily available, such as eosinophils, total serum IgE and allergen-specific IgE. The latter are used to define atopy, which can be accurately, easily and more readily detected by skin prick test. Atopy modestly increases the probability of asthma, but is not essential for diagnosis. Though it is useful to characterise patients, atopy itself is recognised to be heterogeneous, including both "Th2-high" and "Th2-low" phenotypes [5]. Specific sensitisations are useful in clinical practice to suggest clinically relevant allergen avoidance and consider allergen-specific immunotherapy. However, total IgE or allergen-specific IgE quantification cannot predict the response to treatment and are otherwise weak biomarkers in asthma.

Blood eosinophil absolute count has long been associated with asthma and remains a recommended supplemental asthma biomarker [27]. Although it may not reflect the airways and be unspecific, blood eosinophilia supports asthma diagnosis and is an independent risk factor for exacerbations and fixed airflow limitation. Blood eosinophil counts are useful to subphenotype asthma and to monitor systemic biologic effects of pharmacologic interventions in patients with asthma, including (inhaled) corticosteroids, anti-IgE, LT antagonists and 5-lipoxygenase inhibitors [27]. Furthermore, blood eosinophil counts emerged as predictive biomarkers of clinical benefit from IL-5- and IL-13-targeted therapies, being associated with a "Th2 bronchial signature" [82].

Another promising "Th2-high" serum biomarker is the extracellular matrix protein periostin. The expression of periostin is upregulated by IL-13 in bronchial epithelial cells and, unlike IL-13, is abundant and readily detectable in peripheral blood [82]. Interestingly, a multi-centre study collecting matched sputum, bronchoscopy and peripheral blood samples from patients with asthma showed that serum periostin was the best single predictor of airway eosinophilia, with a further advantage of lower intrasubject variability over time than FeNO or blood eosinophilia [82]. However, conflicting results have recently been reported [83, 84]. Nevertheless, periostin levels have been associated with asthma severity and its levels have also been shown to be important to predict lebrikizumab (anti-IL-13) clinical benefit, with greater reduction in severe exacerbations and greater improvement in lung function in the "periostin-high" patients [85]. A greater decrease in exacerbations with anti-IgE therapy has also been reported in "periostin-high" patients. Healthy subjects and lebrikizumab-treated patients still have measurable levels of serum periostin, thus other systemic sources of periostin than IL-13 need to be explored [82].

Overall, blood eosinophils, serum periostin and FeNO reflect "type 2" airway inflammation in different ways and are only weakly correlated; therefore, combinations of these biomarkers obtained with minimally or non-invasive samplings may further enable optimisation of treatment benefit [82, 86, 87].

Recently, application of "omics" technologies to peripheral blood and invasive sampling with unsupervised clustering are yielding crucial data to capture the complexity of various asthma phenotypes and add new insights on asthma endotypes and treatment response. Given its maturity, transcriptomics analysis using microarrays is the current state-of-the-art method for asthma signature discovery [60]. For instance, gene expression profiling of bronchial epithelium identified distinct subtypes of patients with asthma with "Th2-high" or "Th2-low" phenotype [5], supported the involvement of endotoxin and macrophage activation in corticosteroid resistance, and suggested that corticosteroids also exert their beneficial effects through activity on bronchial smooth muscle [60]. "Omics" technologies developments, with data comparison and validation, will lead to the integration of composite signature biomarkers in phenotyping asthma and improvements in our understanding of asthma. Ultimately, breakthroughs in asthma treatment may be reached through the development of innovative targeted therapies [12, 60].

Non-invasive procedures for biomarker analysis form the backbone for day-to-day clinical asthma management. However, invasive tests may provide important information to phenotype and direct therapy in patients with severe refractory asthma [88]. These techniques bring significant additional knowledge in asthma research that needs to be integrated with non-invasive procedures outcomes to allow truly innovative steps in biomarker discovery for asthma management.

## 6. Asthma phenotypes based on cluster analyses

In general, milder asthma phenotypes respond well to standard therapy with corticosteroids (with or without long-acting beta2-agonists), while those with more severe disease urged the development of new therapeutic modalities. To enable the development of effective (targeted) therapies, it is crucial to understand the pathophysiological mechanisms driving these subsets of asthmatic patients. Haldar et al. performed a cluster analysis on baseline data of 184 patients with mild to moderate asthma coming from different general practitioners (GP) and baseline data of 187 patients with refractory disease from specialist settings [3]. Additionally, a third dataset comprised baseline and longitudinal data of 68 patients with refractory disease followed for 12 months. Hierarchical cluster analysis revealed five different clusters, with some overlapping features between patients from GP and specialist origins. Most importantly, patients with concordant symptoms and (eosinophilic) inflammation (based on sputum analysis) were mostly coming from GP and were characterised by overall milder, often atopic, well-controlled disease, with a benign disease course. Alternatively, patients with uncontrolled disease, characterised by either discordant symptoms (i.e. many symptoms, little airway eosinophilia or non-eosinophilic inflammation) or discordant inflammation (few symptoms, prominent airway eosinophilia) mostly originated from the specialist settings. Commonly found confounders consisted of obesity and non-compliance. Overall, these findings supported a symptom-guided management for mild-moderate "concordant"-type asthma, while "discordant"-type refractory asthmatics might benefit from inflammation-guided therapy [78].

Using unsupervised hierarchical cluster analysis in a group of 726 patients from the Severe Asthma Research Program (SARP) revealed five distinct clinical subphenotypes within this population [4], showing some overlap with the findings by Haldar et al. [3]. The results of both cluster analysis studies underscore disease heterogeneity, even in subsets of patients with similar clinical characteristics, with potentially different pathophysiological and immunological mechanisms, requiring different therapeutic approaches.

Further analysis into the molecular mechanisms underlying different asthma phenotypes revealed at least two distinct subsets with a "Th2-high" and a "Th2-low" profile, respectively [5], based on the expression of IL-13 inducible airway epithelial genes (POSTN (periostin), CLCA1 (chloride channel regulator 1) and SERPINB2 (serpin peptidase inhibitor clade B, member2)) as previously described by this research group. Not unexpectedly, patients with Th2-driven asthma responded well to inhaled corticosteroids while those with a "Th2-low" profile did not. Hence, there is an urgent need for effective therapeutic options for "Th2-low" asthmatic patients that appeared to comprise approximately 50% of the study population, and hence, in reality may be larger than originally thought.

Additionally, these findings urged phenotyping of patients (i.e. including an adequate target population) and/or using an appropriate disease model [8], for adequate interpretation of effectiveness data in targeted intervention studies. So far, several applicable (surrogate) biomarkers have been validated to phenotype potential responders and to monitor the effects of currently available (or under development) targeted therapies, i.e. anti-IgE, and Th2-pathway targeted therapies (anti-IL-5, anti-IL-4 and anti-IL-13) [86]. Presently, biomarkers including blood eosinophils, FeNO and serum periostin thus moved the first steps to personalised medicine [87]. Further insight into the heterogeneity of Th2-driven/type 2 asthma, "Th2-low" subsets, as well as further refinement of sensitive (composite) biomarkers should be considered the next steps in this promising direction to optimise and personalise asthma management.

## 7. Conclusions

The complex heterogeneity and dynamics of asthma with varying response to standard treatment is driving the search for distinct asthma phenotypes and endotypes. While inhaled corticosteroids can effectively control asthma, therapeutic responses are individualised (though clinical manifestations may match), can be incomplete in a significant number of patients and no curative treatment exists.

In this setting, biomarkers are needed to innovate asthma management. As indicators of pathophysiologic processes or pharmacologic responses, biomarkers can be useful for asthma diagnosis and phenotyping, prediction of future risk or treatment selection or evaluation of response. Non-invasive sampling has the advantage of being patient-friendly and allowing repeatable measurements across all age and severity groups. More direct airway or distant assessment non-invasive sampling and analysis are currently possible, yielding molecular, cellular, functional and imaging potentially clinically useful biomarkers.

For the promise of delivering valuable new biomarkers to the clinic to come forward, it is mandatory that standard optimised procedures are set for sample collection and analysis, and that resulting data are critically processed, explored and cut-off values are well-defined. This will allow comparison of results and replication, with external validation in different population settings.

Though relevant single biomarkers have been found in asthma, increasing evidence shows that biomarker panels do better and composite signatures may indeed soon be integrated in phenotyping/endotyping of asthma. Multiscale, high-dimensional biological, together with standard clinical measures are adding new relevant knowledge. This systems medicine approach is helping to generate new hypotheses and (re)discover pathways and related biomarkers, linking phenotypes to endotypes and ultimately leading to truly innovative treatments for patients with asthma syndromes.

## Author details

Helena Pite[1,2*], Mário Morais-Almeida[1,3], Tjeert Mensinga[4] and Zuzana Diamant[4,5]

*Address all correspondence to: helenampite@gmail.com

1 Allergy Center, CUF Descobertas Hospital and CUF Infante Santo Hospital, Lisbon, Portugal

2 CEDOC, Chronic Diseases Research Center, NOVA Medical School / Faculdade de Ciências Médicas, Universidade Nova de, Lisboa, Lisbon, Portugal

3 CINTESIS, Center for Research in Health Technologies and Information Systems, Porto, Portugal

4 QPS Netherlands, Hanzeplein 1, GZ Groningen, The Netherlands

5 Department of Respiratory Medicine & Allergology, Institute for Clinical Science, Skane University Hospital, Lund, Sweden

# References

[1]  Diamant Z, Boot JD, Virchow JC. Summing up 100 years of asthma. Respir Med 2007; 101: 378–388.

[2]  Wenzel SE. Asthma: defining of the persistent adult phenotypes. Lancet 2006; 368: 804–813.

[3]  Haldar P, Pavord ID, Shaw DE, et al. Cluster analysis and clinical asthma phenotypes. Am J Respir Crit Care Med 2008; 178: 218–224.

[4]  Moore WC, Meyers DA, Wenzel SE, et al. Identification of asthma phenotypes using cluster analysis in the Severe Asthma Research Program. Am J Respir Crit Care Med 2010; 181: 315–323.

[5]  Woodruff PG, Modrek B, Choy DF, et al. T-helper type 2-driven inflammation defines major subphenotypes of asthma. Am J Respir Crit Care Med 2009; 180: 388–395.

[6]  Wenzel SE. Asthma phenotypes: the evolution from clinical to molecular approaches. Nat Med 2012; 18: 716–725.

[7]  Holgate ST. Innate and adaptive immune responses in asthma. Nat Med 2012; 18: 673–683.

[8]  Zuiker RG, Ruddy MK, Morelli N, et al. Kinetics of TH2 biomarkers in sputum of asthmatics following inhaled allergen. Eur Clin Respir J 2015; 2: 28319.

[9]  Fahy JV. Type 2 inflammation in asthma—present in most, absent in many. Nat Rev Immunol 2015; 15: 57–65.

[10]  Diamant Z, Boot JD, Mantzouranis E, et al. Biomarkers in asthma and allergic rhinitis. Pulm Pharmacol Ther 2010; 23: 468–481.

[11]  Kaminsky DA. Systems biology approach for subtyping asthma; where do we stand now? Curr Opin Pulm Med 2014; 20: 17–22.

[12]  Wheelock CE, Goss VM, Balgoma D, et al. Application of 'omics technologies to biomarker discovery in inflammatory lung diseases. Eur Respir J 2013; 42: 802–825.

[13]  Shaw DE, Sousa AR, Fowler SJ, et al. Clinical and inflammatory characteristics of the European U-BIOPRED adult severe asthma cohort. Eur Respir J 2015; 46: 1308–1321.

[14]  Fleming L, Murray C, Bansal AT, et al. The burden of severe asthma in childhood and adolescence: results from the paediatric U-BIOPRED cohorts. Eur Respir J 2015; 46: 1322–1333.

[15]  Thamrin C, Taylor DR, Jones SL, et al. Variability of lung function predicts loss of asthma control following withdrawal of inhaled corticosteroid treatment. Thorax 2010; 65: 403–408.

[16] Busse WW. The relationship of airway hyperresponsiveness and airway inflammation: airway hyperresponsiveness in asthma: its measurement and clinical significance. Chest 2010; 138: 4S–10S.

[17] Sont JK, Willems LN, Bel EH, et al. Clinical control and histopathologic outcome of asthma when using airway hyperresponsiveness as an additional guide to long-term treatment. The AMPUL Study Group. Am J Respir Crit Care Med 1999; 159: 1043–1051.

[18] ATS/ERS recommendations for standardized procedures for the online and offline measurement of exhaled lower respiratory nitric oxide and nasal nitric oxide, (2005). . Am J Respir Crit Care Med 2005; : –., 171 , 912-930.

[19] Dweik RA, Boggs PB, Erzurum SC, et al. An official ATS clinical practice guideline: interpretation of exhaled nitric oxide levels (FENO) for clinical applications. Am J Respir Crit Care Med 2011; 184: 602–615.

[20] See KC, Christiani DC. Normal values and thresholds for the clinical interpretation of exhaled nitric oxide levels in the US general population: results from the National Health and Nutrition Examination Survey 2007–2010. Chest 2013; 143: 107–116.

[21] Dweik RA, Sorkness RL, Wenzel S, et al. Use of exhaled nitric oxide measurement to identify a reactive, at-risk phenotype among patients with asthma. Am J Respir Crit Care Med 2010; 181: 1033–1041.

[22] Petsky HL, Cates CJ, Li A, et al. Tailored interventions based on exhaled nitric oxide versus clinical symptoms for asthma in children and adults. Cochrane Database Syst Rev 2009: CD006340.

[23] Honkoop PJ, Loijmans RJ, Termeer EH, et al. Symptom- and fraction of exhaled nitric oxide-driven strategies for asthma control: a cluster-randomized trial in primary care. J Allergy Clin Immunol 2015; 135: 682–688 e611.

[24] Powell H, Murphy VE, Taylor DR, et al. Management of asthma in pregnancy guided by measurement of fraction of exhaled nitric oxide: a double-blind, randomised controlled trial. Lancet 2011; 378: 983–990.

[25] Roos AB, Mori M, Gronneberg R, et al. Elevated exhaled nitric oxide in allergen-provoked asthma is associated with airway epithelial iNOS. PLoS One 2014; 9: e90018.

[26] Teague WG. Exhaled nitric oxide in wheezy infants: a marker of inflammation determined by airways acidification and S-nitrosothiol degradation? J Allergy Clin Immunol 2010; 125: 1235–1236.

[27] Szefler SJ, Wenzel S, Brown R, et al. Asthma outcomes: biomarkers. J Allergy Clin Immunol 2012; 129: S9–S23.

[28] Moore WC, Bleecker ER, Curran-Everett D, et al. Characterization of the severe asthma phenotype by the National Heart, Lung, and Blood Institute's Severe Asthma Research Program. J Allergy Clin Immunol 2007; 119: 405–413.

[29]   Paraskakis E, Vergadi E, Chatzimichael A, et al. The role of flow-independent exhaled nitric oxide parameters in the assessment of airway diseases. Curr Top Med Chem 2015. (Epub ahead of print)

[30]   Robroeks CM, van de Kant KD, Jobsis Q, et al. Exhaled nitric oxide and biomarkers in exhaled breath condensate indicate the presence, severity and control of childhood asthma. Clin Exp Allergy 2007; 37: 1303–1311.

[31]   Cavaleiro Rufo J, Madureira J, Oliveira Fernandes E, et al. Volatile organic compounds in asthma diagnosis: a systematic review and meta-analysis. Allergy 2016; 71: 175–88.

[32]   Paredi P, Kharitonov SA, Barnes PJ. Faster rise of exhaled breath temperature in asthma: a novel marker of airway inflammation? Am J Respir Crit Care Med 2002; 165: 181–184.

[33]   Leonardi S, Cuppari C, Lanzafame A, et al. Exhaled breath temperature in asthmatic children. J Biol Regul Homeost Agents 2015; 29: 47–54.

[34]   Popov TA, Dunev S, Kralimarkova TZ, et al. Evaluation of a simple, potentially individual device for exhaled breath temperature measurement. Respir Med 2007; 101: 2044–2050.

[35]   Navratil M, Plavec D, Erceg D, et al. Urates in exhaled breath condensate as a biomarker of control in childhood asthma. J Asthma 2015; 52: 437–446.

[36]   Hamill L, Ferris K, Kapande K, et al. Exhaled breath temperature measurement and asthma control in children prescribed inhaled corticosteroids: a cross sectional study. Pediatr Pulmonol 2016; 51: 13–21.

[37]   Crespo Lessmann A, Giner J, Torrego A, et al. Usefulness of the exhaled breath temperature plateau in asthma patients. Respiration 2015; 90: 111–117.

[38]   Couto M, Santos P, Silva D, et al. Exhaled breath temperature in elite swimmers: the effects of a training session in adolescents with or without asthma. Pediatr Allergy Immunol 2015; 26: 564–570.

[39]   Bijnens E, Pieters N, Dewitte H, et al. Host and environmental predictors of exhaled breath temperature in the elderly. BMC Public Health 2013; 13: 1226.

[40]   Horvath I, Hunt J, Barnes PJ, et al. Exhaled breath condensate: methodological recommendations and unresolved questions. Eur Respir J 2005; 26: 523–548.

[41]   Teng Y, Sun P, Zhang J, et al. Hydrogen peroxide in exhaled breath condensate in patients with asthma: a promising biomarker? Chest 2011; 140: 108–116.

[42]   Thomas PS, Lowe AJ, Samarasinghe P, et al. Exhaled breath condensate in pediatric asthma: promising new advance or pouring cold water on a lot of hot air? a systematic review. Pediatr Pulmonol 2013; 48: 419–442.

[43] Barreto M, Villa MP, Olita C, et al. 8-Isoprostane in exhaled breath condensate and exercise-induced bronchoconstriction in asthmatic children and adolescents. Chest 2009; 135: 66–73.

[44] Baraldi E, Carraro S, Alinovi R, et al. Cysteinyl leukotrienes and 8-isoprostane in exhaled breath condensate of children with asthma exacerbations. Thorax 2003; 58: 505–509.

[45] Biernacki WA, Kharitonov SA, Biernacka HM, et al. Effect of montelukast on exhaled leukotrienes and quality of life in asthmatic patients. Chest 2005; 128: 1958–1963.

[46] Montuschi P, Martello S, Felli M, et al. Liquid chromatography/mass spectrometry analysis of exhaled leukotriene B4 in asthmatic children. Respir Res 2005; 6: 119.

[47] Carraro S, Corradi M, Zanconato S, et al. Exhaled breath condensate cysteinyl leukotrienes are increased in children with exercise-induced bronchoconstriction. J Allergy Clin Immunol 2005; 115: 764–770.

[48] Robroeks CM, van Vliet D, Jobsis Q, et al. Prediction of asthma exacerbations in children: results of a one-year prospective study. Clin Exp Allergy 2012; 42: 792–798.

[49] Loukides S, Kontogianni K, Hillas G, et al. Exhaled breath condensate in asthma: from bench to bedside. Curr Med Chem 2011; 18: 1432–1443.

[50] Paget-Brown AO, Ngamtrakulpanit L, Smith A, et al. Normative data for pH of exhaled breath condensate. Chest 2006; 129: 426–430.

[51] Shin YS, Liu JN, Kim JH, et al. The impact of asthma control on salivary cortisol level in adult asthmatics. Allergy Asthma Immunol Res 2014; 6: 463–466.

[52] Little FF, Delgado DM, Wexler PJ, et al. Salivary inflammatory mediator profiling and correlation to clinical disease markers in asthma. PLoS One 2014; 9: e84449.

[53] Bentur L, Mansour Y, Brik R, et al. Salivary oxidative stress in children during acute asthmatic attack and during remission. Respir Med 2006; 100: 1195–1201.

[54] Watanabe M, Sano H, Tomita K, et al. A nocturnal decline of salivary pH associated with airway hyperresponsiveness in asthma. J Med Invest 2010; 57: 260–269.

[55] Rabinovitch N, Reisdorph N, Silveira L, et al. Urinary leukotriene E(4) levels identify children with tobacco smoke exposure at risk for asthma exacerbation. J Allergy Clin Immunol 2011; 128: 323–327.

[56] Bochenek G, Kuschill-Dziurda J, Szafraniec K, et al. Certain subphenotypes of aspirin-exacerbated respiratory disease distinguished by latent class analysis. J Allergy Clin Immunol 2014; 133: 98–103 e101-106.

[57] Rabinovitch N, Zhang L, Gelfand EW. Urine leukotriene E4 levels are associated with decreased pulmonary function in children with persistent airway obstruction. J Allergy Clin Immunol 2006; 118: 635–640.

[58]   Misso NL, Aggarwal S, Phelps S, et al. Urinary leukotriene E4 and 9 alpha, 11 beta-prostaglandin F concentrations in mild, moderate and severe asthma, and in healthy subjects. Clin Exp Allergy 2004; 34: 624–631.

[59]   Cowan DC, Taylor DR, Peterson LE, et al. Biomarker-based asthma phenotypes of corticosteroid response. J Allergy Clin Immunol 2015; 135: 877–883 e871.

[60]   Wagener AH, Yick CY, Brinkman P, et al. Toward composite molecular signatures in the phenotyping of asthma. Ann Am Thorac Soc 2013; 10 Suppl: S197–S205.

[61]   Gomes-Alves P, Imrie M, Gray RD, et al. SELDI-TOF biomarker signatures for cystic fibrosis, asthma and chronic obstructive pulmonary disease. Clin Biochem 2010; 43: 168–177.

[62]   Ibrahim B, Marsden P, Smith JA, et al. Breath metabolomic profiling by nuclear magnetic resonance spectroscopy in asthma. Allergy 2013; 68: 1050–1056.

[63]   Carraro S, Giordano G, Reniero F, et al. Asthma severity in childhood and metabolomic profiling of breath condensate. Allergy 2013; 68: 110–117.

[64]   Rock F, Barsan N, Weimar U. Electronic nose: current status and future trends. Chem Rev 2008; 108: 705–725.

[65]   Fens N, van der Schee MP, Brinkman P, et al. Exhaled breath analysis by electronic nose in airways disease. Established issues and key questions. Clin Exp Allergy 2013; 43: 705–715.

[66]   van der Schee MP, Palmay R, Cowan JO, et al. Predicting steroid responsiveness in patients with asthma using exhaled breath profiling. Clin Exp Allergy 2013; 43: 1217–1225.

[67]   Carraro S, Rezzi S, Reniero F, et al. Metabolomics applied to exhaled breath condensate in childhood asthma. Am J Respir Crit Care Med 2007; 175: 986–990.

[68]   Motta A, Paris D, D'Amato M, et al. NMR metabolomic analysis of exhaled breath condensate of asthmatic patients at two different temperatures. J Proteome Res 2014; 13: 6107–6120.

[69]   Saude EJ, Skappak CD, Regush S, et al. Metabolomic profiling of asthma: diagnostic utility of urine nuclear magnetic resonance spectroscopy. J Allergy Clin Immunol 2011; 127: 757–764 e751–756.

[70]   Loureiro CC, Duarte IF, Gomes J, et al. Urinary metabolomic changes as a predictive biomarker of asthma exacerbation. J Allergy Clin Immunol 2014; 133: 261–263 e261–265.

[71]   Adamko DJ, Nair P, Mayers I, et al. Metabolomic profiling of asthma and chronic obstructive pulmonary disease: A pilot study differentiating diseases. J Allergy Clin Immunol 2015; 136: 571–580 e573.

[72] Pinkerton M, Chinchilli V, Banta E, et al. Differential expression of microRNAs in exhaled breath condensates of patients with asthma, patients with chronic obstructive pulmonary disease, and healthy adults. J Allergy Clin Immunol 2013; 132: 217–219.

[73] Bloemen K, Van Den Heuvel R, Govarts E, et al. A new approach to study exhaled proteins as potential biomarkers for asthma. Clin Exp Allergy 2011; 41: 346–356.

[74] Willis JC, Lord GM. Immune biomarkers: the promises and pitfalls of personalized medicine. Nat Rev Immunol 2015; 15: 323–329.

[75] Leaker BR, Nicholson GC, Ali FY, et al. Bronchoabsorption; a novel bronchoscopic technique to improve biomarker sampling of the airway. Respir Res 2015; 16: 102.

[76] Bakakos P, Schleich F, Alchanatis M, et al. Induced sputum in asthma: from bench to bedside. Curr Med Chem 2011; 18: 1415–1422.

[77] Petsky HL, Cates CJ, Lasserson TJ, et al. A systematic review and meta-analysis: tailoring asthma treatment on eosinophilic markers (exhaled nitric oxide or sputum eosinophils). Thorax 2012; 67: 199–208.

[78] Green RH, Brightling CE, McKenna S, et al. Asthma exacerbations and sputum eosinophil counts: a randomised controlled trial. Lancet 2002; 360: 1715–1721.

[79] Fleming L, Wilson N, Regamey N, et al. Use of sputum eosinophil counts to guide management in children with severe asthma. Thorax 2012; 67: 193–198.

[80] Fleming L, Tsartsali L, Wilson N, et al. Sputum inflammatory phenotypes are not stable in children with asthma. Thorax 2012; 67: 675–681.

[81] Baines KJ, Simpson JL, Wood LG, et al. Transcriptional phenotypes of asthma defined by gene expression profiling of induced sputum samples. J Allergy Clin Immunol 2011; 127: 153–160, 160 e151–159.

[82] Arron JR, Choy DF, Scheerens H, et al. Noninvasive biomarkers that predict treatment benefit from biologic therapies in asthma. Ann Am Thorac Soc 2013; 10 Suppl: S206–S213.

[83] Wagener AH, de Nijs SB, Lutter R, et al. External validation of blood eosinophils, FE(NO) and serum periostin as surrogates for sputum eosinophils in asthma. Thorax 2015; 70: 115–120.

[84] Kim MA, Izuhara K, Ohta S, et al. Association of serum periostin with aspirin-exacerbated respiratory disease. Ann Allergy Asthma Immunol 2014; 113: 314–320.

[85] Hanania NA, Noonan M, Corren J, et al. Lebrikizumab in moderate-to-severe asthma: pooled data from two randomised placebo-controlled studies. Thorax 2015; 70: 748–756.

[86] Fajt ML, Wenzel SE. Asthma phenotypes and the use of biologic medications in asthma and allergic disease: the next steps toward personalized care. J Allergy Clin Immunol 2015; 135: 299–310; quiz 311.

[87] Bhakta NR, Solberg OD, Nguyen CP, et al. A qPCR-based metric of Th2 airway inflammation in asthma. Clin Transl Allergy 2013; 3: 24.

[88] Good JT, Jr., Kolakowski CA, Groshong SD, et al. Refractory asthma: importance of bronchoscopy to identify phenotypes and direct therapy. Chest 2012; 141: 599–606.

# 7

# Monitoring Asthma in Childhood: Still a Challenge

Patricia W. Garcia-Marcos,
Manuel Sanchez-Solis and Luis Garcia-Marcos

### Abstract

Asthma monitoring should be focused on patient outcomes and goals. Using clinical practice tools allows the clinicians to detect problems such as bad adherence to maintenance therapy, comorbidities, or other external reason for a poorly controlled asthma. To succeed in the process of asthma control, doctors need the participation of the family. Because such educational task requires good agreement between patient environment and doctor, it might be difficult to achieve. However, it is worth to implement because the benefit is a life without symptoms of asthma with a minimum medication.

**Keywords:** Noncontrolled asthma, management, adherence, children, monitoring

## 1. Introduction

Asthma is the most common chronic disease in childhood. It is clinically characterized by episodes of wheezing, dyspnea, cough, and chest tightness with different grades of severity. Most patients are free of symptoms between these episodes or "attacks," either because asthma is well controlled or because it is the natural course of the disease [1, 2]. Although this episodic nature can make patients, parents, and health care professionals interpret asthma as an acute or intermittent disease when episodes are infrequent, asthma is in fact a chronic disease characterized by ongoing inflammation of the airway mucosa, even when the patient is asymptomatic. Successful long-term management of the disease therefore requires careful follow-up and monitoring. However, guidelines on asthma do not provide recommendations that are unanimous [3].

An overwhelming number of 334 million people suffer from asthma worldwide. The most recent global survey calculates that 14% of children experience asthma symptoms [4]. It is difficult to quantify the global economic burden of asthma, but estimates are high enough to encourage active interventions. The indirect costs for children, which are not insignificant, include school Absenteeism; whereas the direct costs are even larger, and include costs from hospitalization, emergency department (ED) visits, unscheduled doctor or nurse visits, and medication. Controlled asthma imposes far less of an economic burden. Strategies towards improving access and adherence to evidence-based therapies are, therefore, likely to be effective in reducing the economic burden of asthma [3, 5]. One of the basics for this goal in developed countries, where access to care and medication is already guaranteed, would be to achieve and maintain asthma control with the least possible medication [6]. In keeping with this paradigm, the concept of problematic severe asthma has been used to describe children who have uncontrolled asthma despite being prescribed multiple controller therapies, including inhaled corticosteroids (ICS), long-acting beta-agonists (LABA), and leukotriene receptor antagonists (LTRA). However, only a minority of children with uncontrolled or problematic severe asthma have true therapy-resistant asthma [7, 8]. Most children with poorly controlled asthma can be in fact well controlled by addressing the basics of asthma management, including patient and parent education, achieving and maintaining correct inhalation technique, avoiding exposure to relevant allergens and irritants, identifying and treating comorbidities, and, perhaps most importantly, identifying poor adherence and helping patients and parents to improve it.

This chapter reviews the recommendations on how to monitor asthma during childhood, focusing on patient outcomes and goals. Using some clinical tools will allow the clinicians to detect situations, such as poor adherence to maintenance therapy, comorbidities, or other external reasons for uncontrolled asthma. To reach a high degree of success, the participation of the whole family in the process of asthma control is needed. Such educational task requires good agreement between the patient, parents, and the health care professionals, which may be difficult to achieve. Despite these difficulties, it is worthwhile to try and implement, as the benefit is a good quality of life for the patient with asthma. We will also search in this chapter for evidence on reliable direct instruments that may be helpful to achieve asthma control.

## 2. Pillars of asthma management

Comprehensive asthma management includes reviewing the following items: adherence to daily controller therapy, teaching and maintaining proper inhalation technique, controlling exposure to main triggers, reconfirming the diagnosis of asthma, and excluding other causes of respiratory symptoms or comorbidities [9]. Addressing these pillars of asthma diligently management will help to ensure asthma control in most cases, without the need of increasing medication [10].

We discuss each of these pillars of asthma management throughout this chapter, but first, we discuss the components of an asthma follow-up and monitoring program.

## 2.1. Asthma follow-up

### 2.1.1. How, when, and who?

Primary care practitioners are usually the first to encounter asthma symptoms in children. Typically, they prescribe medication after a concise education session during a short visit. Parents are encouraged to use the medication at home as long as the child is symptomatic and to come back if they encounter problems in managing the child's symptoms. This results in a relatively high proportion of unscheduled visits [11]. In addition, many parents feel that they are expected to manage their child's asthma on their own [12]. This approach has been characterized as a "reactive" follow-up strategy of asthma [11] and appears to be common in primary care, even though it does not follow national and international guidelines for the management of asthma in children.

The alternative approach to asthma management can be characterized as a proactive approach, following the pillars of asthma management as outlined in international guidelines. This approach includes scheduled follow-up visits, providing repeated tailored education, agreement on treatment goals and methods, ensuring optimal inhalation technique, and addressing patients' and parents' beliefs and concerns; which has shown to help to improve asthma control [13, 14]. This model of management is more common in secondary care centers. The evidence of its effectiveness makes follow-up and monitoring key components of successful asthma management in children [15].

After establishing that a scheduled follow-up plan is more effective, other aspects of these visits, such as who will monitor these patients and how often, need to be determined. One of the proposed models implicates the asthma nurse. This specifically trained health professional is of great importance in a close and time-consuming management. The main role of the asthma nurse is to provide reinforcement of the patient's and parents' knowledge of the disease, to promote adherence to the management plan, to check the inhalation technique, and to adjust the medication according to symptoms of asthma [10]. In fact, the recent evidence suggests that adults with selected chronic diseases can be successfully managed only by nurses [16]. The outpatient management of childhood asthma by asthma nurses has been compared to the one led by pediatricians. Childhood asthma was proven to be successfully managed by an asthma nurse, in close collaboration with a pediatrician [10].

Educational asthma programs are definitely improved if an asthma nurse is included in the team. A follow-up schedule with alternate follow-up visits by asthma nurses and pediatricians implies a follow-up visit every 3 months. Additional follow-up visits can be planned individually if needed, according to the criteria of the pediatrician or of the asthma nurse [10]. Other members of the team would include nutritionists, psychologists, or physiotherapists, when comorbidities are detected.

### 2.1.2. What to monitor?

### 2.1.2.1. Impact of symptoms on life

Symptoms presented since the last visit is the first approach to define asthma control. Although most guidelines provide control scores to establish a degree of asthma control, it is difficult to turn this evaluation into a number because asthma control is a multidimensional concept [6]. The scores of questionnaires on asthma control have several limitations. They only provide information about the situation in the preceding 4 weeks. This makes asthma control scores much variable over time and show little concordance with the risk of exacerbations [17, 18], which is one of the main issues to consider during asthma monitoring. Quality-of-life instruments should help in the task of delimiting asthma control. They share some limitations with asthma scores: children with similar degrees of asthma control or lung function impairment differ considerably in their quality-of-life questionnaire scores, which is partly explained by psychological factors influencing their disease concept [19, 20]. The current consensus is that these instruments provide independent additional information on disease status, complementing other monitoring instruments [19–21].

A way of defining the risk of asthma exacerbation could be the use of reliever medication. However, this information seems to be independent from the risk of exacerbations or other data, such as lung function or inflammation [22]. In fact, the degree of airway narrowing that is perceived as dyspnea of enough severity to prompt the use of reliever medication varies considerably between individuals [23]. Furthermore, other psychological factors influencing this perception can play an important role. Thus, the use of reliever medication is not a reliable way of measuring asthma control.

A practical clinical approach is to review symptoms during follow-up and to consider other factors of the disease. Patients and parents are most concerned about the impact of the disease on daily life [6]. The three things children worry about their asthma control are the need of daily medication, having severe asthma attacks, and not being able to engage in sports and play [24–26]. Follow-up visits should take this into account, starting the clinical interview focusing on patients' outcomes (exacerbations, visits to the ED or hospital admissions; sports limitations or other daily limitations; identified or nonidentified triggers; etc.) and discussing the use of medication, not only the rescue medication but also, most importantly, the daily medication [6].

### 2.1.2.2. Lung function

The latest asthma guidelines do not include lung function as a main way of monitoring asthma control [27–29]. There are different ways of measuring lung function; but the usefulness of lung function measurements in the follow-up of asthma has not been firmly established [1].

The main two ways of studying lung function are measuring forced expiratory volume in one second ($FEV_1$) and measuring its reversibility after administration of a bronchodilator [30]. Reduced lung function is an independent risk factor for future asthma exacerbations [31]. $FEV_1$ levels have shown to improve considerably during treatment with ICS. Normal $FEV_1$

levels are being found in most children with mild-to-moderate asthma, rendering bronchodilator reversibility negative [32]. As a practical approach, most children with stable, controlled asthma and good adherence to ICS therapy have normal values of $FEV_1$ [32–34]. Reduced lung function in asthma is only found when they are measured at the time when asthma symptoms are present, or when adherence to ICS is not achieved [30].

Positive bronchodilator response (PBDR), even in patients with $FEV_1$ >80%, could be another way of monitoring asthma. Children with PBDR have been shown to suffer from poorly controlled asthma, with increased beta2 agonist use, nocturnal symptoms, and exercise limitation [35]. Furthermore, children with consistent PBDR, defined as an increase of 12% or greater in basal $FEV_1$ in every scheduled visit, had more unscheduled Visits, required more systemic corticosteroids, had more nocturnal awakenings, and missed more school days [36]. However, no study has assessed whether the follow-up that includes PBDR helps to better control asthma when compared to the standard follow-up.

Peak expiratory flow (PEF) values are more effort dependent than $FEV_1$. Neither isolated PEF measurements nor home PEF monitoring has been demonstrated to be useful in asthma monitoring, because they are not sufficiently sensitive or reliable to monitor airway obstruction [37–39].

Whether it is possible to recognize reduced lung function relying only on history and physical examination during follow-up and whether lung function measurements are able to detect asthma risk of exacerbation with enough anticipation are yet to be answered. In fact, previous studies have shown that it is possible to predict reduced lung function or increased risk of exacerbation, without requiring objective measurements [40].

Finally, one could think that lung function monitoring would help to improve patients' and parents' adherence and, therefore, to improve asthma control. However, studies testing this hypothesis have failed to support it [38, 39].

In summary, the usefulness of lung function monitoring in asthma management is limited. It may be useful during the follow-up when a diagnosis confirmation is needed or when poorly controlled asthma is suspected [6], mainly in poor perceivers.

### 2.1.2.3. Airway inflammation

Exhaled nitric oxide (FeNO) has been proposed as a noninvasive marker of underlying airway inflammation. FeNO values differ widely among healthy children, which make it difficult to establish reference values. Therefore, FeNO measurement does not appear to be a reliable instrument in asthma diagnosis [41]. FeNO measurements have been thoroughly studied as a monitoring instrument in asthma. Studies in children comparing a standard follow-up with a FeNO-monitored one have shown no evidence of superiority of the FeNO monitoring approach in predicting asthma exacerbation or improving asthma symptoms, while it has been related to higher daily dose of ICS [42]. Similar results are obtained when using sputum eosinophil counts to monitor asthma [6]. As they do not seem to provide further information on asthma control and could favor a step-up of ICS, airway inflammation monitoring should not be recommended in clinical practice to follow-up asthma control.

## 2.1.3. Patient-centered care and self-management concept

There is a wide consensus among experts that getting the basics right in asthma management helps to control the disease in most children with uncontrolled or problematic severe asthma [9]. This starts with a patient-centered follow-up. The self-management concept is probably the best expression of this patient-focused management.

Self-management means that the patient (or in the case of children, the patient and parents) has the ability to manage symptoms, recognize their possible causes and consequences, and can institute appropriate treatment, following the plan previously agreed with the health care professional. This active role from patient/parents is needed to support the pillars of well-controlled asthma: the parents and the patient should know how to use reliever medication properly, recognize and manage exacerbations, avoid or control known triggers, and agree with the decision of giving daily controller medication to their child [43].

Patients and their parents have certain perceptions of their illness and medication, which strongly determine their self-management behavior [25]. These beliefs can be modified by good asthma education [14]. A prerequisite for successful asthma education is to establish an effective patient–physician partnership through the use of appropriate communication skills. However, this is difficult to achieve, because most doctors have not been trained in communication techniques required for this patient-focused care. This consists of discussing illness and medication perceptions of the parents, shared decision making, and motivational interviewing. It has been shown that physicians trained in communication skills obtain better adherence and improve their patients' asthma control [43–46], as patients are more likely to take the steps necessary to improve their asthma control (if they are satisfied with the partnership) [47].

Compared to a doctor-centered consultation, a patient-focused follow-up interview has some differences: approaches must be based on equality, by listening to patients' concerns and preferences showing genuine interest, and offering medical advice based on patients' preferences. This interview should finally arrive to an agreed management plan [48, 49]. Nowadays, asthma guidelines strongly recommend such tailored management plans, as a way of improving asthma control [27]. During follow-up, this agreed plan needs to be reviewed and adapted when necessary. In this sense, starting the follow-up interview letting the patient or their parents talk about their concerns since the last visit, is a good way of reinforcing patient–physician partnership [43]. However, soliciting the patient's agenda (patients' worries and questions) has only limited effects on health outcomes by itself. The beneficial effects of patient-centered care are more pronounced when it includes facilitation of the patient to ask questions, to take the initiative, to provide information, and to be actively involved in controlling the consultation and in disease management [50]. Patients are more forthcoming with questions, opinions, concerns, and preferences when the physician uses partnership building, such as direct question about patient's views and open-ended questions and avoiding interruptions. The process of giving medical advice comprises discussing available options and supported deliberation. After taking in consideration both the medical evidence and the patient's perspective, the deliberation should come to certain point where one of the options appears to be the best possible strategy. Sometimes, patients and parents need time to consider this, discuss it at home, and then come back for a further round of deliberations. The final result of this process of negotiation is a mutually agreed solution, which the patient and parents are happy to embrace and follow [47].

In summary, what patients need for effective self-management is that the medical visit provides understanding of the disease state, the treatment options, the need for lifestyle changes, the need for daily medication, and the willingness to consider changes in the management. These strategies supported on patient concerns and preferences and shared decision making, will cover the patient needs [47]. **Figure 1** shows the process of patient-focused visit and self-management.

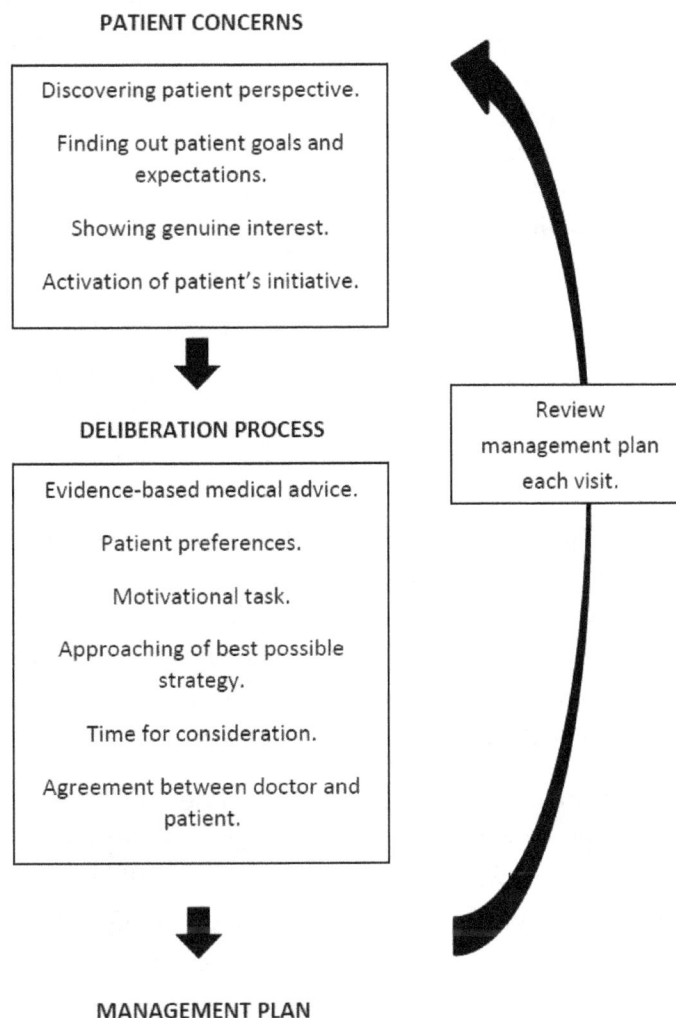

**PATIENT CONCERNS**

Discovering patient perspective.

Finding out patient goals and expectations.

Showing genuine interest.

Activation of patient's initiative.

**DELIBERATION PROCESS**

Evidence-based medical advice.

Patient preferences.

Motivational task.

Approaching of best possible strategy.

Time for consideration.

Agreement between doctor and patient.

Review management plan each visit.

**MANAGEMENT PLAN**

**Figure 1.** Process of the patient-focused visit and self-management.

## 2.2. Adherence to daily therapy

Adherence to daily medication is one of the pillars of successful asthma management. Studies reveal that children with asthma only take between 30% and 70% of the prescribed doses [51]. Poor adherence appears to be the main reason why the patient remains symptomatic despite treatment with ICS [9, 10]. Adherence to controller medication has been strongly linked with better asthma outcomes, making adherence a modifiable factor and a potential target for reducing economic burden of asthma [5]. Adherence should be over 75% of the prescribed doses to influence clinical outcomes [52]. In this section, we will discuss the different kinds of adherence barriers, how to measure them, and how we should manage them.

### 2.2.1. Adherence barriers

A useful model for daily practice divides nonadherence into four categories [53]:

- Unwitting nonadherence: When patients misunderstand medical indications/advice. This usually occurs when there has been a lack of information and can be addressed through proper education. This adherence barrier should be detected by interviewing the parents about the prescribed treatment (what inhalator should be taken, when, and why).

  It could be thought that adherence is directly related to education on the asthma disease, but this is not the case. Consistent evidence shows that adherence to daily medication is not significantly related to knowledge about asthma; therefore, this is neither the only nor the main barrier for asthma control, but it should always be investigated during follow-up [54].

- Intentional nonadherence: This occurs when parental or patient illness perceptions or medication beliefs are in conflict with the medical advice. These cognitions have consistently proved to be a strong determinant of adherence [13, 50, 53]. Illness perceptions are built from earlier experiences and from information collected from the media and people from closer social circles. This modulates their view of necessity for treatment. For example, it is common that a patient with episodic attacks, who is asymptomatic in between attacks, perceives asthma as an intermittent disease for which daily medication is not necessary. However, if parents understand that asthma is a chronic condition with ongoing inflammation even when asymptomatic, they are more likely to recognize daily medication as a way of preventing asthma attacks. On the other hand, fear of ICS side effects could be the reason for adherence resistance [54].

When confronted with poor adherence to the recommendation to give daily ICS, many physicians respond by repeating asthma education and re-emphasizing the importance of daily controller medication. However, as unwitting nonadherence is a minor cause of nonadherence [54], this approach is likely to be ineffective [55, 56]. Dealing with patients' and parents' perceptions is sometimes difficult, but eliciting them during follow-up visits is important to detect poor adherence. After illness or medication beliefs have been explored in a supportive and nonjudgmental way, it could be discovered that they do not correspond to the medical model of asthma. At this point, the physician's task is to discuss these perceptions from the empathy and the genuine interest of the patient's and parents' concerns. Showing this predisposition to listen has been shown to increase patient's satisfaction, which is directly related to their adherence [57]. Although these communication skills require an effort, they are very effective when used during the deliberating process in self-management, and normally an agreement is achieved, resulting in both parts being satisfied with the decision made [47, 57]. This is one of the keys of intentional adherence maintenance, as shaping perception and beliefs have demonstrated to help to a good asthma control [14].

- Unplanned nonadherence: Even if patients have agreed to follow daily ICS, a number of barriers can prevent them from doing so, causing what is called "unplanned" nonadherence. Examples include the lack of family routines, the time for medication competing with important activities on the child's schedule, child raising issues, and social or family complex environment (economic issues, parental psychiatric illnesses, etc.). A recent surprising finding was that excessive responsibility for medication taking was being given to the child at a relatively young age, without proper parental supervision. Self-management should not be expected until 12 years of age [51].

Incorporating behavioral components into educational efforts to improve adherence increases their potential efficacy. Home visits may be an efficient method to collect information on such barriers, specially in patients with severe asthma. It is important to listen to patient's preferences and try to look for some room in the schedule in which remembering and using the daily medication is easy for him/her [54]. All these specifically tailored interventions could be successful and cost-effective; but until now, studies on this subject have just shown to achieve a temporary adherence improvement [58].

- Incorrect inhalation technique: Although it is not the most frequent adherence barrier [9], many patients use their inhaler device incorrectly. The first step for a successful inhalation technique is an adequate device prescription. After this, comprehensive inhaling instructions must be provided [59]. From all ways of checking inhalation technique, the patient-demonstrated technique appears to be the most effective, at least when speaking of metered dose inhaler (MDI) [59]. In the case of MDIs, it is important that the patient or parent actually demonstrates the maneuver himself/herself and to adjust the technique afterwards, if required. Not shaking the canister at the beginning of the maneuver tends to be the most common error in the inhalation technique of patients using an MDI device. On the other hand, patients using a dry powder inhaler (DPI) prepare their inhaler device correctly, but they inhale inadequately through the device, without sufficient peak inspiratory flow (PIF), which is necessary to release medication from the device. Therefore, before prescribing a DPI, it is essential to consider whether the patient will be able to do it forcefully and deeply enough. An inspiration whistle can be used for this purpose, ensuring that the patient is able to achieve a sufficient PIF. It is important to note, however, that sufficient PIF alone is not enough to guarantee for an adequate drug delivery from a DPI [60]. Poor inhalation technique is more frequent in newly referred children using a DPI than in children using an MDI/s device [56]; but there are no significant differences in the correct inhalation technique for the different inhaler devices, when all patients receive repeated inhalation instructions. This means that inhaling technique instructions would not be enough if provided once at the time of prescription. Repeating inhaling instructions can improve correct technique up to 30% [59].

Although the classification in these types of nonadherence is useful from a daily practice point of view, adherence is a complex behavioral process influenced by more interacting conscious and unconscious factors. Therefore, all effective interventions improving adherence to long-term therapies are complex and multidimensional [55]. **Table 1** summarizes patterns of nonadherence and how to manage them.

| Patterns of adherence barrier | Investigate for | How to manage them |
|---|---|---|
| Unwitting non-adherence | • Misunderstanding of medical indications/advice | • Education |
| Intentional non-adherence | • Illness perceptions<br><br>Medication beliefs | • Discussing patient/parents' perceptions<br>• Expressing genuine interest<br>• Partnership between physician and patient/parents<br>• Concordance on treatment and patient/parents' goals<br>• Stressing importance of daily ICS adherence<br>• Self-management |
| Unplanned non-adherence | • Forgetting doses<br>• Child-raising issues<br><br>• Economic issues<br>• Parental psychiatric illnesses<br>• Excess of responsibility relaying on the child | • Establish easy routines<br>• Avoid complicated treatment regimens<br>• Home supervision<br><br>• Child self-management achieved gradually |
| Incorrect inhalation technique | • Check technique<br><br>• Check PIF for DPI device | • Choose suitable device<br>• Provide patient demonstrated technique<br>• Repeat training |

PIF, peak inspiratory flow; DPI, dry powder inhaler.

**Table 1.** Patterns of nonadherence and how to manage them.

A proposed formula to achieve the best adherence to maintenance medication in asthma is the result of a medical team providing evidence-based education, tailored to the patient's (and parents') context, self-management education provided in an organized and repeated way (scheduled follow-up visits), and coupled with goal setting and other behavioral approaches[57].

## 2.2.2. Adherence measurements

Apart from self-reporting during the clinical interview, there are other ways of measuring adherence. More reliable ways could be used when poor adherence is suspected. The Medication Adherence Rating Scale (MARS) is one example. In this case, the patient responds to 10 items of the questionnaire and chooses the answer that best describes their behavior or attitude toward their medication during the past week [61]. This scale has been used previously to assess ICS adherence in adults with asthma [62]. In children, it has only been used to assess medication adherence in other chronic diseases, including pills taking [63]. However, later research has shown that its reliability is not sufficient [64].

Nowadays, validated electronically measured adherence with smart inhalers that register date and time of each ICS actuation is universally accepted to be the most reliable way of measuring adherence [61, 65]. Its use is limited by the high cost of the device, but it is particularly useful with those parents and patients who are not aware of their poor adherence, or in those cases in which the physician is not able to detect whether poor adherence is the problem for uncontrolled asthma.

# Author details

Patricia W. Garcia-Marcos[1], Manuel Sanchez-Solis[1,2] and Luis Garcia-Marcos[1,2*]

*Address all correspondence to: lgmarcos@um.es

1 Pulmonology and Allergy Units, Arrixaca Children's University Hospital, University of Murcia, Spain

2 IMIB Bioresearch Institute, Murcia, Spain

# References

[1] Blanco-Quiros A. Enfermedades Alergicas. Cruz. Tratado de Pediatria. 11 ed. Madrid: Panamericana; 2014. p. 582–584. ISBN: 978-84-9835-725-7

[2] Garcia-Marcos L, Nieto-Garcia A. Asma. Cruz. Tratado de Pediatria. 11 ed. Madrid: Panamericana; 2014. p. 591–596. ISBN: 978-84-9835-725-7

[3] Boluyt N, Rottier BL, de Jongste JC, Riemsma R, Vrijlandt EJ, Brand PL. Assessment of controversial pediatric asthma management options using GRADE. Pediatrics 2012; 130:e658–e668. DOI: 10.1542/peds.2011-3559

[4] Marks G, Pearce N, Strachan D, Asher I. The Global Asthma Report. Auckland: Global Asthma Network; 2014: p. 16–22. ISBN 978-0-473-29125-9

[5] Sadatsafavi M, FitzGerald JM. The Global Asthma Report. 2014. p. 36–38. ISBN 978-0-473-29125-9

[6] Brand PL. The clinician's guide on monitoring children with asthma. Paediatr Respir Rev 2013; 14:119–125. DOI: 10.1016/j.prrv.2012.07.001

[7] Bush A, Saglani S. Management of severe asthma in children. Lancet 2010; 376:814–825. DOI: 10.1016/S0140-6736(10)61054-9

[8] Hedlin G, Bush A, Lødrup Carlsen K, Wennergren G, De Benedictis FM, Melén E, et al. Problematic severe asthma in children, not one problem but many: a GA2LEN initiative. Eur Respir J 2010; 36:196–201. DOI: 10.1183/09031936.00104809

[9] de Groot EP, Kreggemeijer WJ, Brand PL. Getting the basics right resolves most cases of uncontrolled and problematic asthma. Acta Paediatr 2015; 104:916–921. DOI: 10.1111/apa.13059

[10] Kamps AW[1], Brand PL, Kimpen JL, Maillé AR, Overgoor-van de Groes AW, van Helsdingen-Peek LC, et al. Outpatient management of childhood asthma by paediatrician or asthma nurse: randomised controlled study with one year follow up. Thorax 2003; 58:968–973.

[11] Klok T, Kaptein AA, Duiverman E, Oldenhof FS, Brand PL. General practitioners' prescribing behaviour as a determinant of poor persistence with inhaled corticosteroids in children with respiratory symptoms: mixed methods study. BMJ Open 2013; 3:1–8. DOI: 10.1136/bmjopen-2012-002310

[12] Klok T, Brand PL, Bomhof-Roordink H, Duiverman EJ, Kaptein AA. Parental illness perceptions and medication perceptions in childhood asthma, a focus group study. Acta Paediatr. 2011; 100:248–252. DOI: 10.1111/j.1651-2227.2010.02024.x

[13] Brouwer AF, Visser CA, Duiverman EJ, Roorda RJ, Brand PL. Is home spirometry useful in diagnosing asthma in children with nonspecific respiratory symptoms? Pediatr Pulmonol 2010; 45:326–332. DOI: 10.1002/ppul.21183

[14] Klok T, Brand PL, Bomhof-Roordink H, Duiverman EJ, Kaptein AA. Parental illness perceptions and medication perceptions in childhood asthma, a focus group study. Acta Paediatr 2011; 100:248–252. DOI: 10.1111/j.1651-2227.2010.02024

[15] Kuethe MC, Vaessen-Verberne AA, Bindels PJ, van Aalderen WM. Children with asthma on inhaled corticosteroids managed in general practice or by hospital paediatricians: is there a difference? Prim Care Respir J 2010; 19:62–67. DOI: 10.4104/pcrj.2009.00063

[16] Sharples LD, Edmunds J, Bilton D, Hollingworth W, Caine N, Keogan M, et al. A randomised controlled crossover trial of nurse practitioner versus doctor led outpatient care in a bronchiectasis clinic. Thorax 2002; 57:661–666.

[17] Koster ES, Raaijmakers JA, Vijverberg SJ, Koenderman L, Postma DS, Koppelman GH, et al. Limited agreement between current and long-term asthma control in children:

the PACMAN cohort study. Pediatr Allergy Immunol 2011; 22:776–783. DOI: 10.1111/j.1399-3038.2011.01188

[18] Wu AC, Tantisira K, Li L, Schuemann B, Weiss ST, Fuhlbrigge AL. Predictors of symptoms are different from predictors of severe exacerbations from asthma in children. Chest 2011; 140:100–107.

[19] Annett RD, Bender BG, Lapidus J, Duhamel TR, Lincoln A. Predicting children's quality of life in an asthma clinical trial: what do children's reports tell us? J Pediatr 2001; 139:854–861. DOI: 10.1067/mpd.2001.119444

[20] Goldbeck L, Koffmane K, Lecheler J, Thiessen K, Fegert JM. Disease severity, mental health, and quality of life of children and adolescents with asthma. Pediatr Pulmonol 2007; 42:15–22. 10.1002/ppul.20509

[21] Williams J, Williams K. Asthma-specific quality of life questionnaires in children: are they useful and feasible in routine clinical practice? Pediatr Pulmonol 2003; 35:114–118. DOI: 10.1002/ppul.10206

[22] Holt EW, Cook EF, Covar RA, Spahn J, Fuhlbrigge AL. Identifying the components of asthma health status in children with mild to moderate asthma. J Allergy Clin Immunol 2008; 121:1175–1180. DOI: 10.1016/j.jaci.2008.02.015

[23] Brouwer AF, Brand PL, Roorda RJ, Duiverman EJ. Airway obstruction at time of symptoms prompting use of reliever therapy in children with asthma. Acta Paediatr 2010; 99:871–876. DOI: 10.1111/j.1651-2227.2010.01715

[24] Brouwer AF, Brand PL. Asthma education and monitoring: what has been shown to work. Paediatr Respir Rev 2008; 9:193–199. DOI: 10.1016/j.prrv.2008.03.001

[25] Kaptein AA, Klok T, Moss-Morris R, Brand PL. Illness perceptions: impact on self-management and control in asthma. Curr Opin Allergy Clin Immunol 2010; 10:194–199. DOI: 10.1111/pai.12362

[26] Wildhaber J, Carroll WD, Brand PL. Global impact of asthma on children and adolescents' daily lives: the room to breathe survey. Pediatr Pulmonol 2012; 47:346–357. DOI: 10.1002/ppul.21557

[27] Global Initiative for Asthma (GINA). A Pocket Guide for Physicians and Nurses updated 2015. Accessed at: http://www.ginasthma.org/documents/1/Pocket-Guide-for-Asthma-Management-and-Prevention

[28] National Heart LaBI, NHLBI. Guidelines for the Diagnosis and Management of Asthma. 2007. Accessed at: http://www.nhlbi.nih.gov/health-pro/guidelines/current/asthma-guidelines/full-report

[29] N. G. Papadopoulos, H. Arakawa, K.-H. Carlsen, A. Custovic, J. Gern, R. Lemanske et al. International consensus on (ICON) pediatric asthma. Allergy 2012; 67:976–997.

[30] Baatenburg de JA, Brouwer AF, Roorda RJ, Brand PL. Normal lung function in children with mild to moderate persistent asthma well controlled by inhaled corticosteroids. J Allergy Clin Immunol 2006; 118:280–282. DOI: 10.1016/j.jaci.2006.03.013

[31] Fuhlbrigge AL, Weiss ST, Kuntz KM, Paltiel AD. Forced expiratory volume in 1 second percentage improves the classification of severity among children with asthma. Pediatrics 2006; 118:e347–e355. DOI: 10.1542/peds.2005-2962

[32] Adams N, Bestall JM, Lasserson TJ, Jones PW. Inhaled fluticasone versus inhaled beclomethasone or inhaled budesonide for chronic asthma in adults and children. Cochrane Database Syst Rev 2005. DOI: 10.1002/14651858.CD002310

[33] Garcia Garcia ML, Wahn U, Gilles L, Swern A, Tozzi CA, Polos P. Montelukast, compared with fluticasone, for control of asthma among 6- to 14-year-old patients with mild asthma: the MOSAIC study. Pediatrics 2005; 116:360–369. DOI: 10.1542/peds. 2004-1172

[34] Spahn JD, Cherniack R, Paull K, Gelfand EW. Is forced expiratory volume in one second the best measure of severity in childhood asthma? Am J Respir Crit Care Med 2004; 169:784–786. DOI: 10.1164/rccm.200309-1234OE

[35] Galant SP, Morphew T, Newcomb RL, Hioe K, Guijon O, Liao O. The relationship of the bronchodilator response phenotype to poor asthma control in children with normal spirometry. J Pediatr 2011; 158:953–959. DOI: 10.1016/j.jpeds.2010.11.029

[36] Sharma S, Litonjua AA, Tantisira KG, Fuhlbrigge AL, Szefler SJ, Strunk RC, et al.. Childhood asthma management program research group. Clinical predictors and outcomes of consistent bronchodilator response in the childhood asthma management program. J Allergy Clin Immunol 2008; 122:921–928. DOI: 10.1016/j.jaci.2008.09.004

[37] Brand PL, Roorda RJ. Usefulness of monitoring lung function in asthma. Arch Dis Child 2003; 88:1021–1025.

[38] Wensley D, Silverman M. Peak flow monitoring for guided self-management in childhood asthma: a randomized controlled trial. Am J Respir Crit Care Med 2004; 170:606–612. DOI: 10.1164/rccm.200307-1025OC

[39] Yoos HL, Kitzman H, McMullen A, Henderson C, Sidora K. Symptom monitoring in childhood asthma: a randomized clinical trial comparing peak expiratory flow rate with symptom monitoring. Ann Allergy Asthma Immunol 2002; 88:283–291. DOI: 10.1016/ S1081-1206(10)62010-8

[40] Ko FW, Leung TF, Hui DS, Chu HY, Wong GW, Wong E, et al. Asthma Control Test correlates well with the treatment decisions made by asthma specialists. Respirology 2009; 14:559–566. DOI: 10.1111/j.1440-1843.2009.01514

[41] Garcia-Marcos PW, Soriano-Perez MJ, Perez-Fernandez V, Valverde-Molina J, Garcia-Marcos L. Exhaled nitric oxide in school children: in search of the lost variability. Allergol Immunopathol. 2015. DOI: 10.1016/j.aller.2015.06.002. [Epub ahead of print]

[42] Petsky HL, Cates CJ, Lasserson TJ, et al. A systematic review and meta-analysis: tailoring asthma treatment on eosinophilic markers (exhaled nitric oxide or sputum eosinophils). Thorax 2012; 67:199–208. DOI: 10.1136/thx.2010.135574

[43] Klok T, de Groot EP, Brouwer A, Brand P. Follow-up of children with asthma. European Respiratory Monograph 56: Paediatric Asthma 2012; 18:210–223. DOI: 10.1183/1025448x.10018110

[44] Clark NM, Cabana M, Kaciroti N, Gong M, Sleeman K. Long-term outcomes of physician peer teaching. Clin Pediatr (Phila) 2008; 47:883–890. DOI: 10.1177/0009922808319964

[45] de Ridder DT, Theunissen NC, van Dulmen SM. Does training general practitioners to elicit patients' illness representations and action plans influence their communication as a whole? Patient Educ Couns 2007; 66:327–336. DOI: 10.1016/j.pec.2007.01.006

[46] Zolnierek KB, Dimatteo MR. Physician communication and patient adherence to treatment: a meta-analysis. Med Care 2009; 47:826–834. DOI: 10.1097/MLR. 0b013e31819a5acc.

[47] Brand PL, Stiggelbout AM. Effective follow-up consultations: the importance of patient-centered communication and shared decision making. Paediatr Respir Rev 2013; 14:224–228. DOI: 10.1016/j.prrv.2013.01.002.

[48] Janson SL, McGrath KW, Covington JK, Cheng SC, Boushey HA. Individualized asthma self-management improves medication adherence and markers of asthma control. J Allergy Clin Immunol 2009; 123:840–846. DOI: 10.1016/j.jaci.2009.01.053

[49] Weinstein AG. The potential of asthma adherence management to enhance asthma guidelines. Ann Allergy Asthma Immunol 2011; 106:283–291. DOI: 10.1016/j.anai. 2011.01.016

[50] Michie S, Miles J, Weinman J. Patient-centredness in chronic illness: what is it and does it matter? Patient Educ Couns 2003; 51:197–206.

[51] Klok T, Lubbers S, Kaptein AA, Brand PL. Every parent tells a story: why non-adherence may persist in children receiving guideline-based comprehensive asthma care. J Asthma 2014; 51:106–112. DOI: 10.3109/02770903.2013.841191

[52] Williams LK, Peterson EL, Wells K, Ahmedani BK, Kumar R, Burchard EG, et al. Quantifying the proportion of severe asthma exacerbations attributable to inhaled corticosteroid nonadherence. J Allergy Clin Immunol. 2011; 128:1185–1191.doi: 10.1016/ j.jaci.2011.09.011

[53] Bokhour BG, Cohn ES, Cortés DE, Yinusa-Nyahkoon LS, Hook JM, Smith LA, et al. Patterns of concordance and non-concordance with clinician recommendations and parents' explanatory models in children with asthma. Patient Educ Couns 2008; 70:376–385. DOI: 10.1016/j.pec.2007.11.007

[54] Klok T, Kaptein AA, Brand PL. Non-adherence in children with asthma reviewed: The need for improvement of asthma care and medical education. Pediatr Allergy Immunol 2015; 26:197–205. DOI: 10.1111/pai.12362

[55] Dean AJ, Walters J, Hall A. A systematic review of interventions to enhance medication adherence in children and adolescents with chronic illness. Arch Dis Child 2010; 95:717–723. DOI: 10.1136/adc.2009.175125

[56] Kahana SY, Frazier TW, Drotar D. Preliminary quantitative investigation of predictors of treatment non-adherence in pediatric transplantation: a brief report. Pediatr Transplant 2008; 12:656–660.

[57] Brand PL, Klok T, Kaptein AA. Using communication skills to improve adherence in children with chronic disease: the adherence equation. Paediatr Respir Rev 2013; 14:219–223. DOI: 10.1016/j.prrv.2013.01.003

[58] Christakis DA, Garrison MM, Lozano P, Meischke H, Zhou C, Zimmerman FJ. Improving parental adherence with asthma treatment guidelines: a randomized controlled trial of an interactive website. Acad Pediatr 2012; 12:302–311. DOI: 10.1016/j.acap.2012.03.006

[59] Kamps AW, van EB, Roorda RJ, Brand PL. Poor inhalation technique, even after inhalation instructions, in children with asthma. Pediatr Pulmonol 2000; 29:39–42. DOI: 10.1002/(SICI)1099-0496(200001)29:1<39::AID-PPUL7>3.0.CO;2-G

[60] Kamps AW, Brand PL, Roorda RJ. Determinants of correct inhalation technique in children attending a hospital-based asthma clinic. Acta Paediatr 2002; 91:159–163.

[61] Thompson K, Kulkarni J, Sergejew AA. Reliability and validity of a new Medication Adherence Rating Scale (MARS) for the psychoses. Schizophr Res 2000; 42:241–247.

[62] Roy A, Battle K, Lurslurchachai L, Halm EA, Wisnivesky JP. Inhaler device, administration technique, and adherence to inhaled corticosteroids in patients with asthma. Prim Care Respir J 2011; 20:148–154. DOI: 10.4104/pcrj.2011.00022

[63] Wehmeier PM, Dittmann RW, Banaschewski T. Treatment compliance or medication adherence in children and adolescents on ADHD medication in clinical practice: results from the COMPLY observational study. Atten Defic Hyperact Disord 2015; 7:165–174. DOI: 10.1007/s12402-014-0156-8

[64] García-Marcos PW, Brand PL, Kaptain AA, Klok T. Is MARS-5 questionnaire a good predictor of maintenance medication adherence in childhood asthma? Unpublished work.

[65] Ducharme FM. High inhaled corticosteroids adherence in childhood asthma: the role of medication beliefs. Eur Respir J 2012; 40:1072–1074. DOI: 10.1183/09031936.00096912

# 8

# Genetics of Allergic Asthma and Current Perspectives on Therapeutic Management

Mina Youssef, Cynthia Kanagaratham,
Mohamed I. Saad and Danuta Radzioch

## Abstract

Globally, more than 300 million people are asthmatics and this number has been estimated to become 400 million by 2025. Asthma is a chronic inflammatory condition, which, although has no cure, is treatable in most patients. The most common structural alterations in asthmatic airways include thickening of the epithelial and sub epithelial layers, increased airway smooth muscle mass, and angiogenesis. Several genetically controlled factors greatly influence the predisposition and severity of allergic asthma. Twin studies have attributed as much as 75% of asthma susceptibility to heredity. Particularly, genome-wide association studies (GWASs) have discovered several asthma and/or atopy susceptibility genes. Current treatment protocols for managing asthma involve the use of corticosteroids and β-agonists. Over the last 40 years, there has been a marked development-targeted therapy for asthma, such as anti-leukotrienes, anti-immunoglobulin (Ig)E, anti-tumor necrosis factor (TNF)-$\alpha$, and anti-interleukins (ILs) (Th2 cytokines). To identify novel targets and to develop newer drug generations, better understanding of asthma molecular pathophysiology is required. Furthermore, the pharmacogenetic studies, focusing on better understanding of beneficial or/and adverse effects to anti-asthma drugs, will also facilitate the development of more effective and targeted treatments in specific subpopulations of patients suffering from asthma.

**Keywords:** asthma, asthma therapies, genetics, pharmacogenetics

## 1. Introduction

Asthma is an inflammatory chronic condition that has reached globally epidemic levels. Although no cure exists, symptoms are treatable in most patients [1]. Statistically, the number of asthmatic cases has been on the rise over the past 10 years and affecting up to 10% of adults and 20% of children worldwide [2]. Globally, more than 300 million people are asthmatics, and this estimate is predicted to become 400 million by 2025 [3]. The worldwide economic burden caused by asthma is predicted to be more than that of both acquired immunodeficiency syndrome (AIDS) and tuberculosis combined together. For example, in the United States of America, the annual asthma care costs exceed US$6 billion [4]. Moreover, these numbers are due to the fact that more than 50% of asthmatic cases are poorly controlled by medication, since the response to treatments varies considerably among patients despite having similar clinical features [3, 5]. Asthma is characterized by altered and distinct clinical changes in the lung airways obstructing the flow of air into the lungs. The most prominent airway remodeling features include epithelial and subepithelial layer thickening, increased airway smooth muscle (ASM) mass, and angiogenesis [6]. Different classes of asthma therapies address one or more of the phenotypes of asthma; however, the heterogeneous nature of the disease prevents homogeneous clinical outcomes in response to the current treatment guidelines [7].

In the past two decades, the field of human genetics has evolved due to the advancements in the human genome project and high-throughput sequencing technologies [8, 9]. Currently, the advances in genetic, pharmacodynamic, and pharmacokinetic studies, analyzing responsiveness of patients to various therapies, may eventually allow to prescribe personalized treatment and to shift asthma therapies from classical standards, using mostly corticosteroids and β-adrenergic agonists, to a highly tailored approach [10]. Future genetic profiles of the population would form the basis of tomorrow's treatments in order to potentiate the required therapeutic benefits, and to diminish any possible adverse effect risks. Overall, there remains a great need for comprehensive drug research, paralleled with high-throughput genetic profiling, in order to treat asthma in a personalized or stratified manner [11].

## 2. Genetic control of airway hyperresponsiveness, atopy, and allergic asthma

The heritable nature of asthma has been demonstrated through various types of studies over the past decades. Family and twin studies indicate that 60–70% of asthma cases are due to genetic factors. Moreover, it has been proven that the concordance of asthma is greater among monozygotic twins rather than among dizygotic ones. Adoption studies have shown greater disease prevalence within biological relatives of the affected people compared to the adopted family [12].

Higher prevalence of allergic disease phenotypes is observed among relatives of atopic individuals compared to nonatopic individuals. Overall, the heritability estimates remain in between the range of 30–66% for airway hyperresponsiveness, 35–95% for asthma, and 35–84% for total serum IgE levels [13]. It is clear that both the inter-genetic individual differences and the degree of allergen exposure contribute to these variations in heritability. Heritability of asthma is linked to both disease susceptibility and severity. While the main concern of asthma genetic studies has been on disease susceptibility, increasing evidence shows that many genetic variants are important in asthma progression and severity as well [14]. Lung function tests in asthma showed that genes in the T-helper lymphocyte 1 (Th1) pathway affect asthma severity; meanwhile, T-helper lymphocyte 2 (Th2) pathway genes relate to susceptibility [14]. Based on these hypotheses, genes associated with asthma susceptibility differ from those related to asthma severity; hence, it is important to define both groups distinctly.

By knowing the genetic signature associated with allergic asthma, geneticists can help to better understand the molecular mechanism of this disease, and the shared and distinct pathways among other allergic diseases. Moreover, the genetic signature of asthma-associated genes with altered expression during the peak of asthmatic episodes may help predict the severity and response to therapy. Unfavorable response might be identified and, consequently, more targeted and personalized treatments can be considered for this complex trait. The human genome project and the ongoing advancements in sequencing technologies, both, resulted in more successful gene discovery over the last years, even in diseases as complexed as asthma. Since then, dozens of susceptibility genes were identified through a large variety of methods and rationales. *ADAM33* is the first asthma susceptibility gene to be discovered through positional cloning [15]. ADAM33 (also known as Disintegrin and metalloproteinase domain-containing protein 33) is a membrane-bound metalloproteinase enzyme that has been involved in several cellular interactions involving cell-cell and cell-matrix events [16]. Variants in this gene have been correlated to asthma susceptibility and bronchial hyperresponsiveness, but not atopy. Due to its clinical significance, *ADAM33* studies were conducted among 33 different asthmatic population samples all over the world. Additionally, numerous studies have suggested that altered *ADAM33* DNA methylation patterns could result in diversely unbalanced biological effects in the airways [17]. Studies focused on candidate genes have examined a number of genes involved in asthma and highlighted more than 100 interesting genetic spots; however, the role of those loci in asthma susceptibility remains largely unexplored [18].

Genome-wide association studies (GWASs) extensively investigate the unknown genetic bases of many intricate disorders including asthma [19,20]. In the first reported GWAS study for asthma susceptibility, Moffatt et al. [21] identified the 17q21 locus, containing several genes, for example, *ORMDL3* and *GSDMB* as being associated with childhood asthma. Importance of this region was later on replicated in numerous subsequent studies [22–24]. Expression levels of the gene *ORMDL3* are differentially regulated by distinct haplotypes in this region. This gene encodes protein acting as an inhibitor of sphingolipid biosynthesis and in general Orm family proteins were shown to be implicated in the control of sphingolipid homeostasis [25]. Dysregulated sphingolipid formation in the respiratory tract instigates airway hyper-reactivity [26] although exact molecular steps are still not known. The results of these studies suggested that the mechanisms of asthma development are linked with genetically determined abnormalities in some patients resulting in their inability to control balance between oxidative and anti-oxidative reactions. The mechanisms of asthma development are linked with genetically determined abnormalities in the functioning of antioxidant defense enzymes. These alterations seem to be accompanied by a systemic imbalance between oxidative and anti-oxidative reactions with the shift of the redox state toward increased free radical production, oxidation of proteins and phospholipids, and eventually to their selective degradation.

To increase the power of detection of modest alleles due to the large sample size, the results of individual GWAS need to be gathered into a meta-analysis. The scientific literature recognizes two meta-analyses of asthma GWAS. One was done by the GABRIEL Consortium [27] of the European investigators, and the other was conducted by the EVE Consortium of the US investigators [22]. While the EVE meta-analysis included diverse subjects from different ethnic background, US and Mexico population backgrounds, the GABRIEL meta-analysis included only European subjects. Overall, these two thorough meta-analyses present a comprehensive overview of the genetic associations for asthma. Some associations are shared among different populations; by contrast, others are specific to one race. Grouping GWAS in this way increases the power of genetic detection, contrasts different ethnic groups' genotypes, and highlights the worldwide populations' genetic patterns. Overall independent GWASs have identified large number of candidate loci that deserve further testing. Replication studies help to prioritize which genes deserve further study, based on their identification in multiple populations.

Additionally, more loci were identified to be associated with asthma; these include interleukin (IL)-33 (on 9p24), *HLA-DR/DQ* (on 6p21), *IL1RL1/IL18R1* (on 2q12), *TSLP* (on 5q22), and *IL13* (on 5q31) [22,27,28]. Collectively with *ORMDL3/GSDMB* (on 17q21), these are the most remarkable and consistent loci, which are identified for asthma. Since Moffatt et al. had published the first GWAS results for asthma, identifying *ORMDL3* as a candidate gene, numerous other studies have been conducted investigating an array of phenotypes which are observed in allergic diseases. In particular, FCER1A, RAD50, and STAT6 have been associated with total serum IgE levels [29].

## 3. Environmental factors contributing to asthma

Parallel to genetic factors, environmental factors are also involved in the development and progression of asthma (**Figure 1**). The exposure to some environmental factors was shown to contribute not only to asthma but also to other related respiratory disorders, for example, emphysema development. By contrast, there are also some other environmental factors that seem to be solely linked to the development of asthma but not to other inflammatory or/and respiratory disorders [30]. Various studies assessed the risk factors of asthma and found evidence that allergen exposure, respiratory tract infections, gastroesophageal reflux disease (GERD), and physical and psychosocial stress might represent individual risk factors. It is important to keep in mind that some other environmental factors are protective, such as maternal diet, breastfeeding, and farming conditions [31].

Allergen exposure is the major factor impacting sensitization and constitutes the most common cause of asthmatic exacerbations in adults and children. A wide variety of inhaled allergens may trigger asthma symptoms, for example, house dust mite [32], pollens [33], cockroaches [34], and animal fur [35]. Respiratory tract infections have been implicated in asthma occurrence and exacerbation as well. Examples include infection with viruses [36,37], *Mycoplasma* [38], and *Chlamydia species* [39]. Based on the conclusions from the Japanese study, which included 3085 patients, the change in weather followed by smoking was identified as two leading asthma-exacerbating factors [40]. Although (passive) smoking is a predominant contributing factor for the development of asthma [41], one occupational study [42] has shown that nonsmokers might also develop asthma due to occupational air pollutant exposure.

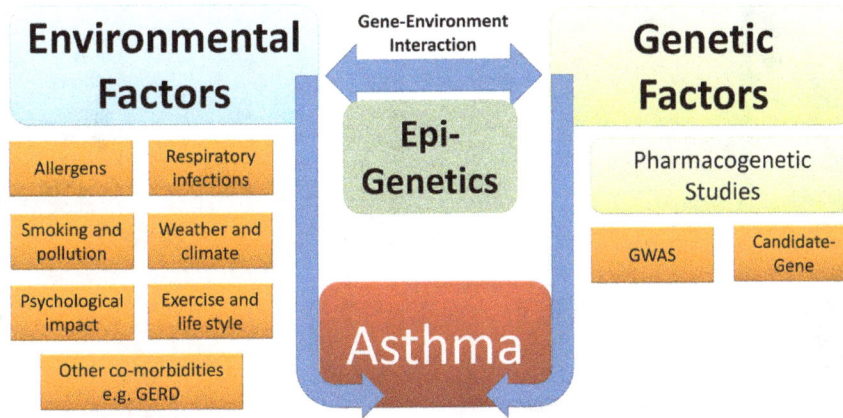

**Figure 1.** Environmental stress, in conjunction with genetic factors, both contribute to the development of asthma exacerbations.

Additionally, a correlation has been observed between the presence of asthma and gastroesophageal reflux-induced disease, with reports showing one-third of asthmatic patients also diagnosed with GERD [43,44]. Although the coexistence of GERD in asthmatic patients did not affect asthma severity, the airway resistance was significantly higher in asthmatic patients with GERD [45]. Some other psychosocial factors such as parental stress during childhood [46] and the socioeconomic status [47] are reported to influence allergic inflammation severity. It is estimated that psychopathology is six times more common among asthmatics, and accordingly it correlates more closely with the asthmatic quality of life, rather than with lung physiological functions [48,49]. In both directions, psychopathology is supposed to precipitate asthma or vice versa; psychopathology may develop as a consequence of asthma [50].

## 4. Asthma pathophysiology

Scientists tried to uncover alterations related to asthma since a long time ago. One of the oldest publications that discussed asthma pathophysiology was in 1873 [51]. Later on, in 1886, F.H. Bosworth concluded a possible relation between asthma and hay fever [52]. Clearly, it is well known that asthmatic patients suffer from reversible airway obstruction resulting from an allergen exposure, consequently releasing multiple broncoconstricting mediators that stimulate airway muscles to contract. Furthermore, airways narrow results from past and current mucus and edema occlusion [53]. The chronic inflammation and associated repair of lung airways leads to structural changes, referred to as *"airway remodeling."* Airway remodeling (**Figure 2**) usually involves lung epithelial layer injury and includes features such as subepithelial thickening, airway smooth muscle hyperplasia, and angiogenesis [6].

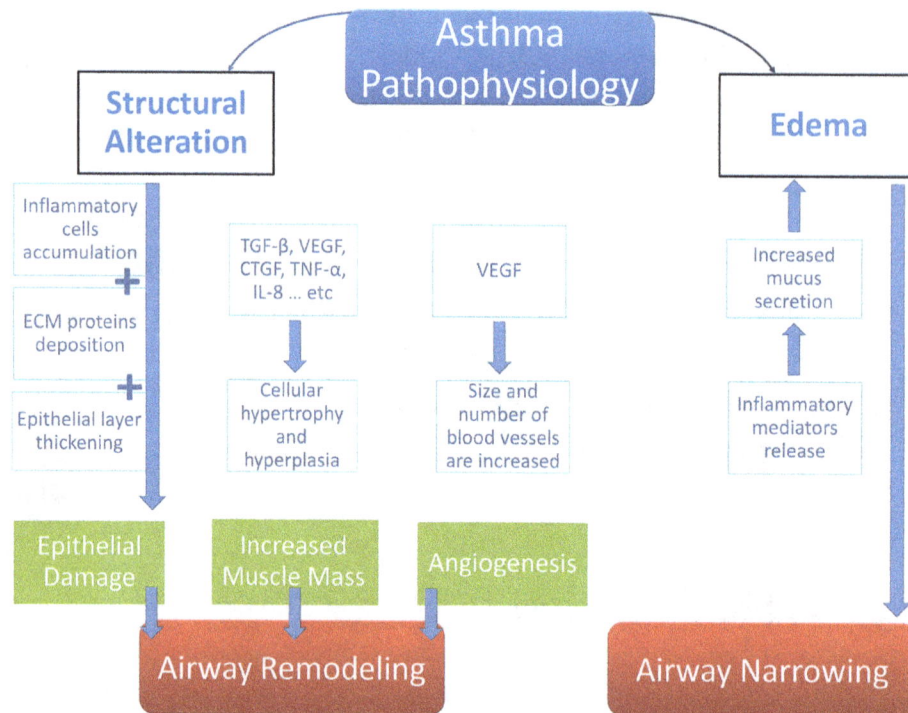

**Figure 2.** Schematic representation of the major events underlying asthma pathophysiology.

Asthma and COPD (chronic obstructive pulmonary disease) are now considered to be discrete respiratory disorders. Although both share several similar underlying mechanisms, driving airway obstruction in COPD, and hyperresponsiveness in asthma, core molecular pathology remains to be mostly different for both [54]. Pauwels et al. [55] defined COPD as "a disease state characterized by airflow limitation that is not fully reversible. The airflow limitation is usually progressive and associated with an abnormal inflammatory response of lungs to noxious particles and gases." One important reason of asthma and COPD overlap is the effect of aging. Asthma-COPD overlap syndrome (ACOS) is a medically recognized coexisting syndrome of both asthma and COPD [56]. Some other health conditions may occur more frequently in asthmatic patients. Rhinosinusitis [57], obstructive sleep apnea [58], or GERD [59] are the most common documented comorbidities. Substantially, they can contribute to the same pathophysiological process, which is already triggered by allergic response or alter asthma phenotype detrimentally. The impact of these diseases on asthma is variable and still not fully clear [60].

## 5. Structural alterations in asthmatic airway walls

### 5.1. Epithelial/subepithelial layer thickening

Epithelial changes are not unique to asthma, they are also observed, in more or less of similar manner, in lungs of smokers and cancer patients [61]. Epithelial layer damage in asthma includes loss of ciliated cell layer, shedding of the epithelium, goblet cell hyperplasia and growth factors, cytokine and chemokine upregulation [62].

One important feature of asthma, which has been routinely used as an asthma severity index, is the thickening of the subepithelial airways layer. The epithelial and subepithelial layer thickening is caused by the overdeposition of extracellular matrix (ECM) proteins [63]. Roche et al. observed that intensive layers of collagen sedimentation contribute to the thickened subepithelial basement membrane. Through immunohistochemistry, they have shown that the commonly involved collagen types are collagen I, III and V, and fibronectin [64]. Additionally, the cells that are responsible for ECM protein production are myofibroblasts and fibroblasts, as both are embedded in the sophisticated ECM which they secrete [65]. Meanwhile, some inflammatory cells, for example, T cells, mast cells, and eosinophils also accumulate in the submucosal layer [66]. Moreover, transforming growth factor-$\beta$ (TGF-$\beta$), and some similar growth factors, is usually secreted by the lung epithelial cells echoing any ongoing lung injury, and consequently directly impress the matrix proteins' production by fibroblasts/myofibroblasts. By increasing the airway rigidity, however, Holgate et al. suggested that the airway thickening due to the ECM proteins precipitation may in fact have a remodeling protective effect via postponing long-term bronchoconstriction events [62]. Collectively, the ECM proteins, the lung structural cells (i.e., epithelial cells and fibroblasts), and the immune system inflammatory cells, all interact together and control the overall airway remodeling and fibrosis [67].

## 5.2. Hyperproliferation of airway smooth muscle mass

Hyperproliferation of airway smooth muscle mass is a common event in asthma and has been suggested to be implicated in its pathophysiology. Hyperplasia and hypertrophy of the ASM in the bronchial airways of asthmatics can be observed by three-dimensional (3D) morphometric studies [68]. Airways smooth muscle layer is estimated to be increased by 25–55% in nonfatal asthma and up to 50–200% in fatal asthma [69]. Meanwhile, in response to some growth factors like TGF-$\beta$, vascular endothelial growth factor (VEGF), and connective tissue growth factor (CTGF), ASM cells actively participate in the remodeling process through the process of ECM synthesis [70]. ASM cells also express cellular adhesion molecules (CAMs), receptors for cytokines (e.g., tumor necrosis factor-$\alpha$), Toll-like receptors, and chemokines (eotaxin, macrophage inflammatory protein 1$\alpha$, and interleukin 8) presenting multiple mechanisms for the inflammatory and remodeling process [71]. Additionally, one characteristic event of the airway remodeling is the ASM cells migration toward the epithelium [72]. Since ASM cells are crucial in asthma, Zuyderduyn et al. suggested that these cells should be targeted, rather than targeting inflammation or dealing with the symptoms [73].

## 5.3. Angiogenesis

Accumulating evidences indicate that there is an abnormal elevation in the size and number of blood vessels, as well as microvessels vascular leakage within the bronchial tissue in remodeled airways [74]. It is assumed that VEGF strongly affects airways remodeling via its angiogenic effects, but the exact molecular mechanism linking the increase in the VEGF expression to remodeling of the airways has not been fully understood [75].

Correlation between angiogenesis and asthma severity has also been documented. Dense vascularity occurs in severe asthmatics, followed by moderate, and then finally mild asthmatics, who experience less angiogenesis events [76]. This pattern was also observed in fatal asthmatics compared with nonfatal asthmatics [77]. While current asthma therapeutics is not directly targeting vascular remodeling, recent trials investigate some anti-angiogenic therapies as a new approach for asthma. Yuksel et al. showed that Bevucizamab, which significantly neutralizes VEGF, results in a reduced thickening of lung epithelium, a reduced ASM, and a reduced basement membrane thickness compared with untreated ovalbumin (OVA)-challenged mice [78].

## 6. Therapies for asthma

Modern treatments for asthma have been tested and used since the early twentieth century [79]. However, the oldest documented drug for asthma dates back to ancient Egypt. Kyphi, an incense mixture drink, was used inside the temples by the priests as a multipurpose lung medicament. There was more than one recipe for Kyphi; each may include as many as 10 herbs [80]. Following this, about 4000 years ago, Atropa Belladonna alkaloids, also called "deadly nightshade" because of their poisonous properties ("Natural Medicinal Herbs"), were derived from the leaves of thorn-apple plant and smoked by the Indians as cough suppressant [82]. Till today, natural and synthesized entities related to the tropane alkaloids class are still widely used. This includes anticholinergics (e.g., natural atropine, hyoscyamine (the levo-isomer of atropine), acopolamine, and the synthetic Ipratropium Bromide and stimulants (e.g., cocaine and hydroxytropacocaine) [83]. In 1872, one of the first papers published on asthma states that rubbing the chest of asthmatics with chloroform liniment can resolve airway constriction [84]. Adrenergic stimulants were in use for asthma over 100 years ago. In 1901, the adrenaline isolated from sheep and oxen adrenal glands was used to treat asthma [85]. The first documented publication of adrenaline as a bronchodilator therapy for asthma was written in 1903 by James Burnett, a physician in Edinburgh [86]. One year later in 1904, adrenaline was synthesized in the laboratories of Friedrich Stolz and Henry Drysdale Dakin, independently [87].

As suggested by the Global Initiative for Asthma (GINA) [88], a five-level step-down approach is widely recognized among the medical practitioners (**Figure 3**). The GINA approach assigns two types of drug classes for managing asthma:

- *Relievers* (bronchodilators) cause immediate dilatation effects on the airways obstruction, mainly by acting on lung's smooth muscle.

- *Controllers* (preventers) provide long-term control of symptoms, mainly by suppressing the underlying disease process.

Legend:
SABA: Short acting beta agonists, ICS: Inhaled corticosteroids (arrow down = low dose, arrow up = high dose), LABA: Long acting beta agoints, LTRA: Leukotriene receptor antagonists, MX: Methylxanthines, OCS: Oral corticosteroids, OZ: Omalizumab

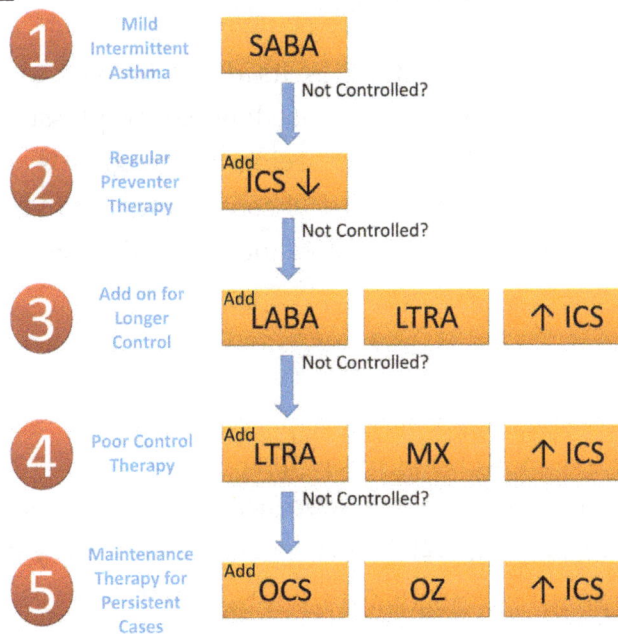

Stepwise approach for controlling asthma symptoms and minimizing future morbidity

**Figure 3.** Stepwise approach for controlling asthma symptoms and minimizing future morbidity.

β2-agonists and anticholinergics are considered to be bronchodilator relievers. Asthma controllers include corticosteroids, anti-leukotrienes, and anti-IgE. Theophylline is casually classified as both a bronchodilator and a reliever. The following book section will briefly discuss each therapeutic class.

## 6.1. Corticosteroids

Nowadays, most popular protocols for managing asthma involve the use of corticosteroids and β-agonists [1]. Anti-inflammatory corticosteroids, which are one of most trusted treatments for asthma, were introduced in mid-twentieth century [79]. The principle mode of action of corticosteroids in asthma is through their direct anti-inflammatory effect in different white blood cells including T cells, mast cells, and eosinophils. Among leukocytes, corticosteroids suppress chemotaxis and adhesion, and prevent inflammatory cytokines recruitment [89]. *In vitro*, corticosteroids reduce human ASM proliferation directly [90] by stimulating p21 gene expression [91], an important regulator of cell cycle progression. Moreover, corticosteroids improve vast majority of vascular remodeling aspects in asthma, reducing angiogenesis, excess blood flow, and vascular leakage [92]. This is mainly mediated by decreasing VEGF activity within the airway wall cells [93].

Various studies describe contradicting effects of corticosteroids on the lung epithelial abnormalities in asthmatics. Dorscheid et al. [94] reported that Dexamethasone treatment resulted in increased epithelial apoptosis and shedding. Similar results were obtained when treating guinea pigs with Budesonide, which did not improve the tracheal epithelium [95]. By contrast, some *in vivo* studies showed that inhaled corticosteroid (ICS) treatment resulted in improvement of epithelial damage in severe asthmatics [96,97].

ICS has been used around for the past couple of decades. Its idea dates back to the nineteenth century when the hand-held glass bulb nebulizer was used; however, pressurized metered-dose inhaler (pMDI) came to the clinic in 1956. After seeing his daughter's suffering while using the hand-held nebulizer, George Maison, a medical consultant at 3M Pharmaceuticals, had advocated the use of pMDI. In 1959, George Maison and Irvine Porush were awarded a patent on the first pMDI [98].

## 6.2 β-adrenergic agonists

Long-acting β-agonists (LABAs), for example, Formoterol [99] and Salmeterol [100], offer a longer period of bronchodilation compared to the short-acting beta agonists (SABAs), for example, Salbutamol [101] and Terbutaline [102]. LABAs persist in the airway tissues for long periods due to their lipophilic nature and they provide a good umbrella of asthma bronchodilation and control, particularly at night [99,100]. However, until recently, the medical literature lacked supporting studies reporting the positive effect of $\beta_2$ agonists on the chronic airway remodeling [103]. Addition of a β-agonist to the corticosteroid therapy allows a "steroid-sparing" effect, that is, maintains asthma control using lower doses of corticosteroids [104]. LABAs are not used as monotherapies anymore and they must be used in combination with ICS [105], because there have been cases of severe exacerbations and death when LABAs are administrated solely.

## 6.3. Antimuscarinic agents

Inhaled antimuscarinic agents, also known as inhaled anticholinergics, are considered another alternative bronchodilator group to β-agonists. The bronchodilation effect is functionally mediated via muscarinic receptor subtypes M1, M2, and M3, although five muscarinic receptors have been revealed in the lungs M1, M2, M3, M4, and M5 [106]. It is widely known that parasympathetic stimulation via the vagus nerve leads to immediate smooth muscle contraction and mucus secretion in the airways [107]. It is also suggested that M receptors interact with β2-adrenergic receptors (ADRB2) on the airways smooth muscle, leading to a reduced bronchodilator response of the β-agonists [108]. For years, in both adults and children, short-acting antimuscarinic agents use, for example, Ipratropium [109], has been limited to acute asthma management, in addition to inhaled SABA [110, 111]. Long-acting antimuscarinic agents, for example, Tiotropium [112], appear to have more benefits in difficult-to-control asthma. Adding Tiotropium to the standard asthma therapy significantly reduces asthma symptoms and highly increases the clinical outcomes [113, 114].

## 6.4. Targeted therapies

Over the last 40 years, there has been a marked increase in the development of targeted treatments for asthma—anti-leukotrienes, anti-IgE, anti-interleukins, and anti-TNF-α [115]. Obviously, as more of the biological basis of asthma is uncovered, more effective targeted asthma treatments might be developed. The list of most recently published clinical trials covering the period from 1 January 2013 to 1 January 2016, as well as the list of currently ongoing registered clinical trials that has started since 2013 for the new asthma medications are summarized in **Tables 1** and **2**, respectively.

| Clinical Trial Identifier | Publication Title | Phase | Drugs | Outcome | Responsible Party | Reference |
|---|---|---|---|---|---|---|
| NCT01147744 | Efficacy, safety, and tolerability of GSK2190915, a 5-lipoxygenase-activating protein inhibitor, in adults and adolescents with persistent asthma: a randomized dose-ranging study. | Phase 2 | GSK2190915 (5-lipoxygenase-activating protein inhibitor) | GSK2190915 30-mg efficacy was demonstrated in day-time symptom scores and day-time SABA use, compared with placebo. No additional improvement on efficacy was gained by administration of greater doses than 30 mg. GSK2190915 was well tolerated. | GlaxoSmithKline | [1] |
| NCT00411814 | A phase 1, randomized, placebo-controlled, dose-escalation study of an anti-IL-13 monoclonal antibody in healthy subjects and mild asthmatics. | Phase 1 | GSK679586 (anti-IL-13) | GSK679586 showed dose-dependent pharmacological activity in the lungs of mild intermittent asthmatic patients. GSK679586 could be a potential therapeutic candidate for treatment of asthma. | GlaxoSmithKline | [2] |
| NCT00659659) | Effects of benralizumab on airway eosinophils in asthmatic patients with sputum eosinophilia. | Phase 1 | Benralizumab (Anti-IL-5) | Single-dose I.V. and multiple-dose S.C. of benralizumab reduced eosinophil counts in airway mucosa/submucosa and sputum and decreases eosinophil counts in bone | MedImmune LLC | [3] |

| Clinical Trial Identifier | Publication Title | Phase | Drugs | Outcome | Responsible Party | Reference |
|---|---|---|---|---|---|---|
| | | | | marrow and peripheral blood in asthmatic patients. | | |
| NCT01007149 | A proof-of-concept, randomized, controlled trial of omalizumab in patients with severe, difficult-to-control, nonatopic asthma. | Phase 3 | Omalizumab (anti-IgE) | Omalizumab may have a therapeutic potential for treatment of severe nonatopic asthma. | Novartis Pharmaceuticals | [4] |
| NCT00971035 | Dose-ranging study of lebrikizumab in asthmatic patients not receiving inhaled steroids. | Phase 2 | Lebrikizumab (anti-IL-13) | Blocking IL-13 alone was insufficient to improve lung function in asthmatic patients. | Genentech, Inc. | [5] |
| NCT00873860 | A phase II placebo-controlled study of tralokinumab in moderate-to-severe asthma. | Phase 2 | Tralokinumab (anti-IL-13) | Safety profile of tralokinumab was acceptable with no serious adverse effects. Although tralokinumab treatment was associated with improved lung function, no improvement in asthma control questionnaire score was observed. | MedImm une LLC | [6] |
| NCT01018186 | Safety and tolerability of the novel inhaled corticosteroid fluticasone furoate in combination with the β2-agonist vilanterol administered once daily for 52 weeks in patients ≥12 years old with asthma: a randomized trial. | Phase 3 | Fluticasone furoate (ICS) + Vilanterol (LABA) | Fluticasone furoate/ Vilanterol (100/25 μg or 200/25 μg) administered once daily over 52 weeks was well tolerated by asthmatic patients aged ≥12 years. The overall safety profile of Fluticasone furoate/ Vilanterol did not reveal any serious adverse effects. | GlaxoSmithKline | [7] |
| NCT00393952 | Efficacy and safety of fluticasone/ formoterol combination | Phase 3 | Fluticasone propionate (ICS) | Fluticasone/formoterol combination therapy was an efficient alternative treatment option for | SkyePharma AG | [8] |

| Clinical Trial Identifier | Publication Title | Phase | Drugs | Outcome | Responsible Party | Reference |
|---|---|---|---|---|---|---|
| | therapy in patients with moderate-to-severe asthma. | | Formoterol fumarate (LABA) | moderate-to-severe asthmatic patients. | | |
| NCT01691521 | Mepolizumab treatment in patients with severe eosinophilic asthma. | Phase 3 | Mepolizumab (anti-IL-5) | Administration of mepolizumab (I.V. or S.C.) significantly reduced asthma exacerbations and is associated with improvements in markers of asthma control. | GlaxoSmithKline | [9] |
| NCT00500539 | Immunogenicity and safety of omalizumab in pre-filled syringes in patients with allergic (IgE-mediated) asthma. | Phase 3 | Omalizumab (anti-IgE) | Pre-filled syringe of omalizumab was not associated with immunogenicity. | Novartis Pharmaceuticals | [10] |
| NCT00781443 | The effects of lebrikizumab in patients with mild asthma following whole lung allergen challenge. | Phase 2 | Lebrikizumab (anti-IL-13) | Lebrikizumab reduced the late asthmatic response in subjects with mild asthma. | Genentech, Inc. | [11] |
| NCT01181895 | Comparison of vilanterol, a novel long-acting beta-2 agonist, with placebo and a Salmeterol reference arm in asthma uncontrolled by inhaled corticosteroids. | Phase 3 | Vilanterol (LABA) | The study failed to show a therapeutic difference between vilanterol and placebo for the primary end point. The magnitude of placebo effect may be due to increased compliance with anti-inflammatory therapy regimen during the treatment period. | GlaxoSmithKline | [12] |

| Clinical Trial Identifier | Publication Title | Phase | Drugs | Outcome | Responsible Party | Reference |
|---|---|---|---|---|---|---|
| NCT01233284 | Tiotropium Respimat® in asthma: a double-blind, randomized, dose-ranging study in adult patients with moderate asthma. | Phase 2 | Tiotropium (LAMA) | Administration of tiotropium Respimat® (Once-daily) add-on to medium-dose ICS improves lung function in symptomatic patients with moderate asthma, and the largest improvement was with a dose of 5 μg. | Boehringer Ingelheim | [13] |
| NCT00983658 | OX40L blockade and allergen-induced airway responses in subjects with mild asthma. | Phase 2 | huMAb OX40L (anti-OX40L) | Anti-OX40L MAb decreased serum total IgE and airway eosinophils at 16 weeks post dosing, but there was no effect on allergen-induced airway responses. This may be due to the treatment duration or dose of antibody was insufficient to have an effect on the airway responses. | Genentech, Inc. | [14] |
| NCT00768079 | A randomized trial of benralizumab, an anti-interleukin 5 receptor α monoclonal antibody, after acute asthma. | Phase 2 | Benralizumab (Anti-IL-5) | A dose of benralizumab—when added to usual care—reduced the rate and severity of asthma exacerbations experienced over 12 weeks by subjects who presented to the emergency department with acute asthma. | MedImmune LLC | [15] |
| NCT01369017 | IL-1 receptor antagonist reduces endotoxin-induced airway inflammation in healthy volunteers. | Phase 1 | Anakinra (Anti-IL-1) | Anakinra effectively reduced airway neutrophilic inflammation with no serious adverse | University of North Carolina, Chapel Hill | [16] |

| Clinical Trial Identifier | Publication Title | Phase | Drugs | Outcome | Responsible Party | Reference |
|---|---|---|---|---|---|---|
| | | | | reactions in a model of inhaled lipopolysaccharide challenge. Anakinra is a potential therapeutic candidate for treatment of asthma. | | |

Abbreviations: **IL**: Interleukin; **IgE**: Immunoglobulin E; **TNF-α**: Tumor necrosis factor – α; **PDE**: Phosphodiesterase enzyme; **ICS**: Inhaled corticosteroids; **OCS**: Oral corticosteroids; **SABA**: Short-acting β-agonists; **LABA**: Long-acting β-agonists; **LAMA**; Long-acting muscarinic antagonists.

**Table 1.** Summary of recent published clinical trials for new drugs used in the treatment of asthma (from 1 January 2013 to 1 January 2016).

| Clinical Trial Identifier | Title | Phase | Drugs | Start Date | Purpose | Study Type | Recruitment Status | Responsible Party |
|---|---|---|---|---|---|---|---|---|
| NCT019 07763 | Phase III study to assess the efficacy and safety of SOTB07 in asthma patients | Phase 3 | Placebo SOTB07 | Jan 2013 | Assessment of the efficacy and safety of SOTB07 in asthma patients. | Interve ntional | Recr uiting | SK Chemicals Co.,Ltd. |
| NCT023 88997 | Treatment with Omalizumab to improve the asthmatic response to an experimental infection with rhinovirus | Phase 2 | Omalizumab (anti-IgE) Rhinovirus (strain 16) | Feb 2013 | Determination of whether anti-IgE therapy will lead to decline in inflammatory biomarkers prior to virus inoculation, and thus reduce the severity of clinical manifestations after an experimental human RV challenge. | Interve ntional | Recr uiting | University of Virginia |
| NCT019 02290 | Study of efficacy and safety of Brodalumab compared | Phase 2 | Placebo Brodalumab (Anti-IL-17) | May 2013 | Determination of the safety and efficacy of Brodalumab (AMG 827). | Interve ntional | Recr uiting | Amgen |

| Clinical Trial Identifier | Title | Phase | Drugs | Start Date | Purpose | Study Type | Recruitment Status | Responsible Party |
|---|---|---|---|---|---|---|---|---|
| | with placebo in inadequately controlled asthma subjects with high bronchodilator reversibility | | | | | | | |
| NCT018 36471 | A study to assess the effect of QAW039 in nonatopic asthmatic patients | Phase 2 | Placebo QAW039 ICS | May 2013 | Assessment of the clinical effect of QAW039 in nonatopic asthmatics taking low-dose ICS as background therapy. | Interve ntional | Recr uiting | Novartis Pharmaceuticals |
| NCT019 55512 | Effect of Clopidogrel on allergen challenge in asthma | Phase 2 | Placebo Clopidogrel (platelets P2Y12 receptor blocker) | May 2013 | Determination if the drug Clopidogrel reduces inflammation following breathing in house dust mite in people with mild asthma. | Interve ntional | Recr uiting | University of Southampton |
| NCT017 05964 | Intramuscular epinephrine as an adjunctive treatment for severe pediatric asthma exacerbation | Phase 4 | Epinephrine (IM) | Jun 2013 | Determination if IM epinephrine is an effective adjunct to inhaled $\beta_2$-agonists for children with severe asthma exacerbation. | Interve ntional | Recr uiting | University of Louisville |
| NCT018 68061 | A study of Lebrikizumab in patients with uncontrolled asthma on inhaled corticosteroids and a second controller medication | Phase 3 | Placebo Lebrikizumab (anti-IL-13) | Jul 2013 | Evaluation of the efficacy and safety of Lebrikizumab in patients with uncontrolled asthma despite daily administration of ICS therapy and at least 1-s controller medication. | Interve ntional | Recr uiting | Hoffmann-La Roche |
| NCT018 67125 | A study of Lebrikizumab in patients with uncontrolled asthma who are on inhaled | Phase 3 | Placebo Lebrikizumab (anti-IL-13) | Jul 2013 | Evaluation of the efficacy and safety of Lebriki zumab in patients with | Interve ntional | Recr uiting | Hoffmann-La Roche |

| Clinical Trial Identifier | Title | Phase | Drugs | Start Date | Purpose | Study Type | Recruitment Status | Responsible Party |
|---|---|---|---|---|---|---|---|---|
| | corticosteroids and a second controller medication | | | | uncontrolled asthma despite daily treatment with ICS therapy and at least 1-s controller medication. | | | |
| NCT018 41281 | L-arginine in severe asthma patients grouped by exhaled nitric oxide levels | Phase 2 | Placebo L-Arginine (Nitric oxide precursor) | Aug 2013 | Identification of the benefit from supplemental L-arginine therapy in adult severe asthma cohort. | Interventional | Recruiting | University of California, Davis |
| NCT019 12872 | Study to assess the efficacy and safety of Omalizumab treatment on ICS reduction for severe IgE-mediated asthma (MEXIC) | Phase 4 | Omalizumab (anti-IgE) Budesonide Formoterol (LABA) | Nov 2013 | Assessment of the efficacy and safety of Omalizumab treatment during 12 months to reduce the use of ICS in pediatric and adult patients with severe IgE-mediated asthma inadequately controlled with high doses of corticosteroids. | Interventional | Recruiting | Novartis Pharmaceuticals |
| NCT020 41221 | Pharmacology study of Sun Pharma Advanced Research Company Limited's S0597 | Phase 1 Phase 2 | Placebo S0597 | Jan 2014 | Evaluation of safety, tolerability, pharmacokinetics, and pharmacodynamics of S0597 by oral inhalation. | Interventional | Not yet recruiting | Sun Pharma Advanced Research Company Limited |
| NCT020 49294 | Study of the prednisone-sparing effect of Xolair (Omalizumab) in patients with Prednisone-dependent asthma with | Phase 2 Phase 3 | Omalizumab (anti-IgE) Placebo Normal Saline | Mar 2014 | Investigation whether addition of Omalizumab enables a reduction in the dose of prednisone in patients with asthma | Interventional | Recruiting | McMaster University |

| Clinical Trial Identifier | Title | Phase | Drugs | Start Date | Purpose | Study Type | Recruitment Status | Responsible Party |
|---|---|---|---|---|---|---|---|---|
| | eosinophilic bronchitis | | | | and eosinophilic bronchitis. | | | |
| NCT019 87492 | A study of Lebrikizumab In patients with severe asthma who depend on oral corticosteroids | Phase 2 | Placebo Lebrikizumab (anti-IL-13) | Mar 2014 | Evaluation of the efficacy of Lebrikizumab compared with placebo as measured by the ability of patients to achieve lower daily doses of OCS in patients with severe corticosteroid-dependent asthma. | Interve ntional | Recr uiting | Hoffmann-La Roche |
| NCT020 75008 | Long-term safety study of QGE031 in patients with allergic asthma who completed study CQGE031 B2201 | Phase 2 | QGE031 | Mar 2014 | Assessment of long-term safety of QGE031 during 12 months of treatment in asthma patients who completed study CQGE031B2201. | Interve ntional | Recr uiting | Novartis Pharmaceuticals |
| NCT020 75255 | Efficacy and safety study of Benralizumab to reduce OCS use in patients with uncontrolled asthma on high-dose inhaled corticosteroid plus LABA and chronic OCS therapy | Phase 3 | Placebo Benralizumab (anti-IL-5) | Apr 2014 | This trial is to confirm if Benralizumab can reduce OCS dependence (after dose optimization) in patients who are uncontrolled on high-dose ICS-LABA, and chronically dependent on OCS as part of their regular asthma controller regimen. | Interve ntional | Recr uiting | AstraZeneca |
| NCT021 35692 | A Phase 3a, repeat dose, open-label, long-term safety study of Mepolizumab in asthmatic subjects | Phase 3 | Mepolizumab (anti-IL-5) Standard of Care | May 2014 | Collection of clinical data for long-term use and further assessment of efficacy in patients | Interve ntional | Recr uiting | GlaxoSmithKline |

| Clinical Trial Identifier | Title | Phase | Drugs | Start Date | Purpose | Study Type | Recruit ment Status | Respon sible Party |
|---|---|---|---|---|---|---|---|---|
| | | | | | with loss of asthma control | | | |
| NCT021 26865 | Multiple rising oral doses of BI 1060469 in healthy subjects and mild asthma patients | Phase 1 | Placebo BI 1060469 | May 2014 | Investigation of the safety and tolerability of repeated rising doses of BI 1060469 in healthy male and female subjects and in asthmatic male and female patients. | Interve ntional | Recr uiting | Boehringer Ingelheim |
| NCT021 61757 | A Phase 3 study to evaluate the efficacy and safety of Tralokinumab in adults and adolescents with uncontrolled asthma (STRATOS1) | Phase 3 | Placebo Tralokinumab (Anti-IL-13) | Jun 2014 | Evaluation of the efficacy and safety of Tralokinumab in adults and adolescents with asthma inadequately controlled on ICS plus long-acting $\beta_2$-agonist. | Interve ntional | Recr uiting | AstraZeneca |
| NCT021 04674 | A study evaluating the efficacy and safety of Lebrikizumab in adult patients with mild to moderate asthma | Phase 3 | Placebo Lebrikizumab (anti-IL-13) Montelukast | Jun 2014 | Assessment of the efficacy and safety of Lebrikizumab in adult patients with mild to moderate asthma treated with SABA therapy alone. | Interve ntional | Recr uiting | Hoffmann-La Roche |
| NCT020 66298 | Steroids In eosinophil-negative asthma (SIENA) | Phase 3 | Placebo Mometasone Tiotropium (LAMA) | Jul 2014 | Determination if patients who are persistently non-eosinophilic differ in their benefit from inhaled corticosteroid treatment compared to patients who are not persistently non-eosinophilic. | Interve ntional | Recr uiting | Milton S. Hershey Medical Center |
| NCT020 | A study | Phase 2 | Placebo | Nov 2014 | Evaluation | Interve | Recr | Hoffmann- |

| Clinical Trial Identifier | Title | Phase | Drugs | Start Date | Purpose | Study Type | Recruitment Status | Responsible Party |
|---|---|---|---|---|---|---|---|---|
| 99656 | evaluating the effects of Lebrikizumab on airway eosinophilic inflammation in patients with uncontrolled asthma | | Lebrikizumab (anti-IL-13) | | of the effects of Lebrikizumab on airway eosinophilic inflammation in patients with uncontrolled asthma on inhaled corticosteroids and a second controller medication. | ntional | uiting | La Roche |
| NCT022 58542 | A safety extension study to evaluate the safety and tolerability of Benralizumab (MEDI-563) in asthmatic adults and adolescents on inhaled corticosteroid plus LABA (BORA) | Phase 3 | Benralizumab (anti-IL-5) | Nov 2014 | Characterization of safety profile of Benralizumab administration in asthma patients who have completed one of the three predecessor studies: D3250C00017, D3250C00018, or D3250C00020. | Interventional | Recruiting | AstraZeneca |
| NCT022 96411 | Efficacy of LAMA added to ICS in treatment of asthma (ELITRA) | Phase 2 | Placebo CHF 5259 Glycopyrrolate bromide (LAMA) | Nov 2014 | Evaluation of the safety and superiority of the glycopyrrolate bromide (CHF 5259 pMDI) versus placebo on top of QVAR® pMDI, in terms of lung functions parameters. | Interventional | Recruiting | Chiesi Farmaceutici S.p.A. |
| NCT022 93265 | Cross-sectional study for identification and description of severe asthma patients | Phase 3 | Mepolizumab (anti-IL-5) Omalizumab (anti-IgE) Reslizumab (anti-IL-5) | Dec 2014 | The potential overlap of patients eligible for treatment with Mepolizumab, Omalizumab and/or Reslizumab will be estimated. | Interventional | Recruiting | GlaxoSmithKline |
| NCT022 81318 | Efficacy and safety | Phase 3 | Placebo Mepolizumab | Dec 2014 | Evaluation of the | Interventional | Recruiting | GlaxoSmithKline |

| Clinical Trial Identifier | Title | Phase | Drugs | Start Date | Purpose | Study Type | Recruitment Status | Responsible Party |
|---|---|---|---|---|---|---|---|---|
| | study of Mepolizumab adjunctive therapy in participants with severe eosinophilic asthma on markers of asthma control | | (anti-IL-5) Standard of Care | | efficacy and safety of Mepolizumab adjunctive therapy in participants with severe eosinophilic asthma on markers of asthma control. | | | |
| NCT023 22775 | Study to evaluate the efficacy and safety of Benralizumab in adult patients with mild to moderate persistent asthma | Phase 3 | Placebo Benralizumab (anti-IL-5) | Feb 2015 | Confirmation of the safety and clinical benefit of Benralizumab administration in asthma patients with mild to moderate persistent asthma. | Interventional | Recruiting | AstraZeneca |
| NCT023 82510 | Multiple ascending dose study of TRN-157 in stable mild and moderate asthmatics | Phase 2 | Placebo TRN-157 Tiotropium (LAMA) | Feb 2015 | Determination of the safety and bronchodilator activity of TRN-157 in approximately 54 mild and moderate asthmatics. | Interventional | Recruiting | Theron Pharmaceuticals, Inc. |
| NCT023 15131 | Study in healthy volunteers and COPD patients to evaluate the efficacy and safety of inhaled TV46017 | Phase 1 | Placebo TV46017 | Mar 2015 | Assessment of the safety profile and duration of bronchodilation of a single dose of inhaled TV46017. | Interventional | Not yet recruiting | Teva Branded Pharmaceutical Products, R&D Inc. |
| NCT021 24226 | Low-dose Methotrexate for reduction GINA 5 medications in chronic severe asthma | Phase 3 | Placebo Methotrexate | Apr 2015 | Investigation of the role of an add-on immunological modifier in patients with chronic severe asthma. | Interventional | Not yet recruiting | Universita degli Studi di Catania |
| NCT023 77427 | Pharmacokinetics and pharmacodynamics of Mepolizumab administered subcutaneously in children | Phase 2 | Mepolizumab (anti-IL-5) | Apr 2015 | Assessment of the pharmacokinetics and pharmacodynamics of Mepolizumab in children aged 6–11 years with severe | Interventional | Not yet recruiting | GlaxoSmithKline |

| Clinical Trial Identifier | Title | Phase | Drugs | Start Date | Purpose | Study Type | Recruitment Status | Responsible Party |
|---|---|---|---|---|---|---|---|---|
| | | | | | eosinophilic asthma. | | | |
| NCT02336425 | Efficacy and safety of QGE031 compared with placebo in patients aged 18–75 years with asthma | Phase 2 | Placebo QGE031 | Apr 2015 | The study will assess the safety and efficacy of different dose levels of QGE031 in asthma patients. | Interventional | Not yet recruiting | Novartis Pharmaceuticals |
| NCT02427165 | Comparison of RPL554 With placebo and Salbutamol in asthmatic patients | Phase 2 | Placebo RPL554 (PDE-3/4 inhibitor) Salbutamol | Apr 2015 | Assessment of the effects of RPL554 compared with Salbutamol and placebo in patients with chronic asthma. | Interventional | Not yet recruiting | Verona Pharma plc |
| NCT02422121 | Effect of RNS60 on the late-phase asthmatic response to allergen challenge | Phase 2 | Placebo RNS60 Budesonide | May 2015 | Evaluation of the effects of multiple doses of inhaled RNS60 and Budesonide on the late-phase asthmatic response to allergen challenge in patients with mild asthma. | Interventional | Not yet recruiting | Revalesio Corporation |
| NCT02571660 | Efficacy of vitamin D on the clinical management of pediatric patients with asthma | Phase 3 | Vitamin D (Low- and high-supplementation doses) | Oct 2015 | Evaluation of vitamin D supplementation on exacerbation and clinical control of asthma. | Interventional | Not yet recruiting | Hospital General Naval de Alta Especialidad - Escuela Medico Naval |

Abbreviations denote: **IL**: Interleukin; **IgE**: Immunoglobulin E; **PDE**: Phosphodiesterase enzyme; **ICS**: Inhaled corticosteroids; **OCS**: Oral corticosteroids; **SABA**: Short-acting β-agonists; **LABA**: Long-acting β-agonists; **LAMA**; Long-acting muscarinic antagonists.

**Table 2.** Summary of recent ongoing clinical trials for new drugs used in the treatment of asthma (started in the past 3 years).

### 6.4.1. Anti-leukotrienes

Leukotrienes are lipid eicosanoids with a wide range of biological activities. They are derived from arachidonic acid through the enzymatic action of 5-lipooxygenase, and play a crucial role in asthma inflammatory pathogenesis, and in other allergic diseases such as allergic rhinitis, rhinosinusitis, atopic dermatitis, and urticaria [116]. Leukotrienes class includes three main types: cysteinyl leukotrienes (CysLTs), LTB4, and LTG4. LTG4 is the metabolite of LTE4 in which the cysteinyl moiety has been oxidized to an $\alpha$ keto-acid [117]. Since, very little is known about the LTG4-putative leukotriene, most clinical research studies focus on CysLTs and LTB4. CysLTs are strong bronchoconstrictors that powerfully affect airway remodeling, whereas LTB4 is a strong chemoattractant for most leukocyte subsets [118]. Over the last 20 years, since leukotriene antagonists were introduced to the clinic for asthma management, Montelukast [119, 120] and Zafirlukast [121] are the most frequently used drugs in this class.

## 6.4.2. Anti-IgE

At the moment, Omalizumab, which is the only approved targeted monoclonal antibody against IgE, is used to treat allergic asthma in clinical practice. It can significantly decrease serum IgE levels (up to 99%) within 2 h following subcutaneous administration, and diminish serum, sputum, and tissue eosinophilia [122]. Recently, Omalizumab has also been reported to have steroid-sparing effect, reducing the rate of asthma exacerbations up to 50%, and hence improving the quality of life [123]. However, nearly 45% of patients treated with Omalizumab had adverse reaction at the local injection site, which is considered the most commonly observed adverse event for Omalizumab. Some other minor upper respiratory tract infections and sinusitis have also been reported as well. Patients treated with Omalizumab display a very low (0.09%) frequency of anaphylaxis reaction. Importantly, there are no data reporting any correlation between cancer and Omalizumab treatment [124].

## 6.4.3. Anti-ILs

Three interleukin pathways are of physiological importance for asthma: IL-5, IL-9, and IL-4/IL-13 pathways. IL-5 is pivotal for both eosinophil differentiation and maturation in the bone marrow. Subsequently, it controls eosinophil mobilization, activation, and survival [125]. Hence, antagonizing IL-5 has been proposed to be beneficial for asthma therapy, particularly for predominantly eosinophilic asthma. A number of anti-IL-5 and anti-IL-5 receptor monoclonal antibodies are in the process of development for allergic diseases: Reslizumab [126], Mepolizumab [127], and Benralizumab [128]. IL-9 is one of the T-helper 2 (Th2) pro-inflammatory cytokines that promote mast cell proliferation and T-cell growth [129]. In mouse models, IL-9 causes several common features of chronic asthma: excessive mucus production, eosinophilic airway inflammation, smooth-muscle cell hyperplasia, and aryl hydrocarbon receptor (AHR) [130]. Currently, a phase IIb clinical trial evaluates the efficacy and safety of subcutaneous Medi-528, a humanized IgG1 anti-IL-9 mAb, in adults with uncontrolled asthma (NCT00968669). Activated mast cells, eosinophils, basophils, and dendritic cells secrete IL-4 and IL-13. IL-4 and IL-13 both play an important role in asthma mainly by enhancing IgE production. They also control mast cells' growth and development, eosinophil recruitment, and AHR [131]. The first trial aimed at antagonizing the IL-4 used a soluble recombinant human IL-4 receptor antagonist (IL-4RA), altrakincept, which blocked the binding of IL-4 to its cellular receptors [132]. Several humanized IL-13-neutralizing antibodies have entered asthma phase I/II clinical trials—anrukinzumab [133], QAX576 [134], and CAT354 [135].

### 6.4.4. Anti-TNF-α

TNF-α, a cytokine produced by Th1 cells and macrophages, has diverse biological functions. TNF-α shows crucial, and previously extensively documented, role in Crohn's disease, rheumatoid arthritis, and psoriasis pathogenesis. The association between TNF-α increase and these disease progressions had inspired studies aiming to extend anti-TNF-α therapies also for the treatment of severe asthma and COPD [136]. Infliximab and Golimumab, two anti-TNF-α mAbs, and Etanercept, a decoy soluble TNF-α receptor, are both able to biologically neutralize TNF-α cytokine, and blunt the immune response, thereby abolishing TNF-α effects in asthma [137].

## 7. Pharmacogenetics of asthma

The US Food and Drug Administration definition for pharmacogenomics is "the study of variations in DNA and RNA characteristics as related to drug response" [138]. "*Pharmacogenomics*" differs from "*Pharmacogenetics*" in that the former is concerned with the whole genome, its components, and regulators, while the latter is focused only on the DNA sequences of individual gene. Thus, in sense, pharmacogenetics is thought to be a subset of pharmacogenomics [139].

Because it is a complex trait, the drug response to asthma is diversely heterogeneous even among patients with apparently similar clinical profiles [7]. It is estimated that up to 50% difference in therapeutic response has been attributed to genetic variations between individuals [140]. Although several possible mechanisms have been postulated, genetic variants affect the pharmacogenetic response to drugs in two different ways:

1. *Pharmacodynamic genetic variations* are variations in which the receptor binding the drug ligand or another member of the drug target pathway is altered resulting in different drug effect. Most of the current pharmacogenetic research fall into this mechanistic category. Populations are stratified into responders and nonresponders, and then analyzed for DNA polymorphisms, which distinguish these two groups apart.

2. *Pharmacokinetic genetic variations* are related to altered uptake, distribution, and/or metabolism of the administered drug. Fewer examples fall in this category; however, the most common research subfield here is the area of investigating drug-catabolizing or -excreting enzymes. An important example here is the cytochrome *P450* (CYP450) family, a widely recognized metabolizing enzyme with several variable pharmacogenetic patterns.

Single nucleotide polymorphism, SNP, denoted by a reference sequence (rs) number, represents a class of polymorphism that is derived from a one-base point mutation in which a single nucleotide is substituted with another one. SNPs may be located in the gene regulatory or coding regions, and so it may affect the gene expression in more than one way; however, in majority of cases, most discovered SNPs do not change the gene function in a significant manner [141]. Consequently, it is essential to investigate whether the DNA sequence variances would actually cause significant functional impacts (i.e., resulting in an altered observed biology), or is a linkage disequilibrium marker of another DNA variant, which is the real cause of the response variability, or is generally nonsignificant. Because of its strong importance, since 15 years, catalogs of SNPs have started to outline the most common genetic polymorphisms among different population groups [141, 142], and this process has attracted more attention during the last couple of years [143].

## Candidate Gene Approach

| Gene | Loci |
|------|------|
| CRHR1 | rs242941, rs1876828 |
| STIP1 | rs2236647, rs6591838, rs1011219 |
| TBX21 | rs2240017 (His$^{33}$Gln) |
| ADCY9 | rs2230739 (Met$^{772}$Ile) |
| CYP3A4 | CYP3A4*22 allele |

| Gene | Loci |
|------|------|
| CRHR2 | rs7793837 |
| ADCY9 | rs2230739 (Ile$^{772}$Met) |
| ADRB2 | rs1042713 (Gly$^{16}$Arg), rs1800888 (Thr$^{164}$Ile), -376 insertion-deletion |
| ARG1 | rs2781659, rs2781667 |
| ARG2 | rs7140310, rs10483801 |
| NOS3 | rs1799983 (Asp$^{298}$Glu) |
| THRB | rs892940 |

| Gene | Loci |
|------|------|
| ALOX5 | Promoter repeat, rs892690, rs2029253, rs2115819 |
| LTC4S | rs272431, rs730012 |
| MRP1 | rs215066, 119774 |
| LTA4H | rs266845 |
| SLCO2B1 | rs12422149 (Arg$^{312}$Gln) |

**Corticosteroids Pathway**

**β-adrenergic Pathway**

**Leukotrienes Pathway**

## GWAS

| Gene | Loci |
|------|------|
| GLCCI1 | rs37972=rs37973 |
| T gene | rs3127412, rs6456042, rs3099266, rs2305089 |

| Gene | Loci |
|------|------|
| SLC24A4 | rs77441273 (Arg$^{585}$Gln) |
| SPATS2L | rs295137 |

**Figure 4.** Pharmacogenetically significant genes with relevance to corticosteroids, β-adrenergic, and leukotriene biological pathways. Left side: Candidate gene approach studies, Right side: GWAS (Genome Wide association studies).

All genes contain huge number of SNPs and copy-number variations (CNVs). CNVs are another form of structural variations, which account for 13% of the human genome bulkiness, and manifest as kilo-to-mega bases of deletions or duplications [144]. Conjointly, it is challenging to outline which polymorphism is influencing the treatment response and which are not relevant. Two major approaches declaiming this challenge have been practiced so far: candidate gene approach and GWAS. As it combines transcriptomic, proteomic and metabolomic profiling traits, a third approach, the integrative system biology approach, had led to a more comprehensive pharmacogenetic view [3]. To differentiate, candidate gene approach is based on a prior evidence according to the knowledge of the drug pharmacodynamics or/and pharmacokinetics, by contrast, GWAS methodology identifies new associations with the null hypothesis being that no associations exist. GWAS picks the variations which are associated with observable phenotypes by scanning SNP markers that tag, via linkage disequilibrium, the complete human genome. GWAS and integrative system biology approaches are modern tools contributing to the recent advancements of genotyping and statistical technologies.

Current pharmacogenetic studies of the corticosteroids, β-adrenergic, and leukotriene pathways are mostly candidate gene studies, with some GWAS, however, altogether have identified several genetic loci in strong association with therapeutic responsiveness to asthma. **Figure 4** summarizes the pharmacogenetically significant genes with relevance to the corticosteroids, β-adrenergic, and leukotriene biological pathways.

### 7.1. Corticosteroid pathway pharmacogenetics

In cytosol, the glucocorticoids bind to their corresponding glucocorticoid receptor, forming a hetero-complex that is activated by ligand binding, and translocate into the nucleus. In the nucleus, this complex binds to the glucocorticoid response elements in some target genes' promoter region resulting in their expression regulation. The core role of glucocorticoids is mediated via activating the transcription of anti-inflammatory genes, and suppressing the transcription of pro-inflammatory genes [145, 146]. The glucocorticoid pharmacogenetic studies formerly focused on candidate gene approach. Those candidate genes covered functions related to the corticosteroid biosynthetic pathway, the hetero-complex receptor formation, and the related chaperone proteins.

Corticotrophin-releasing hormone *(CRHR1)*, stress-inducible protein 1 *(STIP1)*, *TBX21*, *CYP3A4*, *GLCCI1*, T gene, and *FBXL7* are the most up-to-date potential pharmacogenetic biomarker targets for predicting patients' response to ICS [147]. Studies of the corticotrophin-releasing hormone gene are considered to be as one of the oldest and remarkable footsteps in asthma pharmacogenetics. CRHR1 protein, also known as CRF1, is the primary receptor controlling the adrenocorticotropic hormone release; hence, it plays a pleiotropic and vital role in steroid actions. A candidate gene study of *CRHR1* in 1117 asthmatics administrating ICS therapy, from three clinical cohorts, revealed two SNPs (rs242941 and rs1876828) associated with different response in lung functions [148]. Tantisira et al. [148] found that *CRHR1* gene variation was frequently related to augmented therapy response in each of the three studied cohorts. Since 2004, *CRHR1* gene studies opened the doors for all other corticosteroid pharmacogenetics and the possible future therapeutic outcomes.

*STIP1* or *HOP* (abbreviated for Hsp70-Hsp90-Organizing Protein) gene mainly functions to reversibly link Hsp70 and Hsp90 together as a co-chaperone [149]. *STIP1* pharmacogenetic studies in one adult cohort revealed three SNPs (rs2236647, rs6591838, and rs1011219) within this heat shock-organizing protein and related to improved lung response during ICS therapy [150]. *STIP1* rs2236647 variant analysis in healthy and asthmatic children showed that this SNP could serve as an asthma marker for choosing the population who receives corticosteroid therapy[151]; however, further replication studies should be held to confirm those results.

One significant aspect of pharmacogenomics is that it investigates the interactions with genes of other pathways. *TBX21* gene is one good example for observing the ICS response outside the glucocorticoid pathway. *TBX21* is one of the conserved genes of a family sharing a common DNA-binding domain; the T-box encodes T box transcription factor TBx21 protein. Tbx21 protein is a Th1 (T-helper1) transcription factor, which regulates one of the Th1 cytokine expression, interferon-gamma (IFNG). In 2004, a nonsynonymous SNP rs2240017 (His$^{33}$Glu) in the *TBX21* gene was linked to improvements in bronchial hyperresponsiveness or "broncho-protection" in response to ICS in individuals participating in the Child Asthma Management Program (CAMP) cohort [152]. This finding was also observed in an independent Korean cohort in 2009 [153]. Thus, *TBx21* may be an important determinant pharmacogenetic candidate gene for predicting asthmatics' response to inhaled corticosteroid therapies.

In 2005, another example demonstrated the glucocorticoid pathway interactions with one other pathway. *ADCY9*, adenylyl cyclase type 9, gene encodes a membrane-bound enzyme in the β2-adrenergic receptor pathway, which catalyzes the production of cyclic adenosine monophosphate (AMP) from adenosine triphosphate (ATP). This candidate gene contains a pharmacogenetic nonsynonymous SNP, Met$^{772}$Ile, which was correlated to enhanced Salbutamol (SABA) bronchodilator effects only in patients treated with ICS [154]. An independent Korean cohort replicated the trial, using Formoterol (LABA) treatment in combination with ICS, and confirmed those results [155].

Cytochromes P450s belong to a heme cofactor-containing superfamily of metabolizing enzyme proteins that potentially control the metabolism of drug (i.e., pharmacokinetics), and consequently treatment response in many diseases. For asthma, *CYP3A4*, *CYP3A5*, and *CYP3A7* candidate genes have been studied among a retrospective analysis of 413 asthmatic children treated with the ICS Fluticasone propionate [156]. The three candidate CYPs of all subjects were genotyped for nine SNPs. Results showed that asthmatics with the *CYP3A4*22* allele demonstrated a significant symptom control compared with those lacking that allele. This study included a small number of participants ($n = 20$), so further large-scale replication is required.

Tantisira et al. [157] conducted the first pharmacogenetic GWAS for ICS treatment in asthma and identified an SNP (rs37972) in the promoter of the glucocorticoid-induced transcript-1 gene (*GLCCI1*), which significantly associates with lung functions. Replicated in four independent populations (935 persons in total), this candidate SNP was linked to substantial decrements in the response to the ICS in asthmatics. The wild-type allele homozygotes (CC) showed greater forced expiratory volume in 1 s (FEV1) in response to the ICS compared with those identified with the homozygote variant allele (TT). Another functionally correlated SNP (rs37973) in the promoter of the same gene was further validated within *in vitro* studies [157]. Results showed declined luciferase reporter activity in cells with the minor allele. *GLCCI1* GWAS outlines that drug response to asthma treatment is subjected to wide inter-individual variation, and GWAS would uncover more novel pharmacogenetic associations in the future. Tantisira et al. conducted a second GWAS among 418 asthmatics randomized to ICS treatment from the Childhood Asthma Research and Education (CARE), Asthma Clinical Research Network (ACRN), and CAMP trial cohorts. The *T-gene* (encoding the Brachyury transcription factor protein) compromised two SNPs (rs3127412 and rs6456042) that were associated, out of the successfully genotyped 47 SNPs, with altered lung function response to ICS [158].

## 7.2. β-adrenergic receptor pathway pharmacogenetics

β2-adrenergic receptor gene remains to be the most studied pharmacogenetic loci among the beta-agonist pathways. *ADRB2* gene has several polymorphic variants that were discovered in multi-ethnic genetic asthma cohorts [159, 160]. ADRB2 protein is a cell membrane-spanning receptor that binds epinephrine, but not norepinephrine, unlike the other adrenergic receptors, and consequently mediates both smooth muscle relaxation and bronchodilation [161, 162]. Early ADRB2 studies showed that Gly[16]Arg, a prevalent coding variant of the amino acid at position 16 of ADRB2, is associated with altered bronchodilator response to SABAs [163].

The BARGE (Beta-Agonist Response by Genotype) study [164], held by the National Heart, Lung and Blood Institute Asthma Clinical Network, was one of the first genotype "stratified" pharmacogenetic studies for asthma. In this study, only Gly[16]Arg homozygotes for ADRB2 were included (i.e., Arg/Arg and Gly/Gly). Participants were randomly receiving either intermittent or regular albuterol, and then crossed over to receive the alternative treatment dose. For statistical stratification, this study ensured that the Arg[16] homozygotes, who are less frequent, were appropriately randomly distributed to both SABA intermittent and regular protocols. Compared to Gly[16] homozygotes, the BARGE study showed that the Arg[16] homozygotes were good responders only to acute intermittent SABAs rather than to long-term regular treatments, a finding that does not coincide with the current clinical asthma treatment guidelines [165] which recommend SABA as for on-demand intermittent usage. Since the 16th amino acid of ADRB2 controls regular response to albuterol, bronchodilator medications other than SABAs would be more appropriate for Arg/Arg asthmatics.

Collectively, the BARGE study [164], along with some other pharmacogenetic studies [163, 166–168] of Gly[16]Arg and SABAs' exposure, provided insights for further studies [169–171] on LABAs. In contrast to SABAs, a large cohort [169] of 2250 asthmatics, randomly assigned to formoterol plus budesonide, demonstrated no pharmacogenetic action due to *ADRB2* variation on therapeutic response. Furthermore, a multicenter trial [170] showed that asthmatics with both Arg/Arg and Gly/Gly genetic signatures had improved airway functions, if they received combination treatment with Salmeterol and ICS, when compared with ICS therapy alone. Similarly, the results of another prospective trial cohort [171] of 544 subjects, also randomized by genotyping, demonstrated no evidence of any pharmacogenetic action due to *ADRB2* variation in response to Salmeterol. Together, these findings, confirmed among several asthma populations, suggest that in contrast to SABAs, asthmatics can still be treated with LABAs plus ICS irrespective of their genotyping status.

Genetic variants' occurrences among different ethnic groups are quantified by their percentage of allele frequencies. Usually, frequent and common variants have only little or modest impacts on disease susceptibility and, subsequently, therapeutic response. On the other hand, as the variant is characterized to be rare or more "private," its effect size on disease progression and therapeutic response dramatically increases [172]. Early *in vitro* studies had investigated a rare polymorphism of *ADRB2* within the fourth transmembrane domain, the Thr[164]Ile variant. For the Ile[164] genotype, results showed significant lowering in Gs-protein signaling and different SABA- and LABA-binding affinities [173, 174]. While the Thr[164]Ile polymorphism is pointed out to be a rare coding variant (i.e., <5%), population studies showed that this variant is more common in non-Hispanic white populations [159, 160], a finding that requires further pharmacogenetic investigation in different and larger populations. To replicate results, a study of two large Copenhagen population cohorts [175], with more than 55,000 participants, was held to investigate the relation of Thr[164]Ile variation and lung responses. Among the general population, the Copenhagen study reported that the Thr[164] genotype was associated with decreased FEV1, diminished lung function, and increased the overall COPD risk.

In addition to ADRB2 Gly[16]Arg and Thr[164]Ile variants, the (-376 In-Del) polymorphism was extensively studied as another significant pharmacogenetic *ADRB2* variant. Presented primarily among African Americans and Puerto Ricans [159, 160], the 24-bp promoter insertion at −376, related to the start codon, is associated with asthma-related hospitalization in asthmatics treated with LABA [160]. Altogether, these variants, being unique to different populations, highlight the increasing need of personalized-based treatments.

Adenylyl cyclase type 9, encoded in humans by *ADCY9* gene, is a membrane-bound enzyme that catalyzes the formation of cyclic AMP from ATP. ADCY9 is a widely abundant adenylyl cyclase, and it is stimulated via beta-adrenergic receptor activation [176]. Ile[772]Met is a coding variant of *ADCY9* gene that has been associated with both acute FEV1 bronchodilation in response to SABAs [154] and long-term FEV1 response for LABAs [155]. CRHR2 (which is more commonly known as CRF2) is a type-2 G protein-coupled protein receptor for the corticotropin-releasing hormone [177]. Out of the 28 studied SNPs in *CRHR2*, five SNPs were significantly correlated with acute bronchodilator response in one, or frequently more than one, cohort. Among those, variant rs7793837 was associated with altered SABA response in all three cohorts of the *CRHR2* study containing 607, 427, and 152 participants, respectively [178].

Different variants of *ARG1* (Arginase 1) and *ARG2* (Arginase 2) show altered acute response to SABAs, while the endothelial nitric oxide synthase (*NOS3*) shows altered acute response to LABAs. NO (nitric oxide), an endogenous vasorelaxing bronchodilator, is generated by the action of NOS3 on L-arginine. Since ARG1 and ARG2 are metabolizing L-arginine, so it is expected that the entire three genes, *ARG1*, *ARG2*, and *NOS3*, might be implicated in asthma pharmacogenetics. Combined association evidence, surviving Bonferroni correction for multiple testing from the CAMP four asthma cohorts [179], points to SNP rs2781659 in *ARG1*. C-allele homozygotes for SNP rs2781667 in arginase 1 showed significantly less response to the inhaled corticosteroid treatments [180]. Arginase-2 variants rs17249437 and rs3742879 correlated with increased airway obstruction and airway hyperresponsiveness, and lower reversibility of airway constriction following treatment with beta-2 agonists [180]. A small candidate gene study [181] of *NOS3* had revealed one possible variant (Asp[298]Glu) correlated with lung function response to ICS/LABA combined treatment; however, this result still needs to be replicated in larger cohorts. *THRB* [182], *SLC24A4* [183], *SLC22A15* [183], *SPATS2L* [184], and SNPs (rs892940, rs77441273, rs1281748/rs1281743, and rs295137, respectively) show promising loci for further pharmacogenetic investigations.

### 7.3. Leukotriene pathway pharmacogenetics

Relative to the corticosteroid and β-adrenergic pathways, the cysteinyl leukotriene pathway pharmacogenetic studies are generally fewer and have smaller sample sizes. The oldest of these studies [185], held in 1999, had investigated the tandem repeat polymorphism in *ALOX5* promoter. Among 114 asthmatics, it has been shown that the *ALOX5* promoter repeat is associated with altered lung functions in response to a 5-LO inhibitor [185]. It has been shown in children that those who had more or less than five repeats (3, 4, and 6) of the *ALOX5* promoter-binding motif experienced increased urinary leukotriene E4 (the terminal cysteinyl leukotriene metabolite) concentrations and reduced FEV1 baseline than the wild-type genotype with five repeats [186]. Further pharmacogenetic studies revealed that the *ALOX5* promoter polymorphism, along with the *ALOX5* SNPs rs892690, rs2029253, and rs2115819, influences leukotriene pathway antagonist therapy [187–190]. Moreover, variants of *LTC4S*, encoding Leukotriene C4 synthase, and *MRP1* (or *ABCC1*), encoding multidrug resistance-associated protein 1, have been linked to lung function response while treatment with Zileuton and Montelukast [189, 190].

Arg$^{312}$Gln, rs12422149, which is a coding variant in *SLCO2B1* (solute carrier organic anion transporter family member 2B1 gene), has been related to symptom control during Montelukast therapy. This fact was due to the interindividual variability of carrier-mediated Montelukast transport in the intestines, and consequently its plasma levels [191]. By contrast, two other studies, probably due to their small sample sizes, were unable to replicate similar *SLCO2B1* pharmacokinetic effects [192, 193]. Overall, larger replicate cohorts, for the leukotriene pathway identified loci, are still needed.

## 8. Current and future challenges facing asthma pharmacogenetics

As demonstrated above, there has been fundamental progress in the field of asthma pharmacogenetics; however, these efforts have not yet been introduced into clinical practice to guide physician. There are several reasons that account for this gap. Most important is the limited number of asthma pharmacogenetics-focused GWAS, which would compare common candidate gene methodology that would allow combining all patients from small cohorts studied. Small sample sizes prevent any expansion of the pharmacogenetic research of asthma, which needs a large number of subjects for statistical significance. Along with limited cohort size, study defects due to poor ancestry structuring and stratification substantially result in replication inconsistencies. Furthermore, genes interact together in networks; therefore, simply attributing phenotypic variation to individual genes is not appropriate. Epigenetics studies investigate the changes in gene activities, which are heritable to the subsequent generations, but are independent of any DNA sequence alterations [194, 195]. Epigenetic tuning of the genes associated with asthma has a significant impact on determining the drug response. Several mechanisms, related to epigenetics, are currently being investigated for both biomarker tagging and therapeutic innovation intervention [196]. Moreover, epigenetic changes have the ability to override the genetic effects of time, environment, tissue specificity, and other conditions such as age and gender of a patient, nutrition and hygiene, and intestinal microflora, which all highly influence the drug response in addition to the genetic factors. The collective impact of all combination of these factors requires the application of complicated algorithm that could take into consideration each of these factors and their interplay. The prospective genetic profile of an asthmatic should compromise a set of common and rare variants, on ancestral basis, which will be predictive of the pattern of his/her therapeutic responsiveness to different treatment options. The current human variant catalog continues to grow in an exponential manner because of the lower costs associated with whole genomic sequencing. Despite the steep decline in sequencing costs, the technology of sequencing, in terms of speed and quality, enormously increases. The future pharmacogenetic profile would also predict any possible adverse response associated with the chosen line of treatment. Genetic biomarkers are needed to warn the physician about any potential adverse side effects which can be life threatening. It is very important for typical genetic profiling to also consider gene-gene and gene-environment interactions. Gene-gene interactions are predominately crucial in the framework of combination therapies, for example, ICS and β-adrenergic agonists. Interactions between the surrounding environment and the patients' genes are assumed to be an additional element, because environmental stress, apart from the genetic makeup, contributes to the development of asthma exacerbations. Future pharmacogenetic directions need to cover also the pharmacokinetic side of the patient profile. Altered drug absorption, metabolism, distribution, or excretion extensively influence drug dosing and even drug selection. All in all, the complete asthma pharmacogenetic catalog has many aspects to cover, before being introduced into the clinical practice.

## 9. Conclusion

Asthma is a complex respiratory and immune disease. Inadequate (or exaggerated) ability of genetically predisposed individuals to control inflammation, induced by innate and environmental factors, results in asthma. Further, studies using allergic asthma and atopy models enable to better understand several interacting gene products and variable responsiveness of asthmatic subjects to current therapies. Eventually, thorough investigation of the complexity of asthma might lead to successful designing of personalized therapies for patients suffering from allergic asthma.

## Author details

Mina Youssef[1], Cynthia Kanagaratham[1], Mohamed I. Saad[2] and Danuta Radzioch[1,3*]

*Address all correspondence to: danuta.radzioch@mcgill.ca

1 Department of Human Genetics, McGill University, Montreal, Quebec, Canada

2 The Ritchie Centre, Hudson Institute of Medical Research, Monash University, Melbourne, Victoria, Australia

3 Department of Medicine, Division of Experimental Medicine, McGill University, Montreal, Quebec, Canada

# References

[1] Nanzer AM, Menzies-Gow A. Defining severe asthma – an approach to find new therapies. Eur Clin Respir J. 2014;1(5):1–9.

[2] Nakamura Y. Developmental current and future therapy for severe asthma. Inflamm Allergy-Drug Targets. 2013;12(1):54–60.

[3] Park H-W, Tantisira KG, Weiss ST. Pharmacogenomics in asthma therapy: where are we and where do we go? Annu Rev Pharmacol Toxicol. 2015;55(1):129–47.

[4] World Health Organ. (WHO). Bronchial asthma. WHO Fact Sheet 206, World Health Organ. G. No Title [Internet]. Available from: http://www.who.int/mediacentre/factsheets/fs206/en/. Accessed January 2016.

[5] Sossai P, Travaglione AM, Amenta F. Asthma: opinion or evidence based medicine? Clinical Medicine and Diagnositics. 2014;4(2):17-22.

[6] Bergeron C, Boulet L-P. Structural changes in airway diseases. Chest J. 2006;129(4): 1068–87.

[7] Szefler SJ, Martin RJ, King TS, Boushey HA, Cherniack RM, Chinchilli VM, et al. Significant variability in response to inhaled corticosteroids for persistent asthma. J Allergy Clin Immunol. 2002;109(3):410–8.

[8] International HapMap Consortium. The International HapMap Project. Nature. 2003 Dec 18;426(6968):789–96.

[9] International HapMap 3 Consortium, Altshuler DM, Gibbs RA, Peltonen L, Altshuler DM, Gibbs RA, et al. Integrating common and rare genetic variation in diverse human populations. Nature. 2010;467(7311):52–8.

[10] Bleecker E, Ortega V, Meyers D. Asthma pharmacogenetics and the development of genetic profiles for personalized medicine. Pharmgenomics Pers Med. 2015;8(16):9–22.

[11] Meyers DA, Bleecker ER, Holloway JW, Holgate ST. Asthma genetics and personalised medicine. Lancet Respir Med. 2014;2(5):405–15.

[12] Duffy DL, Martin NG, Battistutta D, Hopper JL, Mathews JD. Genetics of asthma and hay fever in Australian twins. Am Rev Respir Dis. 1990;142(6 Pt 1):1351–8.

[13] Ober C, Yao TC. The genetics of asthma and allergic disease: a 21st century perspective. Immunol Rev. 2011;242(1):10–30.

[14] Li X, Ampleford EJ, Howard TD, Moore WC, Torgerson DG, Li H, et al. Genome-wide association studies of asthma indicate opposite immunopathogenesis direction from autoimmune diseases. J Allergy Clin Immunol. 2012;130(4):861–8.e7.

[15] Van Eerdewegh P, Little RD, Dupuis J, Del Mastro RG, Falls K, Simon J, et al. Association of the ADAM33 gene with asthma and bronchial hyperresponsiveness. Nature. 2002;418(6896):426–30.

[16] Yoshinaka T, Nishii K, Yamada K, Sawada H, Nishiwaki E, Smith K, et al. Identification and characterization of novel mouse and human ADAM33s with potential metallo-protease activity. Gene. 2002;282(1–2):227–36.

[17] Tripathi P, Awasthi S, Gao P. ADAM metallopeptidase domain 33 (ADAM33): a promising target for asthma. Mediat Inflamm. 2014;2014:5720–5.

[18] March ME, Sleiman PM, Hakonarson H. Genetic polymorphisms and associated susceptibility to asthma. Int J Gen Med. 2013;6(17):253–65.

[19] Altshuler D, Daly MJ, Lander ES. Genetic mapping in human disease. Science. 2008;322(5903):881–8.

[20] McCarthy MI, Abecasis GR, Cardon LR, Goldstein DB, Little J, Ioannidis JPA, et al. Genome-wide association studies for complex traits: consensus, uncertainty and challenges. Nat Rev Genet. 2008;9(5):356–69.

[21] Moffatt MF, Kabesch M, Liang L, Dixon AL, Strachan D, Heath S, et al. Genetic variants regulating ORMDL3 expression contribute to the risk of childhood asthma. Nature. 2007;448(7152):470–3.

[22] Torgerson DG, Ampleford EJ, Chiu GY, Gauderman WJ, Gignoux CR, Graves PE, et al. Meta-analysis of genome-wide association studies of asthma in ethnically diverse North American populations. Nat Genet. 2011;43(9):887–92.

[23] Karunas AS, Iunusbaev BB, Fedorova II, Gimalova GF, Ramazanova NN, Gur'eva LL, et al. Genome-wide association study of bronchial asthma in the Volga-Ural region of Russia. Mol Biol (Mosk). 2011;45(6):992–1003.

[24] Wan YI, Shrine NRG, Soler Artigas M, Wain L V., Blakey JD, Moffatt MF, et al. Genome-wide association study to identify genetic determinants of severe asthma. Thorax. 2012;67(9):762–8.

[25] Breslow DK, Collins SR, Bodenmiller B, Aebersold R, Simons K, Shevchenko A, et al. Orm family proteins mediate sphingolipid homeostasis. Nature. 2010;463(7284):1048–53.

[26] Worgall TS, Veerappan A, Sung B, Kim BI, Weiner E, Bholah R, et al. Impaired sphingolipid synthesis in the respiratory tract induces airway hyperreactivity. Sci Transl Med. 2013;5(186):186ra67.

[27] Moffatt MF, Gut IG, Demenais F, Strachan DP, Bouzigon E, Heath S, et al. A large-scale, consortium-based genomewide association study of asthma. N Engl J Med. 2010;363(13):1211–21.

[28] Gudbjartsson DF, Bjornsdottir US, Halapi E, Helgadottir A, Sulem P, Jonsdottir GM, et al. Sequence variants affecting eosinophil numbers associate with asthma and myocardial infarction. Nat Genet. 2009;41(3):342–7.

[29] Weidinger S, Gieger C, Rodriguez E, Baurecht H, Mempel M, Klopp N, et al. Genome-wide scan on total serum IgE levels identifies FCER1A as novel susceptibility locus. PLoS Genet. 2008;4(8):e1000166.

[30] Postma DS, Reddel HK, ten Hacken NHT, van den Berge M. Asthma and chronic obstructive pulmonary disease: similarities and differences. Clin Chest Med. Elsevier Inc; 2014;35(1):143–56.

[31] Postma DS, Kerkhof M, Boezen HM, Koppelman GH. Asthma and chronic obstructive pulmonary disease: common genes, common environments? Am J Respir Crit Care Med. 2011;183(12):1588–94.

[32] Celedón JC, Milton DK, Ramsey CD, Litonjua AA, Ryan L, Platts-Mills TAE, et al. Exposure to dust mite allergen and endotoxin in early life and asthma and atopy in childhood. J Allergy Clin Immunol. 2007;120(1):144–9.

[33] Balaban J, Bijelic R, Milicevic S. Hypersensitivity to aeroallergens in patients with nasobronchial allergy. Med Arch. 2014;68(2):86.

[34] Gruchalla RS, Pongracic J, Plaut M, Evans R, Visness CM, Walter M, et al. Inner city asthma study: relationships among sensitivity, allergen exposure, and asthma morbidity. J Allergy Clin Immunol. 2005;115(3):478–85.

[35] Arbes SJ, Gergen PJ, Vaughn B, Zeldin DC. Asthma cases attributable to atopy: results from the third national health and nutrition examination survey. J Allergy Clin Immunol. 2007;120(5):1139–45.

[36] Kelly JT, Busse WW. Host immune responses to rhinovirus: mechanisms in asthma. J Allergy Clin Immunol. 2008;122(4):671–82.

[37] Wu P, Dupont WD, Griffin MR, Carroll KN, Mitchel EF, Gebretsadik T, et al. Evidence of a causal role of winter virus infection during infancy in early childhood asthma. Am J Respir Crit Care Med. 2008;178(11):1123–9.

[38] Darveaux JI, Lemanske RFJ. Infection-related asthma. J Allergy Clin Immunol Pract. 2014;2(6):658–63.

[39] Newcomb DC, Peebles RS. Bugs and asthma: a different disease? Proc Am Thorac Soc. 2009;6(3):266–71.

[40] Koyanagi K, Koya T, Sasagawa M, Hasegawa T, Suzuki E, Arakawa M, et al. An analysis of factors that exacerbate asthma, based on a Japanese questionnaire. Allergol Int. 2009;58(4):519–27.

[41] Beasley R, Semprini A, Mitchell EA. Asthma 1 risk factors for asthma©: is prevention possible©? Lancet. 2015;386(9998):1075–85.

[42] Greer JR, Abbey DE, Burchette RJ. Asthma related to occupational and ambient air pollutants in nonsmokers. J Occup Med. 1993;35(9):909–15.

[43] Havemann BD, Henderson CA, El-Serag HB. The association between gastro-oesophageal reflux disease and asthma: a systematic review. Gut. 2007;56(12):1654–64.

[44] Jaspersen D, Kulig M, Labenz J, Leodolter A, Lind T, Meyer-Sabellek W, et al. Prevalence of extra-oesophageal manifestations in gastro-oesophageal reflux disease: an analysis based on the ProGERD Study. Aliment Pharmacol Ther. 2003;17(12):1515–20.

[45] Sharifi A, Ansarin K. Effect of gastroesophageal reflux disease on disease severity and characteristics of lung functional changes in patients with asthma. J Cardiovasc Thorac Res. 2014;6(4):223–8.

[46] Wright RJ, Cohen S, Carey V, Weiss ST, Gold DR. Parental stress as a predictor of wheezing in infancy: a prospective birth-cohort study. Am J Respir Crit Care Med. 2002;165(3):358–65.

[47] Chen E, Hanson MD, Paterson LQ, Griffin MJ, Walker HA, Miller GE. Socioeconomic status and inflammatory processes in childhood asthma: the role of psychological stress. J Allergy Clin Immunol. 2006;117(5):1014–20.

[48] Moy ML, Lantin ML, Harver A, Schwartzstein RM. Language of dyspnea in assessment of patients with acute asthma treated with nebulized albuterol. Am J Respir Crit Care Med. 1998;158(3):749–53.

[49] Virchow JC, Crompton GK, Dal Negro R, Pedersen S, Magnan A, Seidenberg J, et al. Importance of inhaler devices in the management of airway disease. Respir Med. 2008;102(1):10–9.

[50] Prins LC, van Son MJ, van Keimpema AR, van Ranst D, Pommer A. Psychopathology in difficult asthma. J Asthma. 2015;(19):1–6.

[51] Thorowgood JC. On bronchial asthma. BMJ. 1873;2(673):600–600.

[52] Bosworth FH. Hay fever, asthma, and allied affections. Trans Am Climatol Assoc Meet. 1886;2(1):151–70.

[53] Gerthoffer WT, Solway J, Camoretti-Mercado B. Emerging targets for novel therapy of asthma. Curr Opin Pharmacol. Elsevier Ltd; 2013;13(3):324–30.

[54] Yayan J, Rasche K. Asthma and COPD: Similarities and Differences in the Pathophysiology, Diagnosis and Therapy. In Respiratory Medicine and Science 2015 (pp. 31–38). Springer International Publishing.

[55] Pauwels RA, Buist AS, Calverley PM, Jenkins CR, Hurd SS. Global strategy for the diagnosis, management, and prevention of chronic obstructive pulmonary disease. NHLBI/WHO Global Initiative for Chronic Obstructive Lung Disease (GOLD) Workshop summary. Am J Respir Crit Care Med. 2001;163(5):1256–76.

[56] Chiba S, Tsuchiya K, Nukui Y, Sema M, Tamaoka M, Sumi Y, et al. Interstitial changes in Asthma-COPD Overlap Syndrome (ACOS). Clin Respir J. 2016; (Epub ahead of print). ((Still Epub. Not assigned to issue yet))

[57] Stanley PJ, Wilson R, Greenstone MA, Mackay IS, Cole PJ. Abnormal nasal mucociliary clearance in patients with rhinitis and its relationship to concomitant chest disease. Br J Dis Chest. 1985;79(1):77–82.

[58] Flenley DC. Breathing during sleep. Ann Acad Med Singapore. 1985;14(3):479–84.

[59] Overholt RH, Voorhees RJ. Esophageal reflux as a trigger in asthma. Dis Chest. 1966;49(5):464–6.

[60] Boulet LP. Influence of comorbid conditions on asthma. Eur Respir J. 2009;33(4):897–906.

[61] Auerbach O, Stout AP, Hammond EC, Garfinkel L. Changes in bronchial epithelium in relation to cigarette smoking and in relation to lung cancer. N Engl J Med. 1961;265(1): 253–67.

[62] Holgate ST. Pathogenesis of asthma. Clin Exp Allergy. 2008;38(6):872–97.

[63] Flood-Page P, Menzies-Gow A, Phipps S, Ying S, Wangoo A, Ludwig MS, et al. Anti-IL-5 treatment reduces deposition of ECM proteins in the bronchial subepithelial basement membrane of mild atopic asthmatics. J Clin Invest. 2003;112(7):1029–36.

[64] Roche W, Williams J, Beasley R, Holgate S. Subepithelial fibrosis in the bronchi of asthmatics. Lancet. 1989;1(8637):520–4.

[65] Desmouliere A, Darby IA, Laverdet B, Bonté F. Fibroblasts and myofibroblasts in wound healing. Clin Cosmet Invest Dermatol. 2014;6(7):301–11.

[66] Hamid Q, Song Y, Kotsimbos TC, Minshall E, Bai TR, Hegele RG, et al. Inflammation of small airways in asthma. J Allergy Clin Immunol. 1997;100(1):44–51.

[67] Hostettler KE, Roth M, Burgess JK, Gencay MM, Gambazzi F, Black JL, et al. Airway epithelium-derived transforming growth factor-beta is a regulator of fibroblast proliferation in both fibrotic and normal subjects. Clin Exp Allergy. 2008;38(8):1309–17.

[68]  Ebina M, Takahashi T, Chiba T, Motomiya M. Cellular hypertrophy and hyperplasia of airway smooth muscles underlying bronchial asthma. A 3-D morphometric study. Am Rev Respir Dis. 1993;148(3):720–6.

[69]  Niimi A, Matsumoto H, Takemura M, Ueda T, Chin K, Mishima M. Relationship of airway wall thickness to airway sensitivity and airway reactivity in asthma. Am J Respir Crit Care Med. CRC Press; 2003;168(8):983–8.

[70]  Kazi AS, Lotfi S, Goncharova EA, Tliba O, Amrani Y, Krymskaya VP, et al. Vascular endothelial growth factor-induced secretion of fibronectin is ERK dependent. 2004; (3):L539–45.

[71]  Joubert P, Hamid Q. Role of airway smooth muscle in airway remodeling. J Allergy Clin Immunol. Mosby; 2005;116(3):713–6.

[72]  Al-Muhsen S, Johnson JR, Hamid Q. Remodeling in asthma. J Allergy Clin Immunol. Elsevier Ltd; 2011;128(3):451–62.

[73]  Zuyderduyn S, Sukkar MB, Fust A, Dhaliwal S, Burgess JK. Treating asthma means treating airway smooth muscle cells. Eur Respir J. 2008;32(2):265–74.

[74]  Harkness LM, Ashton AW, Burgess JK. Asthma is not only an airway disease, but also a vascular disease. Pharmacol Ther. 2015;148(1):17–33.

[75]  Smith R. Is VEGF a potential therapeutic target in asthma? Pneumologia. 2013;63(4): 194–7.

[76]  Salvato G. Quantitative and morphological analysis of the vascular bed in bronchial biopsy specimens from asthmatic and non-asthmatic subjects. Thorax. 2001;56(12):902–6.

[77]  Carroll NG, Cooke C, James AL. Bronchial blood vessel dimensions in asthma. Am J Respir Crit Care Med. 1997;155(2):689–95.

[78]  Yuksel H, Yilmaz O, Karaman M, Bagriyanik HA, Firinci F, Kiray M, et al. Role of vascular endothelial growth factor antagonism on airway remodeling in asthma. Ann Allergy Asthma Immunol. 2013;110(3):150–5.

[79]  Chu EK, Drazen JM. Asthma one hundred years of treatment and onward. Am J Respir Crit Care Med. 2005;171(11):1202–8.

[80]  Manniche L. Sacred luxuries: fragrance, aromatherapy, and cosmetics in ancient Egypt. Cornell University Press, Ithaca, USA; 1999. p. 49

[81]  http://www.naturalmedicinalherbs.net/ [Internet]. Available from: http://www.naturalmedicinalherbs.net/ Accessed January 2016

[82]  Lane DJ SA, editor. Bronchodilators. In: Asthma: the facts. 2nd ed. New York, NY: Oxford University Press; 1987. pp. 126–40.

[83]  O'Neil MJ. The Merck index. 15th ed. O'Neil MJ, editor. Merck Sharp & Dohme Corp. Whitehouse Station, N.J., U.S.A.; 2013.

[84]  Gaskoin G. On the treatment of asthma. Br Med J. 1872;1:339.

[85]  Takamine J. The blood-pressure raising principle of the suprarenal gland. J Am Med Assoc. American Medical Association; 1902;38(3):153–5.

[86]  Burnett J. Adrenalin: a short account of its therapeutic applications. Med Times Hosp Gaz. 1903;23(1):385–7.

[87]  Bennett MR. One hundred years of adrenaline: the discovery of autoreceptors. Clin Auton Res. 1999;9(3):145–59.

[88]  Global Initiative for Asthma (GINA) [Internet]. From the Global Strategy for Asthma Management and Prevention. 2015. Available from: http://www.ginasthma.org/ Accessed January 2016

[89]  Heitzer MD, Wolf IM, Sanchez ER, Witchel SF, DeFranco DB. Glucocorticoid receptor physiology. Rev Endocr Metab Disord. 2007;8(4):321–30.

[90]  Stewart AG, Fernandes D, Tomlinson PR. The effect of glucocorticoids on proliferation of human cultured airway smooth muscle. Br J Pharmacol. 1995;116(8):3219–26.

[91]  Cha HH, Cram EJ, Wang EC, Huang AJ, Kasler HG, Firestone GL. Glucocorticoids stimulate p21 gene expression by targeting multiple transcriptional elements within a steroid responsive region of the p21(waf1/cip1) promoter in rat hepatoma cells. J Biol Chem. 1998;273(4):1998–2007.

[92]  Chetta A, Olivieri D. Role of inhaled steroids in vascular airway remodelling in asthma and COPD. Int J Endocrinol. 2012;10(2):397693.

[93]  Feltis BN, Wignarajah D, Reid DW, Ward C, Harding R, Walters EH. Effects of inhaled fluticasone on angiogenesis and vascular endothelial growth factor in asthma. Thorax. 2007;62(4):314–9.

[94]  Dorscheid DR, Low E, Conforti A, Shifrin S, Sperling AI, White SR. Corticosteroid-induced apoptosis in mouse airway epithelium: effect in normal airways and after allergen-induced airway inflammation. J Allergy Clin Immunol. 2003;111(2):360–6.

[95]  Erjefält JS, Erjefält I, Sundler F, Persson CG. Effects of topical budesonide on epithelial restitution in vivo in guinea pig trachea. Thorax. 1995;50(7):785–92.

[96]  Lundgren R, Soderberg M, Horstedt P, Stenling R. Morphological studies of bronchial mucosal biopsies from asthmatics before and after ten years of treatment with inhaled steroids. Eur Respir J. 1988;1(10):883–9.

[97]  Laitinen LA, Laitinen A, Haahtela T. A comparative study of the effects of an inhaled corticosteroid, budesonide, and a beta 2-agonist, terbutaline, on airway inflammation

in newly diagnosed asthma: a randomized, double-blind, parallel-group controlled trial. J Allergy Clin Immunol. 1992;90(1):32–42.

[98]  I . Porush GLM. Self-propelling compositions for inhalation therapy containing a salt of isoproterenol or epinephrine. United States of America; US Patent 2,868,691, 1959. p. US Patent 2,868,691.

[99]  Arvidsson P, Larsson S, Löfdahl CG, Melander B, Wåhlander L, Svedmyr N. Formoterol, a new long-acting bronchodilator for inhalation. Eur Respir J Off J Eur Soc Clin Respir Physiol. 1989;2(4):325–30.

[100]  Johnson M. Salmeterol: a novel drug for the treatment of asthma. Agents Actions Suppl. 1991;34(2):79–95.

[101]  Cullum VA, Farmer JB, Jack D, Levy GP. Salbutamol: a new, selective beta-adrenoceptive receptor stimulant. Br J Pharmacol. 1969;35(1):141–51.

[102]  Persson H, Olsson T. Some pharmacological properties of terbutaline (INN), 1-(3,5-dihydroxyphenyl)-2-(T-butylamino)-ethanol. A new sympathomimetic beta-receptor-stimulating agent. Acta Med Scand Suppl. 1970;512(7):11–9.

[103]  Berair R, Brightling CE. Asthma therapy and its effect on airway remodelling. Drugs. 2014;74(6):1345–69.

[104]  Bowler S. Long acting beta agonists. Aust Fam Phys. 1998;27(12):1115–8.

[105]  Nelson HS, Weiss ST, Bleecker EK, Yancey SW, Dorinsky PM. The salmeterol multicenter asthma research trial: a comparison of usual pharmacotherapy for asthma or usual pharmacotherapy plus salmeterol. Chest. 2006;129(1):15–26.

[106]  Buels KS, Fryer AD. Muscarinic receptor antagonists: effects on pulmonary function. Handb Exp Pharmacol. 2012;208(3):317–41.

[107]  Barnes PJ. Muscarinic receptor subtypes in airways. Life Sci. 1993;52(5–6):521–7.

[108]  Proskocil BJ, Fryer AD. Beta2-agonist and anticholinergic drugs in the treatment of lung disease. Proc Am Thorac Soc. 2005;2(4):305–10; discussion 311–2.

[109]  Engelhardt A, Klupp H. The pharmacology and toxicology of a new tropane alkaloid derivative. Postgrad Med J. 1975;51(7 SUPPL):82–5.

[110]  Powell CV, Cranswick NE. The current role of ipratropium bromide in an acute exacerbation of asthma. J Paediatr Child Health. 2015;51(8):751–2.

[111]  Ward MJ, Fentem PH, Smith WH, Davies D. Ipratropium bromide in acute asthma. Br Med J (Clin Res Ed). 1981;282(6264):598–600.

[112]  Disse B, Reichl R, Speck G, Traunecker W, Ludwig Rominger KL, Hammer R. Ba 679 BR, a novel long-acting anticholinergic bronchodilator. Life Sci. 1993;52(5-6):537–44.

[113] Kerstjens HAM, Engel M, Dahl R, Paggiaro P, Beck E, Vandewalker M, et al. Tiotropium in asthma poorly controlled with standard combination therapy. N Engl J Med. 2012;367(13):1198–207.

[114] Peters SP, Kunselman SJ, Icitovic N, Moore WC, Pascual R, Ameredes BT, et al. Tiotropium bromide step-up therapy for adults with uncontrolled asthma. N Engl J Med. 2010;363(18):1715–26.

[115] Menzella F, Lusuardi M, Galeone C, Zucchi L, Article I, Url A, et al. Tailored therapy for severe asthma. Multidiscip Respir Med. 2015;10(1):1.

[116] Peters-Golden M, Henderson WR Jr. Leukotrienes. N Engl J Med. 2007;357(18):1841–54.

[117] Tomisawa H, Takanohashi Y, Ichihara S, Fukazawa H, Tateishi M. Transamination of LTE4 by cysteine conjugate aminotransferase. Biochem Biophys Res Commun. 1988;155(3):1119–25.

[118] Liu M, Yokomizo T. The role of leukotrienes in allergic diseases. Allergol Int. 2015;64(1):17–26.

[119] Jones TR, Labelle M, Belley M, Champion E, Charette L, Evans J, et al. Pharmacology of montelukast sodium (Singulair), a potent and selective leukotriene D4 receptor antagonist. Can J Physiol Pharmacol. 1995;73(2):191–201.

[120] Reiss TF, Altman LC, Chervinsky P, Bewtra A, Stricker WE, Noonan GP, et al. Effects of montelukast (MK-0476), a new potent cysteinyl leukotriene (LTD4) receptor antagonist, in patients with chronic asthma. J Allergy Clin Immunol. 1996;98(3):528–34.

[121] Spector, Sheldon L. "Management of asthma with zafirlukast." *Drugs*. 1996;52(6):36–46.

[122] Ames SA, Gleeson CD, Kirkpatrick P. Omalizumab. Nat Rev Drug Discov. 2004;3(3):199–200.

[123] Rodrigo GJ, Neffen H, Castro-Rodriguez JA. Efficacy and safety of subcutaneous omalizumab vs placebo as add-on therapy to corticosteroids for children and adults with asthma: a systematic review. Chest. 2011;139(1):28–35.

[124] Polosa R, Casale T. Monoclonal antibodies for chronic refractory asthma and pipeline developments. Drug Discov Today. 2012;17(11–12):591–9.

[125] Leckie MJ, Ten Brinke A, Khan J, Diamant Z, O'Connor BJ, Walls CM, et al. Effects of an interleukin-5 blocking monoclonal antibody on eosinophils, airway hyper-responsiveness, and the late asthmatic response. Lancet. 2000;356(9248):2144–8.

[126] Castro M, Zangrilli J, Wechsler ME, Bateman ED, Brusselle GG, Bardin P, et al. Reslizumab for inadequately controlled asthma with elevated blood eosinophil counts:

results from two multicentre, parallel, double-blind, randomised, placebo-controlled, phase 3 trials. Lancet Respir Med. 2015;3(5):355–6.

[127] Haldar P, Brightling CE, Singapuri A, Hargadon B, Gupta S, Monteiro W, et al. Outcomes after cessation of mepolizumab therapy in severe eosinophilic asthma: a 12-month follow-up analysis. J Allergy Clin Immunol. 2014;133(3):921–3.

[128] Nowak RM, Parker JM, Silverman RA, Rowe BH, Smithline H, Khan F, et al. A randomized trial of benralizumab, an antiinterleukin 5 receptor α monoclonal antibody, after acute asthma. Am J Emerg Med. 2015;33(1):14–20.

[129] Levitt RC, McLane MP, MacDonald D, Ferrante V, Weiss C, Zhou T, et al. IL-9 pathway in asthma: new therapeutic targets for allergic inflammatory disorders. J Allergy Clin Immunol. 1999;103(5 Pt 2):S485–91.

[130] Oh CK, Raible D, Geba GP, Molfino NA. Biology of the interleukin-9 pathway and its therapeutic potential for the treatment of asthma. Inflamm Allergy Drug Targets. 2011;10(3):180–6.

[131] Oh CK, Geba GP, Molfino N. Investigational therapeutics targeting the IL-4/IL-13/ STAT-6 pathway for the treatment of asthma. Eur Respir Rev. 2010;19(115):46–54.

[132] Borish LC, Nelson HS, Lanz MJ, Claussen L, Whitmore JB, Agosti JM, et al. Interleukin-4 receptor in moderate atopic asthma. A phase I/II randomized, placebo-controlled trial. Am J Respir Crit Care Med. 1999;160(6):1816–23.

[133] Reinisch W, Panés J, Khurana S, Toth G, Hua F, Comer GM, et al. Anrukinzumab, an anti-interleukin 13 monoclonal antibody, in active UC: efficacy and safety from a phase IIa randomised multicentre study. Gut. 2015;64(6):894–900.

[134] Rothenberg ME, Wen T, Greenberg A, Alpan O, Enav B, Hirano I, et al. Intravenous anti–IL-13 mAb QAX576 for the treatment of eosinophilic esophagitis. J Allergy Clin Immunol. 2015;135(2):500–7.

[135] Murray LA, Zhang H, Oak SR, Coelho AL, Herath A, Flaherty KR, et al. Targeting interleukin-13 with tralokinumab attenuates lung fibrosis and epithelial damage in a humanized SCID idiopathic pulmonary fibrosis model. Am J Respir Cell Mol Biol. 2014;50(5):985–94.

[136] Russo C, Polosa R. TNF-alpha as a promising therapeutic target in chronic asthma: a lesson from rheumatoid arthritis. Clin Sci (Lond). 2005;109(2):135–42.

[137] Matera MG, Calzetta L, Cazzola M. TNF-alpha inhibitors in asthma and COPD: we must not throw the baby out with the bath water. Pulm Pharmacol Ther. 2010;23(2):121–8.

[138] US Dep. Health Hum. Serv., Food Drug Admin. [Internet]. Guidance for Industry: E15 Definitions for Genomic Biomarkers, Pharmacogenomics, Pharmacogenetics, Genomic Data and Sample Coding Categories. 2008. Available from: http://www.fda.gov/

downloads/drugs/guidancecomplianceregulatoryinformation/guidances/ ucm073162.pdfucm073162.pdf. Accessed January 2016.

[139] Ma Q, Lu AYH. Pharmacogenetics, Pharmacogenomics, and individualized medicine. Pharmacol Rev. 2011;63(2):437–59.

[140] Palmer LJ, Silverman ES, Weiss ST, Drazen JM. Pharmacogenetics of asthma. Am J Respir Crit Care Med. 2002;165(7):861–6.

[141] Gray IC, Campbell DA, Spurr NK. Single nucleotide polymorphisms as tools in human genetics. Hum Mol Genet. 2000;9(16):2403–8.

[142] Palmer LJ, Cookson WO. Using single nucleotide polymorphisms as a means to understanding the pathophysiology of asthma. Respir Res. 2001;2(2):102–12.

[143] Chaudhary R, Singh B, Kumar M, Gakhar SK, Saini AK, Parmar VS, et al. Role of single nucleotide polymorphisms in pharmacogenomics and their association with human diseases. Drug Metab Rev. 2015;47(3):1–10.

[144] Stankiewicz P, Lupski JR. Structural variation in the human genome and its role in disease. Annu Rev Med. 2010;61(2):437–55.

[145] Revollo JR, Cidlowski JA. Mechanisms generating diversity in glucocorticoid receptor signaling. Ann N Y Acad Sci. 2009;1179(4):167–78.

[146] Newton R, Holden NS. Separating transrepression and transactivation: a distressing divorce for the glucocorticoid receptor? Mol Pharmacol. 2007;72(4):799–809.

[147] Ting F Leung, FAAAAI MFT and GWW. Personalized medicine for severe asthma: how far have we achieved? Pharmacogenomics Pharmacoproteomics. 2015;6(2):1.

[148] Tantisira KG, Lake S, Silverman ES, Palmer LJ, Lazarus R, Silverman EK, et al. Corticosteroid pharmacogenetics: association of sequence variants in CRHR1 with improved lung function in asthmatics treated with inhaled corticosteroids. Hum Mol Genet. 2004;13(13):1353–9.

[149] Odunuga OO, Longshaw VM, Blatch GL. Hop: more than an Hsp70/Hsp90 adaptor protein. Bioessays. 2004;26(10):1058–68.

[150] Hawkins GA, Lazarus R, Smith RS, Tantisira KG, Meyers DA, Peters SP, et al. The glucocorticoid receptor heterocomplex gene STIP1 is associated with improved lung function in asthmatic subjects treated with inhaled corticosteroids. J Allergy Clin Immunol. 2009;123(6):1376–83.e7.

[151] Einisman H, Reyes ML, Angulo J, López-Lastra M, Cerda J, JAC-R. Use of steroid receptor related STIP1 gene analysis as an asthma marker. Eur Respir J. 2012;40(56): 1782–5.

[152] Tantisira KG, Hwang ES, Raby BA, Silverman ES, Lake SL, Richter BG, et al. TBX21: a functional variant predicts improvement in asthma with the use of inhaled corticosteroids. Proc Natl Acad Sci U S A. 2004;101(52):18099–104.

[153] Ye Y-M, Lee H-Y, Kim S-H, Jee Y-K, Lee S-K, Lee S-H, et al. Pharmacogenetic study of the effects of NK2R G231E G>A and TBX21 H33Q C>G polymorphisms on asthma control with inhaled corticosteroid treatment. J Clin Pharm Ther. 2009;34(6):693–701.

[154] Tantisira KG, Small KM, Litonjua AA, Weiss ST, Liggett SB. Molecular properties and pharmacogenetics of a polymorphism of adenylyl cyclase type 9 in asthma: interaction between beta-agonist and corticosteroid pathways. Hum Mol Genet. 2005;14(12):1671–7.

[155] Kim SH, Ye YM, Lee HY, Sin HJ, Park HS. Combined pharmacogenetic effect of ADCY9 and ADRB2 gene polymorphisms on the bronchodilator response to inhaled combination therapy. J Clin Pharm Ther. 2011;36(3):399–405.

[156] Stockmann C, Fassl B, Gaedigk R, Nkoy F, Uchida DA, Monson S, et al. Fluticasone propionate pharmacogenetics: CYP3A4*22 polymorphism and pediatric asthma control. J Pediatr. 2013;162(6):1227.e1–2.

[157] Tantisira KG, Lasky-Su J, Harada M, Murphy A, Litonjua AA, Himes BE, et al. Genomewide association between GLCCI1 and response to glucocorticoid therapy in asthma. N Engl J Med. 2011;365(13):1173–83.

[158] Tantisira KG, Damask A, Szefler SJ, Schuemann B, Markezich A, Su J, et al. Genome-wide association identifies the T gene as a novel asthma pharmacogenetic locus. Am J Respir Crit Care Med. 2012;185(12):1286–91.

[159] Hawkins GA, Tantisira K, Meyers DA, Ampleford EJ, Moore WC, Klanderman B, et al. Sequence, haplotype, and association analysis of ADRB2 in a multiethnic asthma case-control study. Am J Respir Crit Care Med. 2006;174(10):1101–9.

[160] Ortega VE, Hawkins GA, Moore WC, Hastie AT, Ampleford EJ, Busse WW, et al. Effect of rare variants in ADRB2 on risk of severe exacerbations and symptom control during longacting B agonist treatment in a multiethnic asthma population: a genetic study. Lancet Respir Med. 2014;2(3):204–13.

[161] Rosenbaum DM, Cherezov V, Hanson MA, Rasmussen SGF, Thian FS, Kobilka TS, et al. GPCR engineering yields high-resolution structural insights into beta2-adrenergic receptor function. Science. 2007;318(5854):1266–73.

[162] Cherezov V, Rosenbaum DM, Hanson M a, Rasmussen SGF, Thian FS, Kobilka TS, et al. High-resolution crystal structure of an engineered human beta2-adrenergic G protein-coupled receptor. Science. 2007;318(5854):1258–65.

[163] Lima JJ, Thomason DB, Mohamed MH, Eberle L V, Self TH, Johnson JA. Impact of genetic polymorphisms of the beta2-adrenergic receptor on albuterol bronchodilator pharmacodynamics. Clin Pharmacol Ther. 1999;65(5):519–25.

[164] Israel E, Chinchilli VM, Ford JG, Boushey HA, Cherniack R, Craig TJ, et al. Use of regularly scheduled albuterol treatment in asthma: genotype-stratified, randomised, placebo-controlled cross-over trial. Lancet. 2004;364(9444):1505–12.

[165] Global Initiative for Asthma (GINA) [Internet]. 2016 Pocket Guide for Asthma Management and Prevention. Available from: http://www.ginasthma.org/. Accessed January 2016

[166] Taylor DR, Drazen JM, Herbison GP, Yandava CN, Hancox RJ, Town GI. Asthma exacerbations during long term beta agonist use: influence of beta(2) adrenoceptor polymorphism. Thorax. 2000;55(9):762–7.

[167] Israel E, Drazen JM, Liggett SB, Boushey HA, Cherniack RM, Chinchilli VM, et al. Effect of polymorphism of the b2-adrenergic receptor on response to regular use of albuterol in asthma. Int Arch Allergy Immunol. 2001;124(1–3):183–6.

[168] Choudhry S, Ung N, Avila PC, Ziv E, Nazario S, Casal J, et al. Pharmacogenetic differences in response to albuterol between Puerto Ricans and Mexicans with asthma. Am J Respir Crit Care Med. 2005;171(6):563–70.

[169] Bleecker ER, Postma DS, Lawrance RM, Meyers DA, Ambrose HJ, Goldman M. Effect of ADRB2 polymorphisms on response to longacting B2-agonist therapy: a pharmacogenetic analysis of two randomised studies. Lancet. 2007;370(9605):2118–25.

[170] Wechsler ME, Kunselman SJ, Chinchilli VM, Bleecker E, Boushey HA, Calhoun WJ, et al. Effect of B2-adrenergic receptor polymorphism on response to longacting B2 agonist in asthma (LARGE trial): a genotype-stratified, randomised, placebo-controlled, crossover trial. Lancet. 2009;374(9703):1754–64.

[171] Bleecker ER, Nelson HS, Kraft M, Corren J, Meyers DA, Yancey SW, et al. Beta2-receptor polymorphisms in patients receiving salmeterol with or without fluticasone propionate. Am J Respir Crit Care Med. 2010;181(7):676–87.

[172] Tsuji S. Genetics of neurodegenerative diseases: insights from high-throughput resequencing. Hum Mol Genet. 2010;19(R1):R65–70.

[173] Green SA, Cole G, Jacinto M, Innis M, Liggett SB. A polymorphism of the human B2-adrenergic receptor within the fourth transmembrane domain alters ligand binding and functional properties of the receptor. J Biol Chem. 1993;268(31):23116–21.

[174] Green SA, Rathz DA, Schuster AJ, Liggett SB. The Ile164 B2-adrenoceptor polymorphism alters salmeterol exosite binding and conventional agonist coupling to Gs. Eur J Pharmacol. 2001;421(3):141–7.

[175] Thomsen M, Nordestgaard BG, Sethi a a, Tybjærg-Hansen A, Dahl M. β2-adrenergic receptor polymorphisms, asthma and COPD: two large population-based studies. Eur Respir J. 2012;39(3):558–66.

[176] Hacker BM, Tomlinson JE, Wayman G a, Sultana R, Chan G, Villacres E, et al. Cloning, chromosomal mapping, and regulatory properties of the human type 9 adenylyl cyclase (ADCY9). Genomics. 1998;50(1):97–104.

[177] Pal K, Swaminathan K, Xu HE, Pioszak A a. Structural basis for hormone recognition by the Human CRFR2{alpha} G protein-coupled receptor. J Biol Chem. 2010;285(51): 40351–61.

[178] Poon AH, Tantisira KG, Litonjua AA, Lazarus R, Xu J, Lasky-Su J, et al. Association of corticotropin-releasing hormone receptor-2 genetic variants with acute bronchodilator response in asthma. Pharmacogenet Genomics. 2008;18(5):373–82.

[179] Litonjua AA, Lasky-Su J, Schneiter K, Tantisira KG, Lazarus R, Klanderman B, et al. ARG1 is a novel bronchodilator response gene: screening and replication in four asthma cohorts. Am J Respir Crit Care Med. 2008;178(7):688–94.

[180] Vonk JM, Postma DS, Maarsingh H, Bruinenberg M, Koppelman GH, Meurs H. Arginase 1 and arginase 2 variations associate with asthma, asthma severity and beta2 agonist and steroid response. Pharmacogenet Genomics. 2010;20:179–86.

[181] Iordanidou M, Paraskakis E, Tavridou A, Paschou P, Chatzimichael A, Manolopoulos VG. G894T polymorphism of eNOS gene is a predictor of response to combination of inhaled corticosteroids with long-lasting β2-agonists in asthmatic children. Pharma-cogenomics. 2012;13(12):1363–72.

[182] Duan QL, Du R, Lasky-Su J, Klanderman BJ, Partch a B, Peters SP, et al. A polymor-phism in the thyroid hormone receptor gene is associated with bronchodilator response in asthmatics. Pharmacogenomics J. 2013;13(2):130–6.

[183] Drake KA, Torgerson DG, Gignoux CR, Galanter JM, Roth LA, Huntsman S, et al. A genome-wide association study of bronchodilator response in Latinos implicates rare variants. J Allergy Clin Immunol. 2014;133(2):370–8.

[184] Himes BE, Jiang X, Hu R, Wu AC, Lasky-Su JA, Klanderman BJ, et al. Genome-wide association analysis in asthma subjects identifies SPATS2L as a novel bronchodilator response gene. PLoS Genet. 2012;8(7):e1002824.

[185] Drazen JM, Yandava CN, Dubé L, Szczerback N, Hippensteel R, Pillari A, et al. Pharmacogenetic association between ALOX5 promoter genotype and the response to anti-asthma treatment. Nat Genet. 1999;22(2):168–70.

[186] Mougey E, Lang JE, Allayee H, Teague WG, Dozor AJ, Wise RA, et al. ALOX5 poly-morphism associates with increased leukotriene production and reduced lung function and asthma control in children with poorly controlled asthma. Clin Exp Allergy. 2013;43(5):512–20.

[187] Telleria JJ, Blanco-Quiros A, Varillas D, Armentia A, Fernandez-Carvajal I, Jesus Alonso M, et al. ALOX5 promoter genotype and response to montelukast in moderate persis-tent asthma. Respir Med. 2008;102(6):857–61.

[188] Klotsman M, York TP, Pillai SG, Vargas-Irwin C, Sharma SS, van den Oord EJCG, et al. Pharmacogenetics of the 5-lipoxygenase biosynthetic pathway and variable clinical response to montelukast. Pharmacogenet Genomics. 2007;17(3):189–96.

[189] Lima JJ, Zhang S, Grant A, Shao L, Tantisira KG, Allayee H, et al. Influence of leukotriene pathway polymorphisms on response to montelukast in asthma. Am J Respir Crit Care Med. 2006;173(4):379–85.

[190] Tantisira KG, Lima J, Sylvia J, Klanderman B, Weiss ST. 5-lipoxygenase pharmacogenetics in asthma: overlap with Cys-leukotriene receptor antagonist loci. Pharmacogenet Genomics. 2009;19(3):244–7.

[191] E. Mougey, H.Feng, M.Castro, C. Irvin JL. Absorption of montelukast is transporter mediated: a common variant of OATP2B1 is associated with reduced plasma concentrations and poor response. Pharmacogenet Genomics. 2009;19(2):129–38.

[192] Kim KA, Lee HM, Joo HJ, Park IB, Park JY. Effects of polymorphisms of the SLCO2B1 transporter gene on the pharmacokinetics of montelukast in humans. J Clin Pharmacol. 2013;53(11):1186–93.

[193] Tapaninen T, Karonen T, Backman JT, Neuvonen PJ, Niemi M. SLCO2B1 c.935G>A single nucleotide polymorphism has no effect on the pharmacokinetics of montelukast and aliskiren. Pharmacogenet Genomics. 2013;23(1):19–24.

[194] Jirtle RL, Skinner MK. Environmental epigenomics and disease susceptibility. Nat Rev Genet. 2007;8(4):253–62.

[195] Jaenisch R, Bird A. Epigenetic regulation of gene expression: how the genome integrates intrinsic and environmental signals. Nat Genet. 2003;33 Suppl:245–54.

[196] Comer BS, Ba M, Singer CA, Gerthoffer WT. Epigenetic targets for novel therapies of lung diseases. Pharmacol Ther. 2015;147:91–110.

[197] Follows RM, Snowise NG, Ho S-Y, Ambery CL, Smart K, McQuade BA. Efficacy, safety and tolerability of GSK2190915, a 5-lipoxygenase activating protein inhibitor, in adults and adolescents with persistent asthma: a randomised dose-ranging study. Respir Res. 2013;14(1):54.

[198] Hodsman P, Ashman C, Cahn A, De Boever E, Locantore N, Serone A, et al. A phase 1, randomized, placebo-controlled, dose-escalation study of an anti-IL-13 monoclonal antibody in healthy subjects and mild asthmatics. Br J Clin Pharmacol. 2013;75(1):118–28.

[199] Laviolette M, Gossage DL, Gauvreau G, Leigh R, Olivenstein R, Katial R, et al. Effects of benralizumab on airway eosinophils in asthmatic patients with sputum eosinophilia. J Allergy Clin Immunol. 2013;132(5):1086–96.e5.

[200] Garcia G, Magnan A, Chiron R, Contin-Bordes C, Berger P, Taillé C, et al. A proof-of-concept, randomized, controlled trial of omalizumab in patients with severe, difficult-to-control, nonatopic asthma. Chest. 2013;144(2):411–9.

[201] Noonan M, Korenblat P, Mosesova S, Scheerens H, Arron JR, Zheng Y, et al. Dose-ranging study of lebrikizumab in asthmatic patients not receiving inhaled steroids. J Allergy Clin Immunol. 2013;132(3):567–74.e12.

[202] Piper E, Brightling C, Niven R, Oh C, Faggioni R, Poon K, et al. A phase II placebo-controlled study of tralokinumab in moderate-to-severe asthma. Eur Respir J. 2013;41(2):330–8.

[203] Busse WW, O'Byrne PM, Bleecker ER, Lötvall J, Woodcock A, Andersen L, et al. Safety and tolerability of the novel inhaled corticosteroid fluticasone furoate in combination with the β2 agonist vilanterol administered once daily for 52 weeks in patients >=12 years old with asthma: a randomised trial. Thorax. 2013;68(6):513–20.

[204] Corren J, Mansfield LE, Pertseva T, Blahzko V, Kaiser K. Efficacy and safety of fluticasone/formoterol combination therapy in patients with moderate-to-severe asthma. Respir Med. 2013;107(2):180–95.

[205] Ortega HG, Liu MC, Pavord ID, Brusselle GG, FitzGerald JM, Chetta A, et al. Mepolizumab Treatment in Patients with Severe Eosinophilic Asthma. N Engl J Med. 2015 Sep 8;372(18):17.

[206] Somerville L, Bardelas J, Viegas A, D'Andrea P, Blogg M, Peachey G. Immunogenicity and safety of omalizumab in pre-filled syringes in patients with allergic (IgE-mediated) asthma. Curr Med Res Opin. 2014;30(1):59–66.

[207] Scheerens H, Arron JR, Zheng Y, Putnam WS, Erickson RW, Choy DF, et al. The effects of lebrikizumab in patients with mild asthma following whole lung allergen challenge. Clin Exp Allergy. 2014;44(1):38–46.

[208] Lötvall J, Bateman ED, Busse WW, O'Byrne PM, Woodcock A, Toler WT, et al. Comparison of vilanterol, a novel long-acting beta2 agonist, with placebo and a salmeterol reference arm in asthma uncontrolled by inhaled corticosteroids. J Negat Results Biomed. 2014;13(1):9.

[209] Beeh K-M, Moroni-Zentgraf P, Ablinger O, Hollaenderova Z, Unseld A, Engel M, et al. Tiotropium Respimat® in asthma: a double-blind, randomised, dose-ranging study in adult patients with moderate asthma. Respir Res. 2014;15(1):61.

[210] Gauvreau GM, Boulet L-P, Cockcroft DW, FitzGerald JM, Mayers I, Carlsten C, et al. OX40L blockade and allergen-induced airway responses in subjects with mild asthma. Clin Exp Allergy. 2014;44(1):29–37.

[211] Nowak RM, Parker JM, Silverman RA, Rowe BH, Smithline H, Khan F, et al. A randomized trial of benralizumab, an antiinterleukin 5 receptor α monoclonal antibody, after acute asthma. Am J Emerg Med. 2015;33(1):14–20.

[212] Hernandez ML, Mills K, Almond M, Todoric K, Aleman MM, Zhang H, et al. IL-1 receptor antagonist reduces endotoxin-induced airway inflammation in healthy volunteers. J Allergy Clin Immunol. 2015;135(2):379–85.

# 9

# Allergen Control in Asthma

Ayfer Ekim

## Abstract

Asthma is one of the most prevalent chronic diseases especially among children so that it continues to be a public health problem. Even though genetics is an important factor for asthma, dramatic increase of the asthma recently is related with environmental triggers and lifestyle factors. Understanding of the interaction of multiple factors causing asthma is absolutely necessary for the planning interventions strategies. Exposure to allergens is a key factor for asthma morbidity. Environmental exposure leads allergen sensitization for genetically predisposed individuals and persisting of exposure is a risk element for asthma and other allergic diseases as well. Evidences suggest that environmental triggers avoidance and control interventions preclude asthma attacks, decrease the frequency of symptoms, and the need for drugs. Thus, environmental control should be focused in the management of asthma. Identifying and controlling of indoor and outdoor environmental triggers is the cornerstone for a successful asthma management. Figuring out the reasoning factors and developing primary preventive precautions are necessary to decrease asthma development frequency throughout the world.

**Keywords:** Allergen, asthma, environment, sensitization, trigger

## 1. Introduction

Asthma and asthma-related allergic diseases are most prevalent chronic diseases in developed countries. In recent years, a dynamic increase has been observed in prevalence of allergic diseases [1–3]. Even though the exact reason for such an increase is not know, home environment design and quality of indoor allergens are thought to be the factors for those diseases [4, 5]. Allergen induced diseases like asthma is an important public health problem and a burden for health resources [6]. Asthma and allergic reactions are life threaten conditions. Additionally, such diseases have negative influence on children and adults [1, 2, 4, 7]. Although increase in asthma for children and adults has been discussed widely in recent years, it is believed that the leading factor for this increase is environmental factors. Genetic heterogeneity and ethnicity variety, lifestyles and changes in the type of accommodation are the key factors for the development of asthma [8, 9]. Since avoidance from allergens is an important part for the management of allergic diseases, taking required precautions to prevent exposing to the allergens is the first step of symptom control. A successful identification and avoidance from environmental triggers might prevent inflammation of diseases. Avoidance from allergens in allergic diseases like asthma is more effective than treatment itself [7, 10]. So international asthma guides recommend environmental control implementations as a part of systematic approach to asthma [2]. This chapter focuses on the importance of allergens and control of allergens for the management of allergic asthma.

In the asthma patogenesis, the role of environment is getting more obvious. Asthma develops through the interaction of genetic agents with environmental exposure [1, 11, 12]. Individual allergen sensitivity is the most important feature and exposing to allergens play the key role to trigger asthma symptoms and inflammation. Asthma management might be controlled by multifaceted interventions since the reasons for asthma are multifactorial. Studies have suggested that combination of different interventions would be much more effective than a single intervention. Thus, it is essential that a successful asthma management should include multiple strategies covering pharmacological and nonpharmacological methods [1].

In allergen control, the risk of exposure should be identified for sensitive individuals, and some interventions should be planned to decrease or to remove the risk, accordingly [4, 6, 13]. In recent years, large number of strategies aiming at reducing of asthma based morbidity and mortality rates have been developed and tested [14, 17]. Within the scope of those strategies, it has been stated in many studies that the education provided for allergen control is not an effective intervention on its own to change environmental control behaviours [18]. To sum up, individual interventions are usually ineffective. Yet, effective allergen avoidance requires a detailed approach.

## 2. Indoor Allergens

Asthma is characterized by chronic airway inflammation caused by genetic-environment interaction [2, 3, 19]. Even though seasons are accepted as triggers for allergens, exposure to indoor allergens and their presence throughout the year means a greater risk for asthma. Many environmental factors might trigger asthma, but the most important ones are indoor allergens [20]. Indoor environment is a source of risk for health, and exposure to indoor allergens occur in indoor areas [11, 21]. Indoor environment means not only the house but also schools, offices, restaurant, and cars [22, 23]. A strong relation between pathogenesis of allergic diseases like asthma and exposure to indoor allergens has been emphasised in many epidemiological cohort studies and population surveys as well. Biological functions of allergens enhance IgE response and cause allergic inflammation directly. Environmental exposure to allergens and atopic predisposition affect the development of IgE and Th2 responses [8].

Modern life conditions and long hours spent indoors leads to high level allergen exposure, enhancing sensitization, and asthma symptoms [24, 25]. Major indoor allergens, which has been proved as triggers of allergy are dust mite, cockroach, mouse, pet dander, and mold [11, 26]. Although major allergens are present in all of the inner city houses, their presence differ in geographic regions due to climatic variety of geographic regions. Controlling of indoor allergens need much more effort compared to seasonal allergens since the presence of indoor allergies continue throughout the year [27]. In studies, it has been suggested that sensitization prevalence of children to indoor allergens is higher and those children with indoor allergen sensitization are also sensitive to outdoor allergens [28, 29].

Poor housing condition is more often the reason for exposure to the triggers and allergen sensitization. Exposure to indoor allergens may produce symptoms for asthmatic individuals [23]. It has been commonly believed that cats and dogs provoke the symptoms. However, high levels dust mites allergens in the house are the majör risk factor for sensitized individuals. Excessive moisture, inappropriate or bad heating/cooling systems, overcrowding, cockroaches, structural problems are the triggers for asthma [26]. Decreasing indoor allergen exposure causes healing in the asthma symptoms, and lessens drug use [22, 26, 27].

## 2.1. Dust mites

Although people have lived with dust mites for centuries, dust mites allergy has increased dramatically in recent times. Such an increase might be explained by the suitable conditions for dust mites due to the modernization of dwellings and long hours being spent in indoor areas. [16]. Dust mites are the first discovered indoor allergens. Two of the most common house dust mites are Dermatophagoides pteronyssinus (Dp), and Dermatophagoides farinae [27, 30, 31]. High levels of mites might be found in from the dust of mattresses, pillows, carpets, upholstered furniture, bed covers, clothes, and soft toys. Ninety percent of children with asthma have IgE sensitization to home dust, this might be attributed to dust mite allergens that are carried by bigger substances and that stays on the air hanging a short while. These mites occupy clothes and they are immobile. Distribution of allergens inside the house differ between rooms, more commonly in the bedroom particularly on the bed [20, 23]. Dust mites can be found in hot and humid places. Dust mites exposure is a risk factor for sensitization, and a trigger for asthma attacks [8, 16, 28, 32]. Asthma development, severity, and morbidity are strongly linked with dust mite allergy [15, 24, 31].

Numerous studies have been carried out to test the effect of dust mites removal on asthma symptoms. The most effective method to remove dust mites on the bed is to cover the bed and pillows with dust resistant clothes [30]. In a clinical study, it has been suggested that seven dust mites allergens are removed due to dust resistant cloth used to cover bed and pillows [18]. However,bed-focused interventions to remove dust mites is not effective enough to decrease the exposure. Instead, interventions focusing on patient's total exposure in a day are much more effective [30, 32]. If possible, carpets should be removed and replaced with *polietilen* coverings. Halken et al. [15] have stated in their study that semipermeable *poliuretan* bed and pillow coverings are important for children and has clinically long-term significant effects. In addition, toys might be a source of mites and constitutes as a serious risk for asthma symptoms. Toys should be cleaned in hot water or kept in deep-frozen once in a week [15].

Acaricides is recommended as a temporary solution to remove dust mites in soft furnishings. However, some studies have suggested that it might be an effective method if combined with allergen-impermeable mattress to remove dust mites [17, 33]. Vacuum cleaning is another effective method for the removal of dust mites. Vacuum cleaners should be equipped with a special bag or high efficiency particulate air (HEPA) filters in order to diminish mites levels in the air. Additionally, wet vacuum cleaning or steam cleaning are beneficial to remove mites. Bedding staff and other items should be wasted in hot water with detergent [11, 17]. Water temperature should be more than $55^0$C because colder water doesn't kill mites. Dry cleaning might be effective to kill the mites [30].

## 2.2. Cockroaches

Cockroach allergens are the second agent of indoor allergic sensitization after dust mites [34, 35]. Urban environment, low socio economic status, old buildings, and multifamily homes are all risk factors for cockroach occupation and high level cockroach allergens [23]. In some geographic regions, sensitization to cockroach allergens are rather common especially for children. In those regions, climate is a determinant factor and spending long hours inside the home during winter months means higher exposure to cockroach allergen. Cockroach allergens might be present in all body including shit or split [27, 34]. The most common cockroach allergens are produced by *Blattella Germanica* and *Periplaneta Americana* [20, 34].

Removing cockroach allergens in closed environments is a long term process. Although it has been considered as the best way to exterminate cockroaches, allergic material stays in the closed environment long after its extermination [28]. Thus, following the extermination of the cockroaches, the material including active allergen proteins should be cleaned with an intense vacuum cleaner. The National Cooperative Inner-City Asthma Study (NCICAS) has recently carried out a phase II study emphasising that a complete extermination of cockroach allergens in closed environments is not an easy task [2]. Education, cleaning and extermination interventions ensure a short term decrease, yet, the quantity of allergens is even higher in long term period. For the extermination of cockroaches allergen reservoirs, all the rooms should be cleaned. Studies have stated that pesticides used by professional pest control teams are highly effective to exterminate cockroach allergens. More effective interventions or chemical agents need to be tested to exterminate cockroach allergens but those agents shouldn't harm human health [10, 34].

## 2.3. Animals

Pet sensitization is an important risk element for asthma and allergic rhinitis. Some studies report that 50–70% of the children with bronchial asthma have sensitivity to pets [34, 36, 37]. Such high rates are the results of the trend of feeding pets at home that leads to high level exposure sensitization [38]. Among pets, cat allergy is the most common type of animal allergy. Sensitized individuals may expose to allergens directly or indirectly. Cats and dogs allergens stay in the form of little particulates and they are very adherent to floor or clothes. People might be exposed to allergens directly by living with them or they might be exposed indirectly in animal-free areas such as schools, hospitals, or transportation vehicles. Preventing exposure to pet allergens completely is not possible. Lower dose indirect exposure to pet allergens might initiate breathing symptoms for sensitized individuals [34, 39].

Ventilation, humidity and regular house cleaning have been shown as the most effective strategies to remove pet allergens. [25]. Utilizing air-filter tools is not useful to remove mites and cockroaches allergens, however, they may constitute as an important means to reduce the quantity of pet allergens on the air – approximately 2–4 times. In the studies conducted on that issue, it has been reported that HEPA filters and vacuum cleaning lead to short term decrease in the cat/dog allergen levels, however, they do not change the levels of dust allergen concentrations [11, 14, 40]. Results of studies have suggested that the removal of pets from house has provided optimal pharmacotherapy reduced airway responsiveness significantly to methacholine, but no significant differences has occurred in the change of FEV1 [37, 38, 41]. Furthermore, it has also been stated in this study that the removal of pets from the house has led to a reduce in the doses of inhaled corticosteroids and in the frequency of follow-up visits. Alternatively, air cleaners and pet washing are other measures when the pets are not removed from the house [31]. Washing cats is aneffective short time intervention. Allergen level of the cat increases dramatically within a week after washing. Past studies have shown that repeated washing progressively decreases the amount of cat allergen, and also reduces the amount of airborne allergens originating from the animal. Animal washing procedure is important to reduce allergens, washing with tap water for at least three minutes and pet shampoo is recommended. Washing is an effective method of reducing allergens, but it is not an effective for a long-term time [14, 31]. Avner et al. [14] indicated that the amount of allergen is significantly reduced after washing, but this reduction could not be maintained for a week. As a results, removal of the pets reduce airway responsiveness in patients with pet allergic asthma more than optimal drug use [37]. Even if the pet is excluded from home environment, allergic material keeps living for several months in the same environment. Thus, removal of carpets, covering of bed and mattresses are necessary for the exclusion of allergens for highly sensitive individuals [11, 42]. For pet allergies, use of HEPA filters , mattress covers, and exclusion of cats from the bedroom leads to airway hyperresponsiveness development, and decrease in peak flow variation [28]. For highly sensitive individuals, removal of carpets and upholstery, and encasement of mattresses might be essential to diminish cat allergen levels to a reduce in allergic symptoms. High proportion of sensitized people are not willing to remove pets from their houses because they accept the pets as a member of their family. In this case, environmental control precautions should be taken seriously, such as keeping the pet outside of the bedroom, room air filtration, washing the pet once a week, keeping it in a separate area inside the home, and using HEPA filters. Nevertheless, presence of pets inside the houses always poses a risk for sensitized people [38].

Even though a consensus is available on the role pet allergens for asthma development, it has been tested by some studies that on early interaction with pets can prevent allergy and asthma development for children [27, 43, 45]. The issue whether pet exposure is a risk factor or a protective factor for allergic symptoms and allergic sensitization has still been under discussion. Studies have focused on the possibility that pet exposure might be beneficial as they can obstacle the development of atopic diseases particularly on the early years of life [43, 46]. Ownby et al. [44] suggested in his study that living with cats and dogs relates to a lower risk of developing atopy during childhood and young adulthood. Collin et al. [36] emphasises in their study that there is no relation between having a pet and bronchial response to metha-choline for an 8 year old child. The relation between exposure to allergens and allergy sensitization is a matter of discussion. The results of recent studies confirms hypothesis that keeping pets at home might lead to development of tolerance in a certain degree [46, 47].

## 2.4. Environmental tobacco smoke

Tobacco smoke is a public health issue and 25-35% of the people with asthma are regular smokers. Approximately 30% of the children has a difficulty to control asthma exposure to environmental tobacco smoke [19]. Environmental tobacco smoke affects individuals at all ages. Negatively, the effect of it on children is stronger, and they can not prevent themselves appropriately [13]. Passive smoking is the most important source of indoor air pollution [48]. Children are exposed to smoke not only at their homes but also in car, other public areas, or restaurants. However, home is the most common place for exposure [49].

The results of exposing to tobacco smoke at pre or postnatal stages are different. Exposure to maternal smoking at prenatal period has long-term effects on the respiratory health of children [50, 51]. Chemical substances available in smoke, transmits to the placenta and affects the health of fetal growth negatively [19]. Prenatal smoke exposure of the baby is associated with deficiency in both functional residual capacity and index of tidal respiratory flow. Furthermore, maternal smoking is associated with increased serum IgE levels, and prevalence of skin-prick test responses in children. Additionally, many studies have suggested that maternal smoking increase the risk of snarling respiration for children under 6–years old [52]. Smoking exposure size at prenatal period and lung irritation are the factors leading allergy development [28, 48, 50].

Children whose parents smoke, experience more severe asthma symptoms and have exacerbations more often [23]. It has been stated in Lang et al.'s [19] study that children exposed in indoor environmental tobacco smoke had more respiratory infections, and significantly worse asthma related quality of life. In addition to its prenatal relation with reduced airway size and its postnatal behavior as a proinflammatory lung irritant, some have proposed that environmental tobacco smoke might also affect allergy development [28].

Tobacco smoke, affecting respiratory and circulatory systems, it the primary reason for many diseases and death, thus, it is a critical issue for public health throughout the world [19]. Although there are several interventions aiming at educating and raising consciousness in people, they are not common enough as desired. Unfortunately, such a public health issue is still waiting for a solution, although lots of strategies has been developed so for. The sole way to prevent children from tobacco smoke is to giving it up inside the house and to inform parents and family members about the mandatory tobacco education programmes helds at school. This is one of the recommended strategies to raise the awareness of environmental tobacco smoke. In addition, strong national and international policies are required for solution of this issue [2, 19, 28, 49, 52].

# 3. Outdoor Allergens

People expose to outdoor allergens directly or indirectly is their life-span [53]. Controlling of outdoor allergens is more difficult than controlling of indoor allergens [1]. The most common sources of outdoor allergens are pollens, fungal spores, and air pollutions. Pollens are important risk factor for allergic rhinitis. Furthermore, they cause asthma through their particules penetrating lower respiratory ways. Some evidences suggest that exposure to pollens and airborne allergens increase asthma exacerbations. In order to reduce the pollen based respiratory symptoms, sensitized people should stay at home with closed windows at certain periods of the day that is an effective method to reduce allergen inhalation. Furthermore, wearing masks in outdoor areas might be useful to reduce exposure [53].

Urbanization is an important contributor for asthma since it increases air pollution. Air pollution is a crucial risk factor for health and quality of life in urban life [54]. Children are more sensitive to air pollution and meteorological factors because their lungs have not completed development and developing immune and respiratory systems make them vulnerable to pathogens [55]. There is a consensus on the idea that air pollution might trigger asthma symptoms but the role of air pollution in the development of asthma is a matter of discussion. Air pollution is associated with asthma inflammation, increasing bronchial sensitivity, admitting to emergency departments and increasing rates in the use of drugs. The effects of air pollutants on lung functions depend on type of pollutants, their environmental concentration and duration of exposure to the pollutants. Airway mucosal induced by air pollutants and ruined mucociliary clearance facilitate transmitting and penetrating of allergens to immune system [56]. Concentration and nature of air pollutants changes among regions while the most common ones are ozone ($O_3$), nitrogen dioxide ($NO_2$), particulate matter (PM), sulfur dioxide ($SO_2$), and carbon monoxide (CO) [53].

Modern lifestyle, emission gases of vehicles and air pollution are important risk factors for respiratory allergy for urban life. Controlling those allergens identified as outdoor is rather difficult however reducing exposure to those allergens might be an ideal approach [3, 38]. Individual efforts to control outdoor allergens might be insufficient since their sources are outdoor environment. Primarily, in order to reduce air-pollution based asthma inflammation high level ozone and PM2*5 levels warning should be done, traffic should be reduced in urban areas, emission rates of vehicles should be controlled by local authorities [54]. On certain days when air-quality is poor patients should avoid outdoor activities and indoor activities should be included in asthma management plan. Air pollution is a global problem and the solution requires local national and international efforts by governments, industries and private sector authorities [55, 56].

## 4. Sensitization

Sensitization is the production of specific IgE antibodies to allergens and immune response begins with sensitization [3]. Asthma prevalence and incidence are affected by many factors. Allergic sensitization is one of the most important factors especially for children and adolescents [9]. Allergic sensitization increases the risk of asthma 4–20 times [23]. The effect of lifestyle factors have still been a matter of debate. On the other hand allergic disease history of the family is doubtlessly an important factor for allergic sensitization [40]. The importance of living conditions and environmental factors exposed at early childhood have been emphasised in many studies [4, 9, 22, 57].

Allergens are a kind of protein and able to penetrate the nasal and respiratory mucosa [58]. Sensitization to inhaler allergens is a major risk factor for asthma however the strength of this factor has still been debated. Furthermore, dose-response relation is another issue that has still been examined. Epidemiological evidences suggest that high level exposure to inhaler allergen is an important risk factor for atopic bronchial asthma especially in the first years of life [13, 20, 57]. It has been reported in many studies that sensitization to allergens is directly related with development of asthma symptoms, exacerbations and severity of asthma symptoms. Childhood asthma, particularly is associated with allergy sensitization and allergy exposure (**Table 1**) [13, 24, 28].

Exposure to high level allergens at early childhoods means a risk for childhood asthma. For the development of sensitization, exposure to indoor allergens at early childhood is an important determinant compared to outdoor allergens. Inner city and urban population studies have indicated that more 80% of school children with asthma sensitized to at least one indoor allergen [4, 23]. Allergic sensitization is a strong determinant for the continuity of disease at later life [40].

Skin prick test, which is the most common method to determine allergic diagnosis, is the basic test procedure to prove IgE based allergic disease sensitization. In the test different allergen extracts is pricked on upper-arm with little quantities and reaction of the person to these extracts is assessed [57]. It provides confirming the type of allergy for sensitization and different allergens can be tested simultaneously as well. The test ensures confirmation of sensitization to allergens objectively [59]. National Asthma Education and Prevention Program (NAEPP) recommends to use the test to assess exposure to allergens besides the patient's history [2]. It is helpful for specific immunotherapy since it makes right interpretation of sensitization children from the birth. As for children, the test can be re-applied if changes in symptoms or new environmental allergens are available. Experienced health professionals perform the test according to international standardized allergens. In test, ≥3 mm swolen tissue is accepted as positive allergen reaction (**Figure 1**) [58].

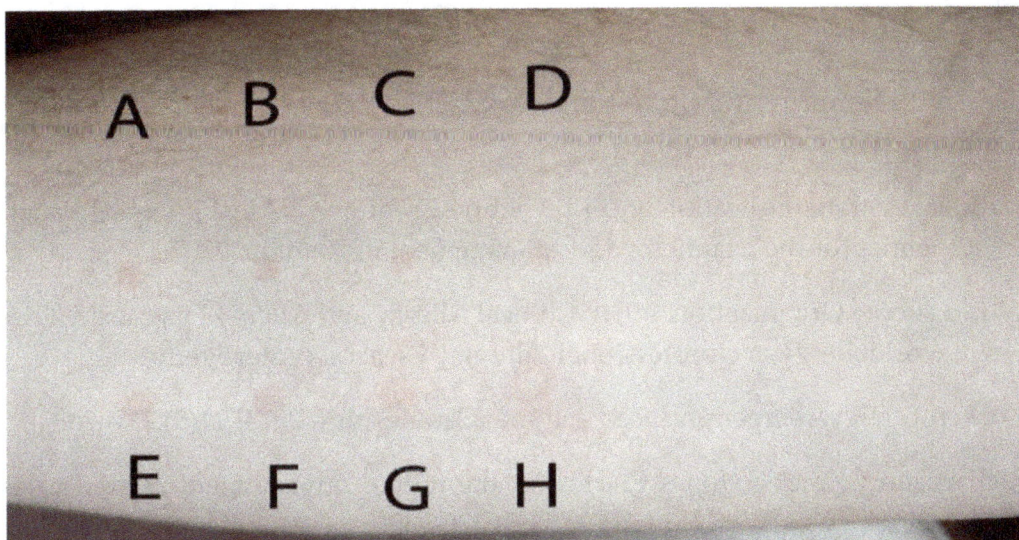

**Figure 1.** Skin prick test. Kwong et al. [60].

Another sensitization test is the measuring of specific IgE antibodies for a certain antigen such as Enzyme-Linked Immunosorbent Assay (ELISA) or Radioallergosorbent test (RAST). ELISA identifies IgE with a colored reaction product whereas RAST uses radioactively labelled allergen [8, 59].

| | |
|---|---|
| Allergy history of family | Genetic influence on allergic sensitization |
| Gender | Underdebate |
| Childhood environment | Rural and farming environment |
| | Close interaction with furry animal at early childhood |
| | Air pollution |
| | Crowded family |
| | Exposure to tobacco smoke |

**Table 1.** Factors affecting allergic sensitization.

# Author details

Ayfer Ekim

Address all correspondence to: ayferekim@hotmail.com

School of Health Sciences, Istanbul Bilgi University, Istanbul, Turkey

# References

[1] Beasley R, Semprini A, Mitchell EA. Risk factors for asthma: Is prevention possible? Lancet. (2015); 386(9998): 1075–1085.

[2] National Asthma Education and Prevention Program (NAEPP). Expert Panel Report 3: Guidelines for the Diagnosis and Management of Asthma, 2007.

[3] World Alergy Organization. IgE in Clinical Allergy and Allergy Diagnosis. 2015. http://www.worldallergy.org/professional/allergic_diseases_center/ige/index.

[4] Cockcroft DW. Allergen-induced asthma. Can Respir J. 2014; 21(5):279–282.

[5] Richardson G, Eick S, Jones R. How is the indoor environment related to asthma?: literature review. J Adv Nurs. 2005; 52(3):328-339.

[6] Arshad SH. Primary prevention of asthma and allergy. J Allergy Clin Immunol. 2005; 116(1):3-14.

[7] World Health Organization. Prevention of Allergy and Allergic Asthma. 2002. Geneva http://www.who.int/respiratory/publications/WHO_NMH_MNC_CRA_03.2.pdf

[8] Milián E, Díaz AM. Allergy to House Dust Mites and Asthma. P R Health Sci J. 2004; 23(1):47-57.

[9] Warm K, Lindberg A, Lundbäck B, Rönmark E. Increase in sensitization to common airborne allergens among adults – two population-based studies 15 years apart. Allergy Asthma Clin Immunol. 2013; 9(1): 20. DOI:10.1186/1710-1492-9-20

[10] Schönberger HJ, Maas T, Dompeling E, Knottnerus JA, van Weel C, van Schayck CP. Compliance of asthmatic families with a primary prevention programme of asthma and effectiveness of measures to reduce inhalant allergens--a randomized trial. Clin Exp Allergy. 2004; 34(7):1024-1031

[11] Matsui EC. Environmental control for asthma: recent evidence. Curr Opin Allergy Clin Immunol. 2013; 13(4);417-425. DOI: 10.1097/ACI.0b013e328362b776.

[12] Sheehan WJ, Phipatanakul W. Difficult to control asthma: Epidemiology and its link with environmental factors. Curr Opin Allergy Clin Immunol. 2005; 15(5): 397–401. DOI:10.1097/ACI.0000000000000195.

[13] Dick S, Doust E, Cowie H, Ayres JG, Turner S. Associations between environmental exposures and asthma control and exacerbations in young children: a systematic review. BMJ Open. 2014; 4:e003827

[14] Avner DB, Perzanowski MS, Platts-Mills TA, Woodfolk JA. Evaluation of different techniques for washing cats: quantitation of allergen removed from the cat and the effect on airborne Fel d 1. J Allergy Clin Immunol. 1997; 100(3):307–312.

[15] Halken S, Høst A, Niklassen U, Hansen LG, Nielsen F, Pedersen S, Osterballe O, Veggerby C, Poulsen LK. Effect of mattress and pillow encasings on children with asthma and house dust mite allergy. J Allergy Clin Immunol. 2003; 111(1):169-176.

[16] Howieson SG, Lawson A, McSharry C, Morris G, McKenzie E, Jackson J. Domestic ventilation rates, indoor humidity and dust mite allergens – are our homes causing the asthma pandemic? Building Services Engineering, Research and Technology. 2003;24(3):137–147.

[17] Mihrshahi S, Marks GB, Criss S, Tovey ER, Vanlaar CH, Peat JK, CAPS Team. Effectiveness of an intervention to reduce house dust mite allergen levels in children's beds. Allergy. 2003;58(8):784–789.

[18] Winn AK, Salo PM, Klein C, Sever ML, Harris SF, Johndrow D, Crockett PW, Cohn RD, Zeldin DC. Efficacy of an in-home test kit in reducing dust mite allergen levels: Results of a randomized controlled pilot study. J Asthma. 2015; 26:1–6

[19] Lang JE, Dozor AJ, Holbrook JT, Mougey E, Krishnan S, Sweeten S, Wise RA, Teague WG, Wei CY, Shade D, Lima JJ, American Lung Association-Asthma Clinical Research Centers. Biologic mechanisms of environmental tobacco smoke in children with poorly controlled asthma: results from a multicenter clinical trial. J Allergy Clin Immunol Pract. 2013;1(2):172-180. DOI: 10.1016/j.jaip.2012.11.006.

[20] Shirai T, Yasueda H, Saito A, Taniguchi M, Akiyama K, Tsuchiya T, Suda T, Chida K. Effect of exposure and sensitization to indoor allergens on asthma control level. Allergol Int. 2012; 61(1):51-56. DOI:10.2332/allergolint

[21] Rhodius R, Wickens K, Cheng S, Crane J. A comparison of two skin test methodologies and allergens from two different manufacturers. Ann Allergy Asthma Immunol. 2002;88(4):374–379.

[22] Eggleston PA. Improving indoor environments: Reducing allergen exposures. J Allergy Clin Immunol. 2005; 116:122–126

[23] Matsui EC, Hansel NN, McCormack MC, Rusher R, Breysse PN, Diette GB. Asthma in the inner city and the indoor environment. Immunol Allergy Clin North Am. 2008; 28(3):665-686, DOI: 10.1016/j.iac.2008.03.004.

[24] Gaffin JM, Phipatanakul W. The role of indoor allergens in the development of asthma. Curr Opin Allergy Clin Immunol. 2009; 9(2):128-135.

[25] Harrison P, Slack R, Bagga S. Indoor Air Pollution. In: Kay AB, Bousquet J, Holt PG, Kaplan AP, editors. Allergy and Allergic Diseases. Volume 1, Second Edition. Wiley-Blackwell, Oxford, UK. 1279-1288.

[26] Krieger J. Home Is Where the Triggers Are: Increasing Asthma Control by Improving the Home Environment. Pediatr Allergy Immunol Pulmonol. 2010; 23(2):139-145. DOI: 10.1089/ped.2010.0022

[27] Surdu S, Montoya LD, Tarbell A, Carpenter DO. Childhood asthma and indoor allergens in Native Americans in New York. Environ Health. 2006; 21:5-22. DOI: 10.1186/1476-069X-5-22

[28] Gold DR. Environmental tobacco smoke, indoor allergens, and childhood asthma. Environ Health Perspect. 2000; 108(Suppl 4): 643-651. DOI:10.2307/3454400

[29] Mortimer K, Neugebauer R, Lurmann F, Alcorn S, Balmes J, Tager I. Early-lifetime exposure to air pollution and allergic sensitization in childrenwith asthma. J. Asthma. 2008;245 (10):874–881. DOI: 10.1080/02770900802195722.

[30] Gøtzsche PC, Johansen HK. House dust mite control measures for asthma: Systematic review. Allergy. 2008; 63: 646–659. DOI: 10.1111/j.1398-9995.2008.01690.x.

[31] Yu SJ, Liao EC, Tsai JJ. House dust mite allergy: environment evaluation and disease prevention. Asia Pac Allergy. 2014;4(4):241-252. DOI: 10.5415/apallergy.2014.4.4.241

[32] Tovey E, Ferro A. Time for new methods for avoidance of house dust mite and other allergens. Curr Allergy Asthma Rep. 2012;12(5):465–477. DOI: 10.1007/s11882-012-0285-0.

[33] National Academy of Sciences Institute of Medicine (NAS). Clearing the Air: Asthma and Indoor Air Exposures. National Academic Press. 2000, Washington, DC.

[34] Liccardi G, Cazzola M, D'Amato M, D'Amato G. Pets and cockroaches: two increasing causes of respiratory allergy in indoor environments. Characteristics of airways sensitization and prevention strategies. Respir Med. 2000; 94:1109–1118.

[35] Salo PM, Xia J, Johnson CA, Li Y, Avol EL, Gong J, London SJ. Indoor allergens, asthma, and asthma-related symptoms among adolescents in Wuhan, China. Ann Epidemiol. 2004;14(8):543-550.

[36] Collin SM, Granell R, Westgarth C, Murray J, Paul ES, Sterne JAC, Henderson AJ. Associations of pet ownership with wheezing and lung function in childhood: Findings from a UK birth cohort. PLoS One. 2015;10(6): e0127756.

[37] Shirai T, Matsui T, Suzuki K, Chida K. Effect of pet removal on pet allergic asthma. Chest. 2005;127:1565–1571.

[38] Phipatanakul W. Animal Allergens and Their Control. Current Allergy Reports. 2001; 1:461–465.

[39] Noertjojo K, Dimich Ward H, Obata H, Manfreda J, Chan-Yeung M. Exposure and sensitization to cat dander. Asthma and asthma-like symptoms among adults. J Allergy Clin Immunol. 1999;103: 60-65.

[40] Platts-Mills TA, Woodfolk JA, Erwin EA, Aalberse R. Mechanisms of tolerance to inhalant allergens: the relevance of a modified Th2 response to allergens from domestic animals. Springer Semin Immunopathol. 2004; 25(3-4):271-279

[41] van der Heide S, van Aalderen WM, Kauffman HF, Dubois AE, de Monchy JG. Clinical effects of air cleaners in homes of asthmatic children sensitized to pet allergens. J Allergy Clin Immunol. 1999;104:447–451.

[42] Francis H, Fletcher G, Anthony C, Pickering C, Oldham L, Hadley E, Custovic A, Niven R. Clinical effects of air filters in homes of asthmatic adults sensitized and exposed to pet allergens. Clin Exp Allergy. 2003; 33:101–105

[43] Hesselmar B, Aberg N, Aberg B, Eriksson B, Bjorksten B. Does early exposure to cat or dog protect against later allergy development? Clin Exp Allergy. 1999; 29:611-617

[44] Ownby DR, Johnson CC, Peterson EL. Exposure to dogs and cats in the first year of life and risk of allergic sensitization at 6 to 7 years of age. JAMA. 2002;288(8):963-972.

[45] Simpson A, Custovic A: Early pet exposure: friend or foe? Curr Opin Allergy Clin Immunol 2003; 3:7-14.

[46] Lødrup Carlsen KC, Roll S, Carlsen KH, Mowinckel P, Wijga AH, Brunekreef B, Torrent M, Roberts G, Arshad SH, Kull I, Krämer U, von Berg A, Eller E, Høst A, Kuehni C, Spycher B, Sunyer J, Chen CM, Reich A, Asarnoj A, Puig C, Herbarth O, Mahachie John JM, Van Steen K, Willich SN, Wahn U, Lau S, Keil T; GALEN WP 1.5 'Birth Cohorts' working group. Does pet ownership in infancy lead to asthma or allergy at school age? Pooled analysis of individual participant data from 11 European birth cohorts. PLoS One. 2012;7(8):e43214. DOI: 10.1371/journal.pone.0043214.

[47] Salo PM., Zeldin DC. Does exposure to cats and dogs decrease the risk of developing allergic sensitization and disease? J Allergy Clin Immunol. 2009; 124(4): 751–752. DOI: 10.1016/j.jaci.2009.08.012.

[48] StosićL, MilutinovićS, LazarevićK, BlagojevićL, TadićL. Household environmental tobacco smoke and respiratory diseases among children in Nis (Serbia). Cent Eur J Public Health. 2012; 20(1):29-32.

[49] NikolićM, NikićD, LazarevićK. Exposure to environmental tobacco smoke and respiratory symptoms in school children of Nis. Srp Arh Celok Lek. 2006;134 (Suppl 2): 104-107.

[50] Gilliland FD, Li YF, Peters JM. Effects of maternal smoking during pregnancy and environmental tobacco smoke on asthma and wheezing in children. Am J Respir Crit Care Med. 2001; 163(2): 429-436. DOI: 10.1164/ajrccm.163.2.2006009

[51] Gilliland FD, Islam T, Berhane K, Gauderman WJ, Mc Connell R, Avol E, Peters JM. Regular smoking and asthma incidence in adolescents. Am J Respir Crit Care Med. 2006; 174:1094–1100.

[52] Stapleton M, Thompson AH, George C, Hoover RM, Self TH. Smoking and asthma. J Am Board Fam Med (JABFM). 2011; 24:313–322. DOI:10.3122/jabfm.2011.03.100180

[53] Burge HA, Rogers CA. Outdoor allergens. Environmental Health Perspectives. 2000; 108(Sup 4): 653-659.

[54] Guarnieri M, Balmes JR. Outdoor air pollution and asthma. Lancet. 2014; 383(9928): 1581-92. DOI: 10.1016/S0140-6736(14)60617-6.

[55] Kurt OK, Zhang J, Pinkerton KE. Pulmonary health effects of air pollution. Curr Opin Pulm Med. 2016; 22(2):138-143. DOI: 10.1097/MCP.0000000000000248.

[56] Wang IJ, Tung TH, Tang CS, Zhao ZH. Allergens, air pollutants, and childhood allergic diseases. Int J Hyg Environ Health. 2016; 219(1):66-71. DOI: 10.1016/j.ijheh.2015.09.001.

[57] Leung TF, Li AM, Ha G. Allergen sensitisation in asthmatic children: consecutive case series. Hong Kong Med J. 2000;6(4):355-360.

[58] Heinzerling L, Mari A, Bergmann KC, Bresciani M, Burbach G, Darsow U, Durham S, Fokkens W, Gjomarkaj M, Haahtela T, Bom AT, Wöhrl S, Maibach H, Lockey R. The skin prick test - European standards. Clin Transl Allergy. 2013; 3(1):3. DOI: 10.1186/2045-7022-3-3.

[59] Raun LH, Ensor KB, Persse D. Using community level strategies to reduce asthma attacks triggered by outdoor air pollution: a case crossover analysis. Environmental Health. 2014; 13:58

[60] Kwong KYC, Jean T, Redjal N. Variability in Measurement of Allergen Skin Testing Results among Allergy-Immunology Specialists. J Allergy Ther. 2014; 5:1 DOI: 10.1016/j.jaci.2013.12.767

# Permissions

All chapters in this book were first published in ASTHMA, by InTech Open; hereby published with permission under the Creative Commons Attribution License or equivalent. Every chapter published in this book has been scrutinized by our experts. Their significance has been extensively debated. The topics covered herein carry significant findings which will fuel the growth of the discipline. They may even be implemented as practical applications or may be referred to as a beginning point for another development.

The contributors of this book come from diverse backgrounds, making this book a truly international effort. This book will bring forth new frontiers with its revolutionizing research information and detailed analysis of the nascent developments around the world.

We would like to thank all the contributing authors for lending their expertise to make the book truly unique. They have played a crucial role in the development of this book. Without their invaluable contributions this book wouldn't have been possible. They have made vital efforts to compile up to date information on the varied aspects of this subject to make this book a valuable addition to the collection of many professionals and students.

This book was conceptualized with the vision of imparting up-to-date information and advanced data in this field. To ensure the same, a matchless editorial board was set up. Every individual on the board went through rigorous rounds of assessment to prove their worth. After which they invested a large part of their time researching and compiling the most relevant data for our readers.

The editorial board has been involved in producing this book since its inception. They have spent rigorous hours researching and exploring the diverse topics which have resulted in the successful publishing of this book. They have passed on their knowledge of decades through this book. To expedite this challenging task, the publisher supported the team at every step. A small team of assistant editors was also appointed to further simplify the editing procedure and attain best results for the readers.

Apart from the editorial board, the designing team has also invested a significant amount of their time in understanding the subject and creating the most relevant covers. They scrutinized every image to scout for the most suitable representation of the subject and create an appropriate cover for the book.

The publishing team has been an ardent support to the editorial, designing and production team. Their endless efforts to recruit the best for this project, has resulted in the accomplishment of this book. They are a veteran in the field of academics and their pool of knowledge is as vast as their experience in printing. Their expertise and guidance has proved useful at every step. Their uncompromising quality standards have made this book an exceptional effort. Their encouragement from time to time has been an inspiration for everyone.

The publisher and the editorial board hope that this book will prove to be a valuable piece of knowledge for researchers, students, practitioners and scholars across the globe.

# List of Contributors

**Bei-Yu Wu and Chun-Ting Liu**
Department of Chinese Medicine, Kaohsiung Chang Gung Memorial Hospital and School of Traditional Chinese Medicine, Chang Gung University College of Medicine, Kaohsiung, Taiwan

**Yu-Chiang Hung**
Department of Chinese Medicine, Kaohsiung Chang Gung Memorial Hospital and School of Traditional Chinese Medicine, Chang Gung University College of Medicine, Kaohsiung, Taiwan
School of Chinese Medicine for Post Baccalaureate, I-Shou University, Kaohsiung, Taiwan

**Wen-Long Hu**
Department of Chinese Medicine, Kaohsiung Chang Gung Memorial Hospital and School of Traditional Chinese Medicine, Chang Gung University College of Medicine, Kaohsiung, Taiwan
Kaohsiung Medical University College of Medicine, Kaohsiung, Taiwan
Fooyin University College of Nursing, Kaohsiung, Taiwan

**Irina Diana Bobolea**
Department of Allergology Hospital Doce de Octubre Institute for Health Research (i+12), Madrid, Spain
Highly-specialized Severe Asthma Unit Hospital Doce de Octubre Institute for Health Research (i+12), Madrid, Spain

**Carlos Melero**
Highly-specialized Severe Asthma Unit Hospital Doce de Octubre Institute for Health Research (i+12), Madrid, Spain
Department of Pulmonology Hospital Doce de Octubre Institute for Health Research (I +12), Madrid, Spain

**Jesús Jurado-Palomo**
Department of Allergology Nuestra Señora del Prado General Hospital, Talavera de la Reina, Spain

**Irina Bobolea**
Allergy Department, Hospital 12 de octubre Institute for Health Research (i+12), Madrid, Spain

**Luis Alejandro Pérez de Llano**
Head of the Pulmonology Department, Hospital Lucus Augusti, Lugo, Spain

**Katarzyna Grzela, Agnieszka Strzelak, Wioletta Zagórska and Tomasz Grzela**
The Medical University of Warsaw, Department of Paediatrics, Pneumonology and Allergology (KG, AS, WZ), and Department of Histology and Embryology (TG), Poland

**Yousser Mohammad**
Department of Pulmonary and Family Medicine, Syrian Private University, Damascus, Syria
Department of Pulmonary, Damascus University, Damascus, Syria
Center for Research and Training for CRD, Tishreen University, Latakia, Syria

**Basim Dubaybo**
Department of Internal Medicine, Wayne State University School of Medicine, Detroit, Michigan, USA

**Helena Pite**
Allergy Center, CUF Descobertas Hospital and CUF Infante Santo Hospital, Lisbon, Portugal
CEDOC, Chronic Diseases Research Center, NOVA Medical School / Faculdade de Ciências Médicas, Universidade Nova de, Lisboa, Lisbon, Portugal

**Mário Morais-Almeida**
Allergy Center, CUF Descobertas Hospital and CUF Infante Santo Hospital, Lisbon, Portugal
CINTESIS, Center for Research in Health Technologies and Information Systems, Porto, Portugal

**Tjeert Mensinga**
QPS Netherlands, Hanzeplein 1, GZ Groningen, The Netherlands

**Zuzana Diamant**
QPS Netherlands, Hanzeplein 1, GZ Groningen, The Netherlands
Department of Respiratory Medicine & Allergology, Institute for Clinical Science, Skane University Hospital, Lund, Sweden

**Patricia W. Garcia-Marcos**
Pulmonology and Allergy Units, Arrixaca Children's University Hospital, University of Murcia, Spain

**Manuel Sanchez-Solis and Luis Garcia-Marcos**
Pulmonology and Allergy Units, Arrixaca Children's University Hospital, University of Murcia, Spain
IMIB Bioresearch Institute, Murcia, Spain

**Mina Youssef and Cynthia Kanagaratham**
Department of Human Genetics, McGill University, Montreal, Quebec, Canada

**Danuta Radzioch**
Department of Human Genetics, McGill University, Montreal, Quebec, Canada
Department of Medicine, Division of Experimental Medicine, McGill University, Montreal, Quebec, Canada

**Mohamed I. Saad**
The Ritchie Centre, Hudson Institute of Medical Research, Monash University, Melbourne, Victoria, Australia

**Ayfer Ekim**
School of Health Sciences, Istanbul Bilgi University, Istanbul, Turkey

# Index

www.ingramcontent.com/pod-product-compliance
Lightning Source LLC
Chambersburg PA
CBHW080636200326
41458CB00013B/4644

* 9 7 8 1 6 3 2 4 2 7 9 6 0 *

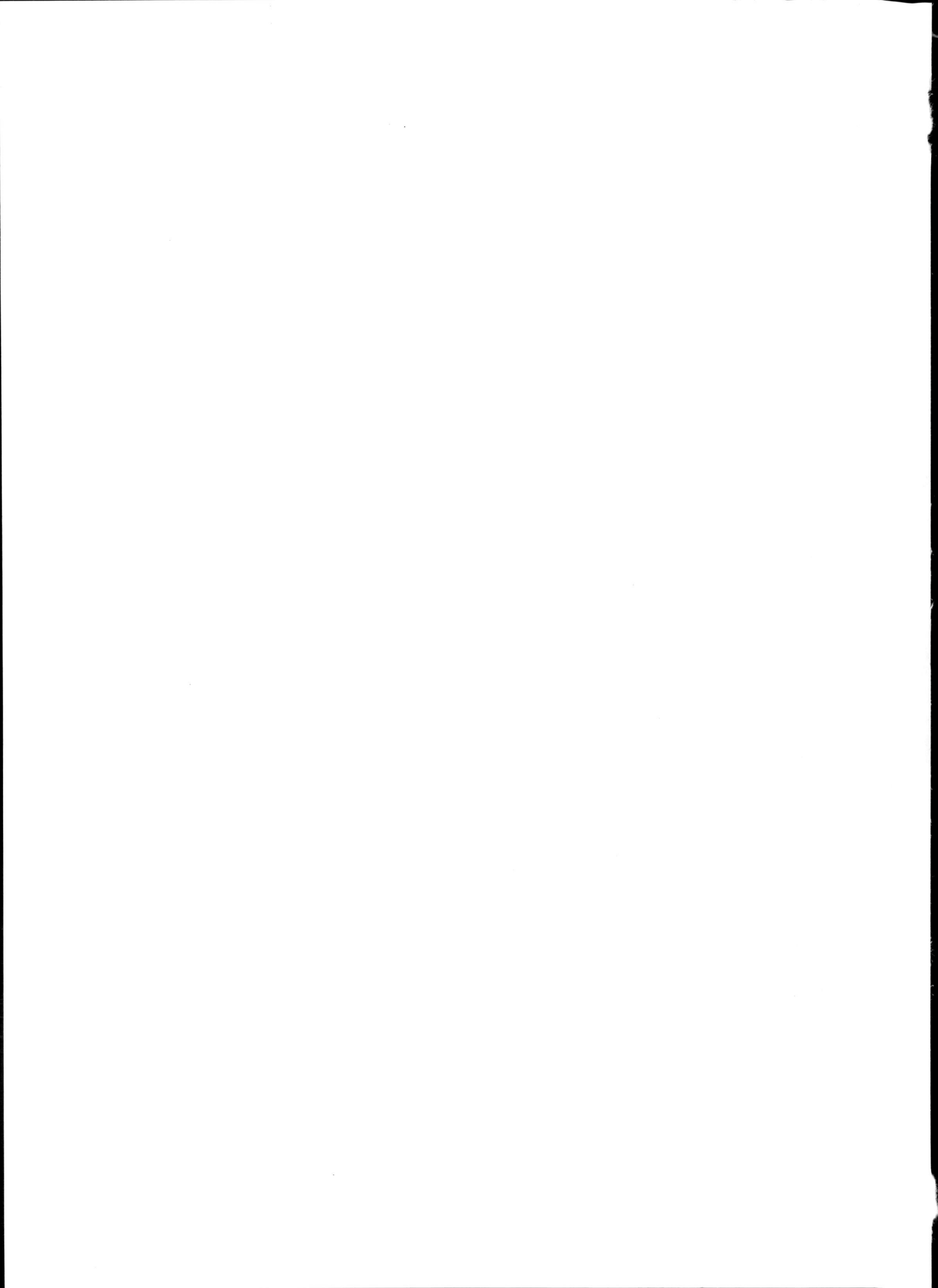